Advances in Experimental Medicine and Biology

Volume 1061

More information about this series at http://www.springer.com/series/5584

Jun Yu
Editor

Obesity, Fatty Liver and Liver Cancer

Springer

Editor
Jun Yu
Institute of Digestive Disease and Department of Medicine
& Therapeutics State Key Laboratory of Digestive Disease
LKS Institute of Health Sciences
The Chinese University of Hong Kong
Hong Kong, Hong Kong

ISSN 0065-2598 ISSN 2214-8019 (electronic)
Advances in Experimental Medicine and Biology
ISBN 978-981-10-8683-0 ISBN 978-981-10-8684-7 (eBook)
https://doi.org/10.1007/978-981-10-8684-7

Library of Congress Control Number: 2018943896

Printed on acid-free paper

This Springer imprint is published by the registered company Springer Nature Singapore Pte Ltd.
The registered company address is: 152 Beach Road, #21-01/04 Gateway East, Singapore 189721, Singapore

Foreword

Obesity has become a prevalent disorder due to various factors such as opulent meals, unhealthy eating habits and sedentary lifestyle. More than two-thirds of the adult population in developed countries is considered overweight and more than a third of them are obese. In addition to the well-known association of obesity with type II diabetes and cardiovascular diseases, emerging evidence suggests that obesity represents a major risk factor for fatty liver diseases, hepatocellular carcinoma (HCC) and other solid tumours. Non-alcoholic fatty liver disease (NAFLD) is becoming the most common cause of chronic liver disease in the West and in Asia. Its incidence in obese individuals can be extremely high. NAFLD can progress from relatively benign, simple steatosis to more aggressive diseases such as non-alcoholic steatohepatitis (NASH) and HCC. Given that obesity, fatty liver and fatty liver-associated HCC are increasingly prevalent in developed countries and in particular in children, this book is an important endeavour. It offers a comprehensive overview on these diseases and provides an outlook on future strategies for their detection, prevention and treatment.

The purpose of this book is to provide both medical professionals and research scientists with an expert update on NAFLD, NASH and fatty liver disease-associated HCC. In particular, it focusses on the recent advances as well as unresolved challenges in the field of fatty liver research. The book begins with the description of the epidemiology and etiology of NAFLD and associated HCC, and highlights their rising trend in the developed countries. The role of inflammation in the pathogenesis of NAFLD and HCC is explored in the subsequent chapters because accumulating evidence suggests that inflammation is a key for the transition from simple steatosis to NASH and fibrosis. Immune mediators, such as cytokines, adipokines and chemokines, play a pivotal role in the development of NAFLD and NASH. In these chapters, the underlying molecular mechanisms and the potential of the immune system in the pathogenesis of NAFLD are being discussed. Furthermore, the authors elucidate the pathogenesis of NAFLD-related HCC and the underlying role of the metabolic syndrome. Recent advances in the utilization of clinical and genetic biomarkers for patient stratification and disease detection are summarized.

Gut microbiota disorder has been established recently as a novel contributor to obesity and liver cancer. In addition to outlining the influence of gut microbiota-derived metabolites on the pathogenesis of NAFLD, this book illustrates the interaction between obesity and microbiota, as well as its contribution to the development of NAFLD. Microbiota dysfunction in HCC is then discussed, highlighting its potential role in the transition from NAFLD to HCC. The last part of the book focuses on established therapies and future therapeutic strategies for the prevention and treatment of NAFLD, NASH and HCC, respectively.

In this up-to-date book, researchers and clinicians from different regions share their expertise in NAFLD, NASH and NASH-associated HCC. Supported by clinical studies and experimental data, the authors' insights into current challenges and future perspectives will help shed light on the development in the field. The authors and the editor are to be congratulated for their work. This book does enrich our knowledge on fatty liver diseases.

Alexander L. Gerbes

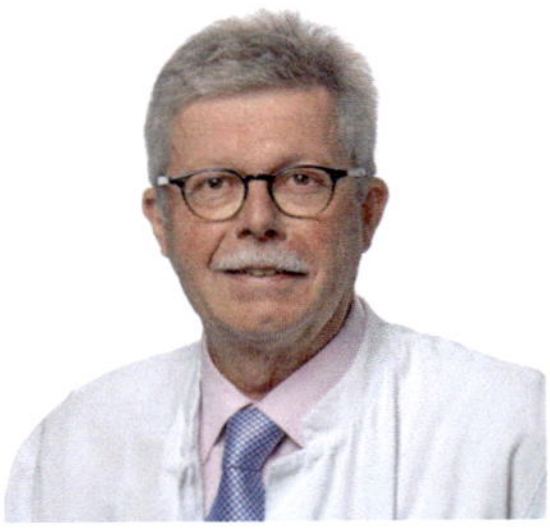

Dr. Alexander L. Gerbes is a Professor of Internal Medicine in Medizinische Klinik und Poliklinik II, Klinikum der Universität München, FRG. He earned his MD degree following study at University of Munich, UCSF at San Francisco and the Royal Hallamshire Hospital, Sheffield, UK, from the Ludwig-Maximilians-University Munich in 1981. He began his professional career as staff physician at the Department of Medicine, University of Munich where he was appointed as assistant professor in 1990. Following a research stay at University of Montreal, Canada, 1991–1992, he was granted lifetime full professorship (C3) in 1995. In 2001, he was appointed as deputy chief of the Department of Medicine 2 of the Munich University Hospital where he founded the Liver Center Munich in 2008. Currently, he is acting chief of the Department of Gastroenterology and Hepatology at the Munich university hospital and is medical director of the Munich liver transplantation program. From the start of his academic career, Alexander Gerbes has focused his research on pathophysiology, diagnosis and treatment of liver diseases with emphasis on complications of cirrhosis. He is a Fellow of the European Board of Gastroenterology, Fellow of the AGA and Inaugural Fellow of AASLD. Since 2010, he has served as deputy editor of GUT, a leading journal of gastroenterology and hepatology. He has co-authored over 200 articles in acknowledged journals including *N Engl J Med*, *Lancet*, *Gastroenterology*, *Gut*, *Hepatology* and *J Hepatol*.

Contents

1 **Introduction** 1
Chi Chun Wong and Jun Yu

2 **Epidemiology and Etiologic Associations of Non-alcoholic Fatty Liver Disease and Associated HCC** 3
Ken Liu and Geoffrey W. McCaughan

3 **Pathogenesis of NASH: How Metabolic Complications of Overnutrition Favour Lipotoxicity and Pro-Inflammatory Fatty Liver Disease** 19
Geoffrey C. Farrell, Fahrettin Haczeyni, and Shivakumar Chitturi

4 **Chemokines and Chemokine Receptors in the Development of NAFLD** 45
Yoon-Seok Roh and Ekihiro Seki

5 **NAFLD Related-HCC: The Relationship with Metabolic Disorders** 55
Xiang Zhang

6 **Hepatocellular Carcinoma in Obesity: Finding a Needle in the Haystack?** 63
György Baffy

7 **Dysregulated Epigenetic Modifications in the Pathogenesis of NAFLD-HCC** 79
Fung Zhao

8 **The Influence of Gut Microbial Metabolism on the Development and Progression of Non-alcoholic Fatty Liver Disease** 95
Wei Jia and Cynthia Rajani

9 **Microbiota, Obesity and NAFLD** 111
Louis H. S. Lau and Sunny H. Wong

10 Autophagy, NAFLD and NAFLD-Related HCC 127
William K. K. Wu, Lin Zhang, and Matthew T. V. Chan

11 Animal Models of Non-alcoholic Fatty Liver Diseases and Its Associated Liver Cancer 139
Jennie Ka Ching Lau, Xiang Zhang, and Jun Yu

12 Current Prevention and Treatment Options for NAFLD 149
Vincent Wai-Sun Wong

Contributors

György Baffy Department of Medicine, VA Boston Healthcare System and Brigham and Women's Hospital, Harvard Medical School, Boston, MA, USA

Matthew T. V. Chan Department of Anaesthesia and Intensive Care, The Chinese University of Hong Kong, Hong Kong, Hong Kong

Shivakumar Chitturi Australian National University Medical School, and Gastroenterology and Hepatology Unit, The Canberra Hospital, Woden, ACT, Australia

Geoffrey C. Farrell Australian National University Medical School, and Gastroenterology and Hepatology Unit, The Canberra Hospital, Woden, ACT, Australia

Fahrettin Haczeyni Australian National University Medical School, and Gastroenterology and Hepatology Unit, The Canberra Hospital, Woden, ACT, Australia

Wei Jia University of Hawaii Cancer Center, Honolulu, HI, USA

Shanghai Jiao Tong University School of Medicine, Shanghai, China

Jennie Ka Ching Lau Institute of Digestive Disease and Department of Medicine & Therapeutics, State Key Laboratory of Digestive Disease, LKS Institute of Health Sciences, The Chinese University of Hong Kong, Hong Kong

SHHO College, The Chinese University of Hong Kong, Hong Kong, Hong Kong

Louis H. S. Lau Institute of Digestive Disease, State Key Laboratory of Digestive Diseases, Department of Medicine & Therapeutics and LKS Institute of Health Sciences, The Chinese University of Hong Kong, Hong Kong, Hong Kong

Ken Liu AW Morrow Gastroenterology and Liver Centre, Royal Prince Alfred Hospital, Sydney, NSW, Australia

Faculty of Medicine, University of Sydney, Sydney, NSW, Australia

Centenary Institute, University of Sydney, Sydney, NSW, Australia

Geoffrey W. McCaughan AW Morrow Gastroenterology and Liver Centre, Royal Prince Alfred Hospital, Sydney, NSW, Australia

Faculty of Medicine, University of Sydney, Sydney, NSW, Australia

Centenary Institute, University of Sydney, Sydney, NSW, Australia

Cynthia Rajani University of Hawaii Cancer Center, Honolulu, HI, USA

Yoon-Seok Roh Department of Pharmacy, Chungbuk National University College of Pharmacy, Cheongju, Chungbuk, South Korea

Ekihiro Seki Division of Digestive and Liver Diseases, Department of Medicine, Cedars-Sinai Medical Center, Los Angeles, CA, USA

Chi Chun Wong Institute of Digestive Disease and Department of Medicine & Therapeutics, State Key Laboratory of Digestive Disease, LKS Institute of Health Sciences, The Chinese University of Hong Kong, Hong Kong, Hong Kong

Sunny H. Wong Institute of Digestive Disease, State Key Laboratory of Digestive Diseases, Department of Medicine & Therapeutics and LKS Institute of Health Sciences, The Chinese University of Hong Kong, Hong Kong, Hong Kong

Vincent Wai-Sun Wong Department of Medicine and Therapeutics and State Key Laboratory of Digestive Disease, The Chinese University of Hong Kong, Hong Kong, Hong Kong

William K. K. Wu Department of Anaesthesia and Intensive Care, The Chinese University of Hong Kong, Hong Kong, Hong Kong

State Key Laboratory of Digestive Diseases, Department of Medicine & Therapeutics and LKS Institute of Health Sciences, The Chinese University of Hong Kong, Hong Kong, Hong Kong

Jun Yu Institute of Digestive Disease and Department of Medicine & Therapeutics, State Key Laboratory of Digestive Disease, LKS Institute of Health Sciences, The Chinese University of Hong Kong, Hong Kong, Hong Kong

Lin Zhang Department of Anaesthesia and Intensive Care, The Chinese University of Hong Kong, Hong Kong, Hong Kong

State Key Laboratory of Digestive Diseases, Department of Medicine & Therapeutics and LKS Institute of Health Sciences, The Chinese University of Hong Kong, Hong Kong, Hong Kong

Xiang Zhang Institute of Digestive Disease and Department of Medicine & Therapeutics, State Key Laboratory of Digestive Disease, LKS Institute of Health Sciences, The Chinese University of Hong Kong, Hong Kong, Hong Kong

Fung Zhao Institute of Digestive Disease, Department of Medicine and Therapeutics, The Chinese University of Hong Kong, Hong Kong, Hong Kong

About the Editor

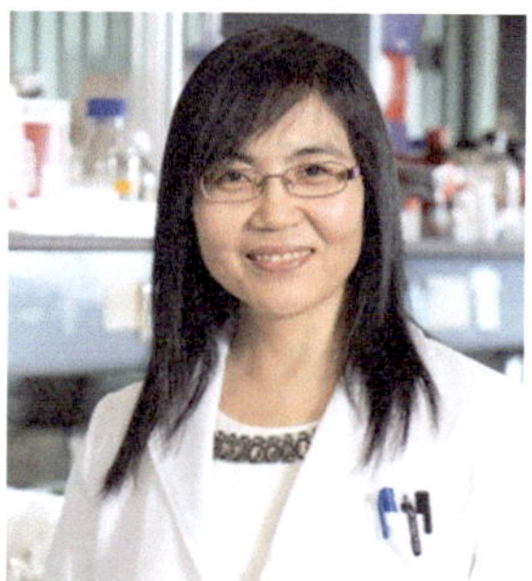

Dr. Jun Yu is a Professor at Department of Medicine and Therapeutics, Director of the Research Laboratory of Institute of Digestive Disease, and Associate Director of State Key Laboratory of Digestive Disease, The Chinese University of Hong Kong (CUHK). She is a Council Member of American Gastrointestinal Association (AGA) oncology USA; Member of International Cancer Genome Consortium (ICGC) USA; President of Hong Kong Immunology Association; Vice-chairman of Hong Kong Scientist Association. She is serving as Associate Editor for *Oncogene* and *Life Science* (2007–2015); Editor for *Gut*, *Scientific Reports*, *J Gastroenterol Hepatol*, etc. over 10 peer-reviewed journals.

Prof Yu earned her MD and PhD at Tongji Medical University in 1994. Then she embarked on gastrointestinal specialist in Beijing University, followed by a postdoctoral fellowship in University of Dresden and University of Magdeburg, Germany, and CUHK, Hong Kong. She has worked as a Senior Research Officer at the University of Sydney and has been a CUHK faculty member since 2005. She is also the visiting or honorary professor of over 10 universities including Beijing University, University of Hong Kong, Sun Yat-Sen University, Shanghai Jiaotong University, Zhejiang University, etc.

Her research interests are mainly on gastrointestinal cancers (colon, liver and stomach) in relation to the genomic/epigenomic alterations, gut microbiota dysbiosis, molecular mechanisms and cancer biomarkers. She has over 340 publications (57 papers IF>10, h index=57) in international peer-reviewed journals including *Nature*, *Nature Biotechnology*, *Cancer Cell*, *Cell Metabolism*, *J Clin Oncol*, *J Clin Invest*, *Gastroenterology*, *Gut*, *Nature Communication*, *Hepatology*, *Cancer Res*, and *Oncogene*, and 9 book or book chapters. Her contributions to the advancement of medical sciences have been recognized with 17 prestigious awards, including American Gastroenterology Association (AGA) Council Oncology Research Mentor Award, USA, May 2017; The State Natural Science Award (second class) 2016; The State Scientific and Technological Progress Award (Innovation Team) 2016; Croucher Senior Research Fellowship 2016; The State Science and Technology Progress Award (second class) 2012; First-Class of Higher

Education Outstanding Scientific Research Output Awards (Natural Science) 2014; First-Class Higher Education Outstanding Scientific Research Output Awards (Scientific and Technological Progress Award) 2012; First-Class of Higher Education Outstanding Scientific Research Output Awards (Natural Science) 2010.

1 Introduction

Chi Chun Wong and Jun Yu

Abstract

Obesity is fast becoming a major disorder for mankind. Numerous lifestyle factors play a role in the rising obesity epidemic, including changes in the diet and the lack of physical activity. Unfortunately, more than two-thirds of the adult population in developed countries is considered overweight and more than a third of them are obese. In addition to the well-publicized association of obesity with type II diabetes and cardiovascular diseases, emerging evidence indicates that obesity represents a major risk factor for fatty liver diseases and fatty liver disease-associated hepatocellular carcinoma (HCC).

Keywords

Obesity · Non-alcoholic steatohepatitis · Hepatocellular carcinoma · Microbiota · Therapy

C. C. Wong · J. Yu (✉)
Institute of Digestive Disease and Department of Medicine & Therapeutics, State Key Laboratory of Digestive Disease, LKS Institute of Health Sciences, The Chinese University of Hong Kong, Hong Kong, Hong Kong
e-mail: chichun.wong@cuhk.edu.hk; junyu@cuhk.edu.hk

Obesity is fast becoming a major disorder for mankind. Numerous lifestyle factors play a role in the rising obesity epidemic, including changes in the diet and the lack of physical activity. Unfortunately, more than two-thirds of the adult population in developed countries is considered overweight and more than a third of them are obese. In addition to the well-publicized association of obesity with type II diabetes and cardiovascular diseases, emerging evidence indicate that obesity represents a major risk factor for fatty liver diseases and fatty liver disease-associated hepatocellular carcinoma (HCC).

Non-alcoholic fatty liver disease (NAFLD), defined by the collective features of obesity, diabetes, insulin resistance and dyslipidemia, is the most common cause of chronic liver disease in the West and in Asia. This is particularly true among obese individuals, where its incidence can be as high as 98%. Pathologically, NAFLD comprise of a full spectrum of liver conditions ranging from relatively benign, simple steatosis to more aggressive disease such as non-alcoholic steatohepatitis (NASH). NASH often progresses to cirrhosis, which in turn, predisposes HCC. In fact, NASH is increasingly considered as an important causative factor of HCC. Whilst a relatively small proportion of patients with NAFLD eventually develop cirrhosis and progress to HCC, the rising incidence of obesity coupled with metabolic syndrome means that to a large

J. Yu (ed.), *Obesity, Fatty Liver and Liver Cancer*, Advances in Experimental Medicine and Biology 1061, https://doi.org/10.1007/978-981-10-8684-7_1

proportion of the general population are susceptible to NASH or NASH-associated HCC.

In the past decade, there has been an enormous research efforts studying the pathogenesis of hepatitis B/C (HBV/HCV)-associated HCC, which broadened our understanding of HBV/HCV-associated HCC. NASH-associated HCC has received less attention thus far; however, we are now beginning to understand its pathogenesis and molecular mechanism of action. One key unifying theme between NASH and NASH-associated HCC is chronic inflammation. Induction of inflammation is a hallmark of NAFLD and plays an important role in disease progression to NASH and cirrhosis. Moreover, chronic inflammation has been casually linked to the development of multiple malignancies. With advances in both basic sciences and biotechnology, much progress has been made in the development of therapeutic targets and drugs in the prevention and treatment of inflammatory conditions and inflammation-associated cancer, and they hold great promise for targeting NASH and NASH-associated HCC.

In this book, we invited researchers and clinicians from different regions to share their expertise in NAFLD, NASH and NASH-associated HCC, to shed new insights and future perspectives on the development of the field. In this regard, this book begins with the description of the epidemiology and etiology of NAFLD and its associated HCC to highlight their rising trend in the developed countries as a result of the obesity epidemic. Inflammation is a key player in the pathogenesis of NAFLD and HCC. The next two chapters describe the role of immune mediators and inflammatory pathways, including cytokines, adipokines and chemokines, which contribute to the development of NAFLD and NASH. Next, an up-to-date overview on the pathogenesis of NAFLD-related HCC is given and the underlying role of metabolic syndrome in the transition of steatosis to NASH, fibrosis and HCC is discussed. Surveillance of NAFLD-related HCC is a major challenge as only a small portion of patients will eventually progress to HCC. Recent advances in the utilization of clinical and genetic biomarkers for the cost effective patient stratification and disease detection is therefore summarized. The first part of the book concludes with a discussion on the role of epigenetic changes, heritable changes in gene expression that are not resulted from alterations in DNA sequence, in NAFLD and HCC, and how might these epigenetic alterations be used for disease diagnosis and prognosis.

The second part of the book focuses on in-depth reviews on current hot topics in NAFLD, NASH and HCC. The gut microbiota is an emerging environmental factor that triggers a multitude of diseases. Intensive efforts have established the microbiota dysfunction as a novel contributor to obesity and liver cancer, and these studies are reviewed to emphasize their diverse roles in disease development. The influence of gut microbiota-derived metabolites on the pathogenesis of NAFLD is first outlined with a focus on microbiota-derived bile acids. This is followed by an overview on the interaction between obesity and microbiota contributing to development of NAFLD. Microbiota dysfunction in HCC is then discussed, highlighting its potential role in the transition from NAFLD to HCC. Another key research area is the role of autophagy in HCC. Autophagy represents a cell survival mechanism that mediates the recycling of dysfunctional cellular components, and impairment of autophagy has a contributory role in NAFLD. As such, targeting autophagy processes will be a novel therapeutic strategy for treating inflammation and cancer in the liver.

The third part of the book aims to capture latest developments in established therapies and future therapeutic strategies for the prevention and treatment of NAFLD, NASH and HCC. It begins with an extensive overview of pre-clinical experimental animal models of NAFLD and NAFLD-associated HCC that can be used for efficacy evaluation of novel therapeutics or treatment modalities, and the pros and cons of each model. This is followed by an up-to-date review of prevention and treatment options for NAFLD, with a focus on management of NAFLD in order to minimize disease progression to cirrhosis and HCC. The current therapies and future therapeutic strategies for the treatment of obesity related HCC is also discussed. Given that obesity, fatty liver and fatty liver-associated HCC are increasingly prevalent in developed countries, this book offers a timely and comprehensive overview on these diseases, and provides perspectives on future strategies for their detection, prevention and treatment.

Epidemiology and Etiologic Associations of Non-alcoholic Fatty Liver Disease and Associated HCC

2

Ken Liu and Geoffrey W. McCaughan

Abstract

Non-alcoholic fatty liver disease (NAFLD) is the most common chronic liver disease in the world and will soon become the number one cause of hepatocellular carcinoma (HCC), liver transplantation and liver-related mortality. The disease often occurs in the setting of metabolic conditions such as obesity and type II diabetes mellitus. These same metabolic drivers are also risk factors for NAFLD associated HCC which can occur even in the absence of cirrhosis or advanced fibrosis and appears to be phenotypically different to HCCs arising from other chronic liver diseases. The frequencies of liver-related events and HCC among NAFLD patients is low, especially when compared to cardiovascular disease and extrahepatic malignancies. However, the large denominator of total patients affected with NAFLD means that these events will impose an enormous clinical and economic burden on our society. Moreover, this burden is expected to rise further in the future. Therefore, the global NAFLD epidemic has arrived at our doorstep and demands our attention.

Keywords

Non-alcoholic fatty liver disease · Non-alcoholic steatohepatitis · Hepatocellular carcinoma · Epidemiology · Metabolic syndrome · Economic burden

K. Liu · G. W. McCaughan (✉)
AW Morrow Gastroenterology and Liver Centre, Royal Prince Alfred Hospital, Sydney, NSW, Australia

Faculty of Medicine, University of Sydney, Sydney, NSW, Australia

Centenary Institute, University of Sydney, Sydney, NSW, Australia
e-mail: Ken.Liu@sydney.edu.au; G.McCaughan@centenary.usyd.edu.au

2.1 Introduction

In the face of a global obesity epidemic, non-alcoholic fatty liver disease (NAFLD) has become the major cause of chronic liver disease worldwide [1, 2]. With continuing improvements in global hepatitis B virus (HBV) vaccination coverage and effective therapies to either control or eradiate chronic viral hepatitis, the proportional burden of NAFLD and its complications is set to rise dramatically. Accordingly, NAFLD is the fastest growing indication for liver transplantation (LT) in the United States (U.S.) over the past decade and is expected to surpass chronic hepatitis C virus (HCV) infection as the leading indication in next 5 years [3, 4]. In particular, the number of patients undergoing LT for hepatocellular carcinoma (HCC) secondary to NAFLD has increased by nearly fourfold to 13.5% of HCC-

J. Yu (ed.), *Obesity, Fatty Liver and Liver Cancer*, Advances in Experimental Medicine and Biology 1061, https://doi.org/10.1007/978-981-10-8684-7_2

related LT. Although the absolute risk of HCC and liver-related mortality among NAFLD patients is low, the high (and rising) global prevalence of these patients translates into substantial numbers. Thus, on current trends, the future burden of NAFLD and associated HCC (NAFLD-HCC) will be staggering.

2.2 Epidemiology of NAFLD

2.2.1 Definitions

Non-alcoholic fatty liver disease is typically regarded as the hepatic manifestation of metabolic syndrome, a condition characterized by the presence of at least three of the following criteria: elevated body mass index (BMI) and waist circumference, dyslipidemia, insulin resistance and/or type II diabetes and hypertension [5]. NAFLD is defined as the presence of hepatic steatosis seen on imaging or histology (exceeding 5% of total liver weight) to the exclusion of secondary causes of hepatic fat accumulation [6]. It can be further classified into non-alcoholic fatty liver (also known as simple steatosis) or non-alcoholic steatohepatitis (NASH) based on the absence or presence of significant hepatic inflammation, respectively. The latter is considered a more aggressive form of disease which can progress to hepatic fibrosis, cirrhosis and NAFLD-HCC (Fig. 2.1).

2.2.2 Prevalence of NAFLD

The reported prevalence of NAFLD varies widely depending on the population studied and the diagnostic method used. In a landmark meta-analysis of 86 studies across 22 countries over 26 years, Younossi et al. estimated the global prevalence of NAFLD diagnosed on imaging to be 25.2% (range 22.1%–28.7%) [7]. Alternatively, when the prevalence of NAFLD was estimated using blood tests (elevated liver enzymes or other indices), only 9.3%–12.0% of individuals were diagnosed with the condition across the world. Indeed, the level of liver enzymes fluctuates throughout the course of NAFLD and may be normal in the vast majority of patients [8]. Hence blood tests, although simple and easily accessible, are thought

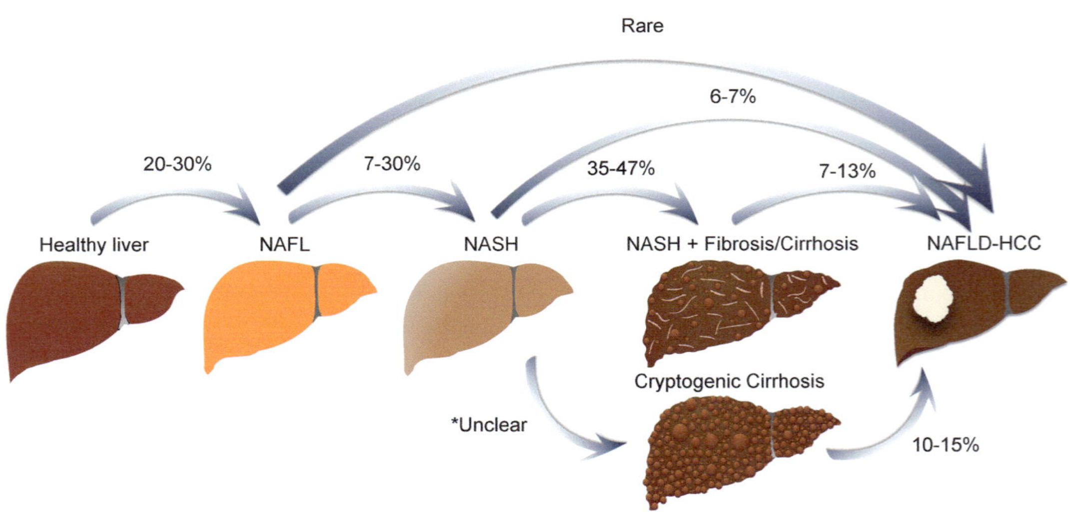

Fig. 2.1 The natural history of non-alcoholic fatty liver disease (NAFLD)
Although NASH accounts for up to half of cryptogenic cirrhosis cases, the proportion of NASH-cirrhosis patients misclassified as cryptogenic cirrhosis is not known

NAFL non-alcoholic fatty liver or simple steatosis, *NASH* non-alcoholic steatohepatitis, *NAFLD-HCC* non-alcoholic fatty liver disease-associated hepatocellular carcinoma
Figure courtesy of Dr. Weiqi Xu, Institute of Digestive Disease, The Chinese University of Hong Kong, Hong Kong

to underestimate the true prevalence of NAFLD. Liver histology is considered the most accurate yet least practical and most invasive method for diagnosing NAFLD. Autopsy series reveal a NAFLD prevalence of 13.0–15.8%, while liver biopsies obtained from potential living liver donors showed 20% of patients in the U.S. and 10.4% in South Korea had >30% steatosis [9].

Although the majority of literature arises from the North America and Europe where obesity and type II diabetes mellitus are epidemic, NAFLD has never been just a "Western disease" [1]. Indeed, it is highly prevalent in all continents. The highest prevalences of NAFLD are found in the Middle East (31.8%), South America (30.5%) and Asia (27.4%) where the prevalence rates of obesity are correspondingly high [7, 10]. The prevalence in U.S. and Europe are reported to be 24.1% and 23.7%, respectively while the lowest prevalence is reported in studies from Africa (13.5%). Hence the problem of NAFLD is just as common and important in other parts of the world as it is in the West [1].

2.2.3 Incidence

Compared to prevalence studies, NAFLD incidence studies are limited. The earliest study by Suzuki et al. showed the incidence of suspected NAFLD (as indicated by elevated serum transaminases) was 31 cases per 1000 person-years in a cohort of Japanese government employees without previous liver disease [11]. Most studies which used ultrasonography to diagnose NAFLD found an incidence rate of 18–27 cases per 1000 patient-years [12–15], although one Japanese study documented an incidence rate of 86 cases per 1000 patient-years [16]. A study of 565 community Chinese patients without NAFLD who underwent serial intrahepatic triglyceride content measurements with proton-magnetic resonance spectroscopy reported the incidence of NAFLD to be 34 per 1000 patient-years [17]. Finally, a population-based study of hepatology referrals in the United Kingdom showed a much lower incidence rate of 29 cases per 100,000 person-years [18], suggesting only a fraction of NAFLD patients are actually seen by hepatologists. Almost all incidence studies found that metabolic syndrome, or its components were strong predictors for NAFLD development. Regression of NAFLD is also known to occur, especially in the setting of weight loss. In the studies which also followed up patients with NAFLD at baseline, the regression rate was found to vary widely between 12 and 140 cases per 1000 patient-years [12–14, 16]. The average amount of weight loss in patients who demonstrated regression of NAFLD was small (2–3 kg) [12, 16].

2.2.4 Trends Over Time

In the past three decades, there has been a two to threefold increase in obesity across the Americas, Europe and Asia [2]. A parallel increase in the number of people with NAFLD has also been observed over this period of time. For instance, the prevalence of NAFLD has more than doubled in the U.S., Japan and some areas of China during the last two decades, while the prevalence of other chronic liver diseases has either remained stable or decreased [19–21]. However, recent pooled worldwide NAFLD prevalence estimates suggest a milder upward trend from 20.1% to 23.8% to 26.8% during 2000–2005, 2006–2010, and 2011–2015, respectively. This trend is also seen in patients at the severe end of the NAFLD spectrum. The percentage of NAFLD patients undergoing LT in the U.S. increased from 1.2% in 2001 to 9.7% in 2009 [22].

2.2.5 NASH

NASH is defined histologically by the presence of hepatic steatosis and two additional features: lobular inflammation and hepatocyte injury (ballooning) [1]. The global prevalence of NASH among biopsied NAFLD patients is estimated to be 59.1% (range 47.6%–69.7%) [7]. Since the condition can only be diagnosed by liver histology, NAFLD patients suspected of having it may undergo liver biopsy for the purpose of diagnosing NASH (with or without fibrosis), thus creating a selection bias. Comparatively, NASH prevalence estimates among NAFLD patients without an indication for liver biopsy (e.g. elevated liver enzymes or clinical signs of liver disease) are much lower (6.7%–29.9%) [7]. The prevalence of NASH in the general population has been estimated to be between 3% and 5% [9]. However, in the obese population the median prevalence of NASH is 33% (range 10%–56%).

2.3 Risk Factors for NAFLD and Its Progression

2.3.1 Age and Gender

The prevalence of NAFLD increases with age. Pooled data show adult patients aged 30–39 years old have a prevalence of 22.4% which increments with each decade of life to 34.0% in those >70 years old [7]. In one population study by Wong et al., the prevalence of NAFLD in patients older than 60 years was >50% [23]. The same group also demonstrated older age was an independent predictor of incident NAFLD [17]. The prevalence of NAFLD in the pediatric general population (5–10%) is lower than adults, although still considerable especially in children with obesity (>30%) [24]. Unsurprisingly, the metabolic risk factors associated with NAFLD, including obesity, diabetes and hyperlipidemia and hypertension similarly, increase with age [9].

Data on the effect of gender on NAFLD are conflicting. Early reports published prior to 1990 suggested both NAFLD and NASH were more common in women [25]. However, most subsequent studies have consistently demonstrated a male predominance [9, 26]. The gender distribution also varies with age and race as NAFLD appears to be more common in Asian or black women than their male counterparts after the age of 50 [23, 26].

2.3.2 Race and Genetics

Considerable variation in NAFLD prevalence is observed around the world and in subjects of different ethnicities residing in the same country [7, 26]. Hispanics have the highest prevalence of NAFLD, while African Americans appear to be protected despite substantially higher rates of obesity and diabetes compared to other ethnicities in the U.S. [2, 9]. These disparities can be partially explained by variations in genetic polymorphisms associated with NAFLD. In the Dallas Heart Study cohort where 2287 subjects underwent proton-magnetic resonance spectroscopy, the frequency of hepatic steatosis was 45% in Hispanics, 33% in whites and 24% in blacks [8]. Using genome-wide association studies in 2008, Romeo et al. showed that two alleles of the patatin-like phospholipase domain containing protein 3 (*PNPLA3*) gene could account for 72% of ethnic differences in hepatic fat content seen in the Dallas Heart Study cohort [27]. The I148M allele which predisposes individuals to NAFLD is prevalent in Hispanics, while the S453I which is protective is commonly found in African Americans. The *PNPLA3* genotype can explain 10%–12% of the variance in the NAFLD trait overall. Since then, genetic variants in *APOC3, NCAN, GCKR, LYPLAL1, PPP1R3B, TM6SF2* and other genes have been discovered as significant NAFLD contributors [28–30] with both similarities and differences in frequency observed across ethnicities [1]. While genetic predisposition contributes to individual susceptibility to NAFLD and family clustering is known to occur [31], twin and family studies estimate the heritability of NAFLD to be roughly 39%–52% [32, 33]. Clearly environmental factors also play a big role.

2.3.3 Metabolic Factors

A strong relationship exists between the components of metabolic syndrome and prevalence of NAFLD. From a cohort of 12,454 adults, Lazo et al. calculated the age-, sex- and ethnicity-adjusted NAFLD prevalence ratios for patients with obesity, insulin resistance, diabetes, hypertension and hypercholesterolemia to be 3.93, 2.54, 2.40, 1.57 and 1.26, respectively compared to those without these conditions (26). The prevalence ratios for obesity, insulin resistance and diabetes remained significant even after further adjustment for the other metabolic abnormalities and lack of physical activity. Furthermore, effect of these metabolic risk factors appears to be additive. Wong et al., demonstrated that each additional component of the metabolic syndrome increased the risk of NAFLD in a dose-dependent manner (prevalence of 4.5% in subjects without any component to 80.0% in those with all components) [23].

Indeed, the prevalence of NAFLD is exceedingly high in patients with features of metabolic syndrome. An Italian study of 187 young adult (age 18–50 years) non-diabetic obese patients detected hepatic steatosis on ultrasound in all but four patients, or 98% of patients [34]. The prevalence of histologically-proven NAFLD in those undergoing bariatric surgery similarly exceeds 90% [35]. In particular, central obesity as evidenced by increased waist circumference and/or waist-to-hip ratio has been shown to be a greater predictor of NAFLD than general obesity (BMI $\geq$30 kg/m^2) [36]. It should be noted that the distribution of visceral adipose tissue and percentage of fat for a given body mass differs between Asian and European subjects [1]. Previous studies conducted in Asian countries have reported non-obese individuals in 15–21% of NAFLD patients even after applying ethnic-specific anthropometric criteria [37]. These patients typically have a history of weight gain above their ideal body mass (but not reaching obese levels) and/or presence of other metabolic factors. It has been suggested that Asians may express the clinical phenotype associated with the metabolic syndrome at a lower BMI threshold than white populations [2]. However, pooled regional estimates of obesity prevalence among NAFLD patients (using a BMI cut-off of $\geq$25kg/m^2 for Asians and $\geq$30 kg/m^2 for others) are actually the highest in Asia (64.0%) followed by the U.S. (57.0%) and Europe (36.8%). Overall, obesity is present in 51.3% of NAFLD patients and 81.8% of NASH patients [7].

Insulin resistance is key in the pathogenesis of NAFLD and its progression, hence strong associations exist between NAFLD and diabetes. Up to 60–70% of individuals with type II diabetes exhibit ultrasonography evidence of NAFLD [38, 39]. In one study, 70.8% of diabetic patients with fatty infiltration seen on ultrasound underwent liver biopsy and NAFLD was confirmed in 86.7% of patients [39]. These ultrasound studies are supported by a prospective cohort study which screened diabetics for NAFLD using controlled attenuation parameter and found a prevalence of 72.8% [40]. Significant liver fibrosis was also detected by liver stiffness measurement in 17.7% of patients in this study. Furthermore, studies have shown that the risk of developing diabetes increases by three- to fourfold within 3 years of NAFLD diagnosis in patients without diabetes at baseline [1].

Hyperlipidemia or dyslipidemia is present in 69.2% of NAFLD patients [7] and diffuse fatty liver on ultrasound is seen in half of the individuals with hyperlipidemia [41]. In particular, hypertriglyceridemia may have a closer association with NAFLD than hypercholesterolemia. The above associations have led to changes to some international guidelines which now recommend screening for NAFLD in patients with obesity, insulin resistance or metabolic syndrome [42].

2.3.4 Progression to Fibrosis

As previously mentioned, approximately 7%–30% of NAFLD patients have NASH. Of these, up to 39.1%–40.8% will progress to develop fibrosis which occurs at a mean rate of 0.09–0.14 fibrosis stages per year [7, 43]. The incidence of advanced fibrosis in NASH patients is estimated to be 70.0 in 1000 person-years. Patients with simple steatosis have also been reported to develop fibrosis progression, although this is considered uncommon [9]. Factors associated with progressive or advanced fibrosis include older age, features of metabolic syndrome, elevated liver enzymes (especially aspartate aminotransferase [AST]) and low platelet count [44–47]. In terms of metabolic syndrome components, increased waist circumference, BMI, presence of diabetes (as well as insulin resistance or glucose intolerance), hyperlidemia and hypertension have all been associated with worsened fibrosis stage [1, 9, 43, 48, 49]. Multiple predictive scoring systems using clinical and laboratory variables have been developed to identify NAFLD patients at risk of advanced liver fibrosis with area under the receiver operating characteristics curves (AUROCs) of 0.80–0.94 [50]. Almost all the risk factors mentioned above feature as a variable in one or more of these scoring systems. The *PNPLA3* I148M polymorphism has also been shown to favor NAFLD progression and liver fibrosis [51]. In terms of histological predictors, two studies observed that patients with higher steatosis grade were more likely to develop progressive fibrosis while no association was found between baseline severity of necroinflammation and risk of progressive fibrosis [43].

2.4 Epidemiology of NAFLD-HCC

Hepatocellular carcinoma is the fifth most common cancer in men and ninth most common in women globally [52]. The disease carries a high mortality rate and represents the second most frequent cause of cancer death worldwide accounting for 746,000 deaths in 2012. The median survival following diagnosis is poor, ranging from four to 20 months [53, 54]. Patients with NAFLD are at increased risk for developing HCC, however this risk is typically limited (but not exclusive) to those with advanced fibrosis or cirrhosis [6].

Since the first report of NAFLD-HCC in 1990 [55], the global incidence and prevalence of NAFLD-HCC has been steadily increasing [3, 56]. NAFLD is currently the third leading cause of HCC in the U.S. [56], however it is poised to become the leading cause of HCCs in the future [2, 57]. Indeed, a retrospective study of 162 HCC patients between 2007 and 2008 from one German center has already demonstrated that NAFLD was the most common underlying etiology of HCC [58]. A study of 632 consecutive HCC cases in the United Kingdom reported that between 2000 and 2010, there was a greater than tenfold increase in NAFLD-HCC compared to only a two to threefold increase in HCCs due to other liver diseases [59]. Changes are also occurring in non-Western countries, where the majority of the world's HCCs (>80%) currently arises mainly in the setting of chronic infection with HBV or HCV [60]. In particular, China contributes half of the world's HCC deaths, of which up to 80% are attributable to HBV [61]. However, since 1990 China has seen a 30% reduction in the rate of deaths due to HBV-related HCC [62]. A study from South Korea, another HBV endemic area, reported the proportion of patients with NAFLD-HCC increased from 3.8% in 2001–2005 to 12.2% in 2006–2010 while HBV-related HCC dropped from 86.6% to 67.4% during the same periods [63]. Similar trends have also been recorded in Japan [20].

The aforementioned rise in NAFLD-HCC burden is driven by the increase in proportion of NAFLD patients, since progression to HCC in NAFLD patients remains uncommon. The cumulative incidence of NAFLD-HCC has been reported across the world as 0.5%–2.3% after of 7.6–13.7 years of follow-up [44, 64–66]. Higher percentages of 6.7–7.6% after 5–10 years are seen in studies of NASH patients [67, 68]. In a large meta-analysis of 86 studies, Younossi et al. calculated that the HCC incidence rate is up to 12-fold higher in NASH patients as compared with NAFLD patients overall [7]. The rate in those with NASH-related cirrhosis is even higher still. The cumulative incidence of HCC in this group of patients is quoted at 6.7%–12.8% with follow-up times of between 3.2 and 10 years [64, 68–70]. One international cohort of 247 NAFLD patients across four Western countries found an HCC incidence of only 2.4% in patients with at least advanced fibrosis and 3.1% in patients with cirrhosis after a median follow-up of 7.2 years [71]. However, only patients with Child-Pugh class A liver disease were enrolled in this study.

Studies have consistently shown a lower rate of HCC development in patients with NAFLD compared to other chronic liver diseases. In particular, NAFLD patients have a 15- to 35-fold lower HCC incidence than that of chronic HBV [7]. Differential susceptibility to HCC was also seen in a retrospective study of 3200 Japanese elderly patients (>60 years old) with either NAFLD or HCV [66]. After a mean follow-up of 8.2 years, the cumulative incidence of HCC was 0.6% in the NAFLD group compared to 17% in the HCV group. Two separate prospective studies from the U.S. comparing patients with NASH-related cirrhosis and HCV-related cirrhosis both recorded a lower incidence of HCC in the NASH group: 12.8% vs. 20.3%, respectively after 3.2 years of follow-up [70] and 6.7% vs. 17.0%, respectively after 10 years of follow-up [68]. However, a Japanese study of 157 cirrhotic patients including 72 with NASH and 85 with alcoholic liver disease found similar rates of HCC development in the two groups after 5 years (10.5% vs. 12.3%, respectively) [69].

The estimation of NAFLD-HCC is further made difficult by HCC cases in patients with cryptogenic cirrhosis which accounts for 15–30% of cirrhosis and 30–40% of HCCs worldwide [3, 72]. Growing evidence suggests that "burned-out" NASH accounts for a large proportion (up to half) of cryptogenic cirrhosis [3, 73, 74]. Indeed, some cryptogenic cirrhosis patients demonstrate histological features of NASH, however these features may also be lost over time with the development of cirrhosis [6]. Patients with cryptogenic cirrhosis and associated HCC also share many characteristics with patients with NAFLD and NAFLD-HCC, respectively. In particular, those with cryptogenic liver disease and NAFLD are older with an increased occurrence of metabolic risk factors and less aggressive tumors when HCCs arise compared to patients with other chronic liver diseases [75–77]. In a prospective study of 105 consecutive HCC patients in the U.S., up to half of patients with cryptogenic cirrhosis and HCC had histologic or clinical features of NAFLD [78]. The authors concluded at least 13% of HCCs in the study were NAFLD-HCC. Hence, studies which do not account for the proportion of NAFLD patients in those with HCC arising from cryptogenic cirrhosis may be underestimating the true prevalence of NAFLD-HCC.

2.5 Risk Factors for NAFLD-HCC

While the classic risk factors associated with HCC, such as older age, male sex and cigarette smoking also apply in NAFLD-HCC, the following risk factors deserve mention.

2.5.1 Fibrosis

The majority of NAFLD-HCC, like other HCCs, occurs in the setting of cirrhosis [2]. The cumulative incidence of HCC in NASH-related cirrhosis is up to 25-fold higher than the overall NAFLD population. Advanced fibrosis is also an important risk factor for HCC. In a prospective cohort of 382 Japanese patients with biopsy-proven NASH, 34 patients were found to have HCC [67]. Of the NAFLD-HCC patients, 88% had advanced fibrosis, compared to only 31% in NASH patients without HCC. On multivariate analysis, the authors found that advanced fibrosis was the strongest independent risk factor for NAFLD-HCC with an odds ratio of 4.2 (95% confidence interval [95% CI] 1.8–9.7). In another Japanese study, 6508 patients with NAFLD diagnosed by ultrasonography were retrospectively studied for a median of 5.6 years. Since few patients in the study underwent a liver biopsy (<2%), the AST to platelet ratio index (APRI) was used to separate patients with significant fibrosis (F3-F4). The study reported a significantly higher cumulative rate of HCC in patients with significant fibrosis compared to those without (hazard ratio 25.0, 95% CI 9.0–69.5) [65]. However, NAFLD-HCC has also been well documented to occur without cirrhosis or advanced fibrosis in one third to one half of cases [79, 80]. HCC has even been demonstrated in patients with simple steatosis (without steatohepatitis or fibrosis) [81]. Despite the contribution by metabolic risk factors such as obesity and diabetes, hepatopcarcinogenesis in non-cirrhotic NAFLD patients remains complex and the precise molecular pathways are still not fully understood.

2.5.2 Obesity

Obesity is recognized as a significant risk for the development of several malignancies, including HCC [82]. A meta-analysis of 11 cohort studies from the U.S., Europe and Asia evaluated the association between being overweight (BMI $\geq$25 kg/m^2) or obese (BMI $\geq$30 kg/m^2) and HCC. The study found relative risks of 1.2 (95% CI 1.02–1.3) and 1.9 (95% CI 1.5–2.4) for HCC in overweight and obesity patients, respectively [83]. These findings were supported by a larger meta-analysis of 26 prospective studies which demonstrated similar relative risks of 1.5 (95% CI 1.3–1.7) and 1.8 (95% CI 1.6–2.1) for primary liver cancer in overweight and obese patients, respectively [84]. Of note on subgroup analyses, these associations were independent of geographic locations, alcohol consumption, history of diabetes or viral hepatitis status. Like in NAFLD, central obesity may be particularly important. A prospective multicenter European cohort study of over 350,000 subjects showed that among all anthropometric measures of obesity, waist-to-hip ratio had the strongest association with a relative risk of 3.5 (95% CI 2.1–5.9) when comparing first and third tertiles [85]. Obesity also increases the risk of HCC-related mortality. HCC is now the leading cause of obesity related cancer deaths in middle-aged males in the U.S. [3]. In a prospective study of more than 900,000 adults in the U.S. followed up for 16 years, Calle et al. reported that HCC mortality rates were 4.5-fold higher in men with BMI $\geq$35 kg/m^2 than men with normal BMI [86]. Among obese men, the relative risk of cancer death from HCC was the highest compared to all other cancers (4.5 vs. 1.3–2.6). Multiple obesity-mediated mechanisms are believed to play a role in development of HCC with and without NAFLD including low-grade chronic inflammatory response, increased lipid storage and lipotoxicity, and alteration of gut microbiota with increased levels of lipopolysaccharide [87]. In particular, there is accumulating evidence which links alterations in gut microbiota with obesity, NAFLD and HCC. A recent study of obese mice found the gut microbiome metabolite deoxycholic acid promoted obesity-associated HCC, while treatment of the mice with vancomycin inhibited deoxycholic acid production and HCC development [88].

2.5.3 Diabetes Mellitus

Type II diabetes mellitus and insulin resistance with associated hyperinsulinemia and increased insulin-like growth factor levels may also contribute to HCC development. Cohort and case-controlled studies report patients with diabetes have a two to fourfold increased risk of developing HCC, independent of viral hepatitis and alcohol use [89–91]. Similarly systematic reviews and meta-analyses estimate the increased risk of HCC in diabetic patients to be 1.9–2.2-fold [92, 93]. In addition, diabetes has also been shown to increase the incidence of HCC recurrence after curative therapy [94]. Indeed, in up to 70% of patients with diabetes there is associated NAFLD [40] which is itself a risk factor for HCC. However, a large prospective cohort study of 257,649 diabetes and 772,947 non-diabetics showed that the increased risk of HCC in diabetics persisted even after excluding patients diagnosed with NAFLD (adjusted hazard ratio 2.13, 95% CI 1.99–2.28) [89], thus suggesting an independent effect. Furthermore, the use of anti-diabetic medications, in particular metformin and possibly thiazolidinediones has been associated with a decreased risk of HCC among patients with diabetes [95, 96].

Since obesity, diabetes and NAFLD often coexist, the independent contributions of each factor to HCC risk are not known. Notably, it appears obesity and diabetes synergistically increase the risk of HCC development. A 14-year prospective follow up study of 23,820 Taiwanese residents showed that obesity was associated with a 3.3-fold increase in HCC among HCV-positive patients while diabetes increased HCC risk in both HBV-positive and HCV-positive patients, by 2.2-fold and 3.5-fold respectively [97]. However, in HBV or HCV chronic carriers with both obesity and diabetes, the risk of HCC was increased by more than 100-fold compared with patients without these factors. A multicenter Italian case-control study also demonstrated a progressive increase in HCC with the number of components of metabolic syndrome [98]. In particular, the odds ratio for HCC in patients with obesity, diabetes and both were 2.0, 4.3 and 4.8, respectively. Hepatocarcinogenesis in NAFLD is multifactorial and clearly a complex interplay exists between the components of the metabolic syndrome.

2.5.4 Iron

Hepatic iron accumulation is thought to be involved in oxidative DNA damage, NASH, fibrosis and potentially HCC [99–101]. Increased iron absorption through up-regulation of divalent metal transporter 1 has been demonstrated in NASH patients compared to those with simple steatosis and control subjects [102]. Sorrentino et al. retrospectively studied the hepatic iron content in 153 patients with NASH-cirrhosis (51 patients with HCC and 102 age- and sex-matched patients without HCC) and showed that iron deposition was more frequent in the HCC group, thus implicating it as a cofactor in the pathogenesis of NAFLD-HCC [103]. Conversely, iron depletion has been shown to reduce oxidative damage in NASH patients and lower the risk of HCC in patients with chronic HCV [104, 105]. Further studies are needed to better understand the role of iron accumulation in NASH and HCC.

2.6 Characteristics of NAFLD-HCC

Until recently, inferences on the characteristics of NAFLD-HCC have largely been made based on summations of case reports or case series [80, 106, 107]. Typically, patients with NAFLD-HCC tend to be male, older, and have one or more features of metabolic syndrome (Table 2.1).

Table 2.1 Characteristics of patients with NAFLD-HCC and patients with HCC secondary to other chronic liver diseases

Characteristic	NAFLD-HCCs	Other HCCs
Dominant gender	Male	Male
Age at diagnosis (years)	65–70	60–65
Metabolic syndrome (%)	45–58	14–18
Type II diabetes mellitus	54–74	12–49
Obesity	48–66	12–37
Hypertension	47–60	18–52
Dyslipidemia	28–35	6–14
Cirrhosis at presentation (%)	51–62	78–97
Liver function	Largely preserved	Worse
Average tumor size (cm)	≥3	≤3
Tumor differentiation	Well-differentiated	Well- to moderately-differentiated

2.6.1 Sex, Age and Initial Presentation

The male predominance seen with HCCs overall is also observed in NAFLD-HCC. Males make up 62.0%–88.9% of NAFLD-HCC patients [58, 65, 80, 106–108]. However, data are conflicting on whether differences in sex distribution exist between NAFLD-HCC and HCCs related to other diseases. In a large Italian multicenter prospective study by Piscaglia et al. comparing 145 NAFLD-HCC patients with 611 HCV-related HCC patients, significantly more males were seen in the NAFLD-HCC group (79.3% vs. 61.2%) [108]. On the contrary, Reddy et al. showed that in the subset of HCC patients undergoing curative treatments, females were more common in those with NASH relative to HCV or alcoholic liver disease (48.1% vs. 16.7%) [77]. Female gender was similarly more common in a Japanese nationwide cross-sectional study comparing NAFLD-HCC with alcoholic liver disease-related HCC (38% vs. 4%) [109]. Data are also conflicting on the age of HCC diagnosis in

NAFLD with respect to other chronic liver diseases. Published literature reports a mean and median age of NAFLD-HCC diagnosis at 66.7–74.7 years and 65–72 years, respectively [56, 58, 77, 80, 106–110]. While most studies demonstrate NAFLD-HCC patients are 5–8 years older at presentation compared to other HCC patients [56, 58, 75, 77, 110], the aforementioned Italian study found NAFLD-HCC patients were younger than patients with HCV-related HCC (67.8 vs. 71.1 years). However, the HCV-related HCC patients in this study were older than the typical age distribution for this disease [111]. Further prospective studies are needed to clarify these sex and age demographic associations observed in NAFLD-HCC.

One explanation for the older age of NAFLD-HCC patients is that fibrosis progression in NASH is slow (~0.1 fibrosis stages per year) and not universal (~40%) [7]. Although significant fibrosis is not essential for NAFLD-HCC development, it remains an important risk factor in 50% or more of patients. Furthermore, NAFLD-HCC patients tend to present late in the course of their disease. Up to half of patients who develop NAFLD-HCC have HCC diagnosed at time of initial referral [107]. Compared to HCV-related HCC, almost twice as many NAFLD-HCC patients at first presentation are symptomatic (7.4% vs. 13.8%), which is typically a late event in the course of HCC [108]. Correspondingly, patients with HCV-related HCC were more likely to receive surveillance prior to diagnosis (86.7% vs. 43.3%) and more likely to have their HCC picked up by surveillance programs (63.3% vs. 47.6%) than NAFLD-HCC patients [108, 110], hence facilitating earlier detection of HCC in non-NAFLD patients. Indeed, international guidelines for HCC surveillance in non-cirrhotic NAFLD patients are currently lacking.

2.6.2 Metabolic Syndrome

Metabolic syndrome and its constituents such as obesity and type II diabetes commonly co-exist with NAFLD and are independent risk factors for both NAFLD and NAFLD-HCC. It is therefore unsurprising that patients with NAFLD-HCC exhibit a higher prevalence of metabolic features compared to HCCs arising from other etiologies [58, 77, 106, 108]. Almost all patients (>98%) with NAFLD-HCC have at least one feature of metabolic syndrome while most (>75%) have two or more features [106]. Type II diabetes (54%–74%) and obesity (62%–66%) are most prevalent followed by hypertension (47%–60%) and dyslipidemia (28%–35%) [67, 77, 80, 109]. A retrospective study of 214 patients undergoing curative treatment for HCC found the presence of metabolic syndrome was three times more common in NAFLD-HCC compared to HCV- or alcoholic liver disease-related HCC (45.1% vs. 14.8%) [77]. Tokushige et al. found similar disparities in rates of metabolic syndrome with 58% seen in NAFLD-HCC patients and only 18% in patients with HCC due to alcoholic liver disease [109]. Clearly these metabolic features and their associated pathways play a key role in hepatocarcinogenesis.

2.6.3 Liver Function

Patients with NAFLD-HCC tend to have less severe liver dysfunction compared with other causes of HCC. Reddy et al. reported lower median model for end-stage liver disease (MELD) scores in NAFLD-HCC than those with HCC secondary to HCV or alcoholic liver disease (9 vs. 10) [77]. Using another measure of liver function, Piscaglia et al. showed proportionately more NAFLD-HCC patients with Child-Pugh class A (compensated) cirrhosis when compared to patients with HCV-related HCC (82.3% vs. 61.8%) [108]. Consistently, both studies found higher serum albumin levels, lower serum bilirubin and international normalized ratio values and lower rates of ascites in the NAFLD group. These differences are likely influenced by the substantial proportion (up to half) of NAFLD-HCC patients who do not have cirrhosis or advanced fibrosis.

Hepatic injury as reflected by elevation in transaminase levels appears to be less in NAFLD-HCC compared with other HCCs, especially AST levels [77]. The predictive value of AST level for NAFLD-HCC was evaluated in two separate cohort studies of Japanese NAFLD patients. Interestingly, the studies reached opposing conclusions with one identifying elevated AST as risk factor for HCC [65] and the other showing it was protective [67]. The predictive value of AST level for NAFLD-HCC therefore remains uncertain.

2.6.4 Tumor Characteristics

Emerging data suggest NAFLD-HCCs may be phenotypically different to HCCs resulting from other liver diseases [3]. Most NAFLD-HCCs present as a well-differentiated, solitary lesion with an average size of 3–4 cm [79, 80, 107]. Up to 70%–78% of NAFLD-HCCs are solitary lesions [67, 75, 80, 106]. One study found that in patients eligible for curative treatments, those with NAFLD-HCC had a fewer tumor nodules compared to HCC secondary to HCV or alcoholic liver disease [77]. This finding was not supported by Piscaglia et al. however, the authors did document fewer small HCCs (Barcelona Clinic Liver Cancer Stage 0) and more advanced-stage HCCs (Barcelona Clinic Liver Cancer stage C) in NAFLD versus HCV groups [108]. NAFLD-HCCs were also more likely to be infiltrative and outside the Milan criteria for liver transplantation, while extrahepatic metastases were less likely. The same study demonstrated larger tumors from NAFLD-HCC compared to other HCCs (4.1 cm vs 3.3 cm) [108]. In another study, HCC patients with metabolic syndrome as their sole risk factor (a surrogate for NAFLD-HCC) also exhibited larger tumors compared to HCC patients with other chronic liver diseases (8.8 cm vs. 7.8 cm), although this fell just short of statistical significance [75]. These larger tumors seen with NAFLD-HCC may be a reflection of their aforementioned delayed presentation [107].

Tumor marker expression may also differ. Levels of α-fetoprotein (AFP) appear to be raised less often in NAFLD-HCC patients than in those with HCC due to other chronic liver diseases [3, 110]. In a Japanese prospective study of 34 patients with NAFLD-HCC, only 26.5% had an elevated AFP [67]. With regards to AFP levels, some studies have demonstrated lower levels in HCC patients with NAFLD versus non-NAFLD etiologies [75, 108], while others found no significant differences [77, 109]. Finally, a greater proportion of NAFLD-HCCs appear well-differentiated on histology compared to other HCCs [75, 77].

Similar to the clinical features of NAFLD-HCC, these tumor characteristics have been confirmed by most but not all studies. This highlights that HCC is still a heterogeneous disease even among the subset of NAFLD-HCC patients.

2.7 Cost and Economic Burden

The cost and economic burden of NAFLD and associated HCC deserves mention. In a study assessing economic burden of NAFLD, Younossi et al. estimated the annual cost to be US$103 billion in the U.S and €35 billion across four European countries – expenditures similar to that of diabetes and heart disease [112]. Based on recent trends, these costs associated with resource utilization are set to rise further in both inpatient and outpatient settings [113, 114]. Although a fraction of these costs may be mediated by comorbid diseases such as diabetes mellitus or angina pectoris [115], their economic impact is huge.

Furthermore, NAFLD patients consistently demonstrate lower health-related quality of life scores as measured by SF-36 or Chronic Liver Disease Questionnaire compared to the general population and patients with other chronic liver diseases [116]. NAFLD patients also experience higher levels of fatigue, physical inactivity and day-time somnolence than healthy controls [117]. These impairments result in loss of work productivity and reflect the unmeasured impact of psychological and psychiatric issues such as depression and anxiety associated with NAFLD. Therefore, NAFLD also imposes significant indirect costs on patients and society. The above study by Younossi et al. approximated that after adding the societal costs of quality-adjusted life-years lost due to NAFLD, the annual burden of NAFLD in the U.S. and four European countries increases by two to sixfold to US$292.19 billion and €227.84 billion, respectively [112].

The economic cost associated with HCC are similarly considerable and higher than that of other cancers [118, 119]. In particular, the annual cost of NAFLD-HCC was quoted to be US$522.7 million in the United States and €90.2 million in Germany, France, Italy and United Kingdom combined [112]. Significant burdens have also been reported in other countries [118]. Therefore, NAFLD and associated HCC imposes a severe human and economic burden on patients, their families, and society. Of concern, the relative recency and ongoing rise of the obesity epidemic along with the lag period required for NAFLD to develop into cirrhosis and/or HCC has meant that the full impact of NAFLD-related advanced liver disease has not yet been felt [110].

While NAFLD is associated with increased liver-related mortality and HCCs [120], its clinical burden should be tempered by perspective. Indeed, non-liver-related death remains far more common than liver-related death or NAFLD-HCC combined [7]. Consistently, liver disease has been shown to be the third common cause of death in NAFLD patients behind cardiovascular disease and malignancies [64, 121–123]. For every 100 patients with NAFLD, only one to two will die from liver-related death [57]. Even in patients with NASH [44] including those with advanced fibrosis [121], cardiovascular disease remains the top cause of mortality. Therefore, the non-liver-related outcomes of NAFLD patients should not be neglected.

2.8 Conclusion

NAFLD is the most common chronic liver disease in the world and will soon become the number one cause of HCC, liver transplantation and liver-related mortality. The disease often occurs in the setting of metabolic conditions such as obesity and type II diabetes mellitus. These same metabolic drivers are also risk factors for NAFLD-HCC which can occur even in the absence of cirrhosis or advanced fibrosis and appears to be phenotypically different from HCCs arising from other chronic liver diseases. The frequencies of liver-related events and HCC among NAFLD patients is low, especially when compared to cardiovascular disease and extrahepatic malignancies. However, the large denominator of total patients affected with NAFLD means that these events will impose an enormous clinical and economic burden on our society. Moreover, this burden is expected to rise further in the future. Therefore, the global NAFLD epidemic has arrived at our doorstep and demands our attention.

References

1. Farrell GC, Wong VWS, Chitturi S. NAFLD in Asia – as common and important as in the west. Nat Rev Gastroenterol Hepatol. 2013;10:307–18.
2. Loomba R, Sanyal AJ. The global NAFLD epidemic. Nat Rev Gastroenterol Hepatol. 2013;10:686–90.
3. Michelotti GA, Machado MV, Diehl AM. NAFLD, NASH and liver cancer. Nat Rev Gastroenterol Hepatol. 2013;10:656–65.
4. Wong RJ, Cheung R, Ahmed A. Nonalcoholic steatohepatitis is the most rapidly growing indication for liver transplantation in patients with hepatocellular carcinoma in the U.S. Hepatology. 2014;59:2188–95.
5. Executive Summary of the third report of the National Cholesterol Education Program (NCEP) expert panel on detection, evaluation, and treatment of high blood cholesterol in adults (adult treatment panel III). JAMA 2001;285:2486–97.
6. Chalasani N, Younossi Z, Lavine JE, et al. The diagnosis and management of non-alcoholic fatty liver disease: practice guideline by the American Association for the Study of Liver Diseases, American College of Gastroenterology, and the American Gastroenterological Association. Hepatology. 2012;55:2005–23.
7. Younossi ZM, Koenig AB, Abdelatif D, Fazel Y, Henry L, Wymer M. Global epidemiology of nonalcoholic fatty liver disease – metaanalytic assessment of prevalence, incidence, and outcomes. Hepatology. 2016;64:73–84.
8. Browning JD, Szczepaniak LS, Dobbins R, et al. Prevalence of hepatic steatosis in an urban population in the United States: impact of ethnicity. Hepatology. 2004;40:1387–95.
9. Vernon G, Baranova A, Younossi ZM. Systematic review: the epidemiology and natural history of

non-alcoholic fatty liver disease and non-alcoholic steatohepatitis in adults. Aliment Pharmacol Ther. 2011;34:274–85.
10. Sayiner M, Koenig A, Henry L, Younossi ZM. Epidemiology of nonalcoholic fatty liver disease and nonalcoholic steatohepatitis in the United States and the rest of the world. Clin Liver Dis. 2016;20:205–14.
11. Suzuki A, Angulo P, Lymp J, et al. Chronological development of elevated aminotransferases in a nonalcoholic population. Hepatology. 2005;41:64–71.
12. Zelber-Sagi S, Lotan R, Shlomai A, et al. Predictors for incidence and remission of NAFLD in the general population during a seven-year prospective follow-up. J Hepatol. 2012;56:1145–51.
13. Bedogni G, Miglioli L, Masutti F, et al. Incidence and natural course of fatty liver in the general population: the Dionysos study. Hepatology. 2007;46:1387–91.
14. Sung KC, Wild SH, Byrne CD. Development of new fatty liver, or resolution of existing fatty liver, over five years of follow-up, and risk of incident hypertension. J Hepatol. 2014;60(5):1040.
15. Xu C, Yu C, Ma H, Xu L, Miao M, Li Y. Prevalence and risk factors for the development of nonalcoholic fatty liver disease in a nonobese Chinese population: the Zhejiang Zhenhai study. Am J Gastroenterol. 2013;108:1299–304.
16. Hamaguchi M, Kojima T, Takeda N, et al. The metabolic syndrome as a predictor of nonalcoholic fatty liver disease. Ann Intern Med. 2005;143:722–8.
17. Wong VW, Wong GL, Yeung DK, et al. Incidence of non-alcoholic fatty liver disease in Hong Kong: a population study with paired proton-magnetic resonance spectroscopy. J Hepatol. 2015;62:182–9.
18. Whalley S, Puvanachandra P, Desai A, Kennedy H. Hepatology outpatient service provision in secondary care: a study of liver disease incidence and resource costs. Clin Med. 2007;7:119–24.
19. Younossi ZM, Stepanova M, Afendy M, et al. Changes in the prevalence of the most common causes of chronic liver diseases in the United States from 1988 to 2008. Clin Gastroenterol Hepatol. 2011;9:524–30.
20. Okanoue T, Umemura A, Yasui K, Itoh Y. Nonalcoholic fatty liver disease and nonalcoholic steatohepatitis in Japan. J Gastroenterol Hepatol. 2011;26(Suppl 1):153–62.
21. Fan JG, Farrell GC. Epidemiology of non-alcoholic fatty liver disease in China. J Hepatol. 2009;50:204–10.
22. Charlton MR, Burns JM, Pedersen RA, Watt KD, Heimbach JK, Dierkhising RA. Frequency and outcomes of liver transplantation for nonalcoholic steatohepatitis in the United States. Gastroenterology. 2011;141:1249–53.
23. Wong VW, Chu WC, Wong GL, et al. Prevalence of non-alcoholic fatty liver disease and advanced fibrosis in Hong Kong Chinese: a population study using proton-magnetic resonance spectroscopy and transient elastography. Gut. 2012;61:409–15.
24. Anderson EL, Howe LD, Jones HE, Higgins JP, Lawlor DA, Fraser A. The prevalence of non-alcoholic fatty liver disease in children and adolescents: a systematic review and meta-analysis. PLoS One. 2015;10:e0140908.
25. Sanyal AJ. AGA technical review on nonalcoholic fatty liver disease. Gastroenterology. 2002;123:1705–25.
26. Lazo M, Hernaez R, Eberhardt MS, et al. Prevalence of nonalcoholic fatty liver disease in the United States: the Third National Health and Nutrition Examination Survey, 1988–1994. Am J Epidemiol. 2013;178:38–45.
27. Romeo S, Kozlitina J, Xing C, et al. Genetic variation in PNPLA3 confers susceptibility to nonalcoholic fatty liver disease. Nat Genet. 2008;40:1461–5.
28. Richart C, Auguet T, Terra X. Apolipoprotein C3 gene variants in nonalcoholic fatty liver disease. N Engl J Med. 2010;363:193–4.
29. Speliotes EK, Yerges-Armstrong LM, Wu J, et al. Genome-wide association analysis identifies variants associated with nonalcoholic fatty liver disease that have distinct effects on metabolic traits. PLoS Genet. 2011;7:e1001324.
30. Kozlitina J, Smagris E, Stender S, et al. Exome-wide association study identifies a TM6SF2 variant that confers susceptibility to nonalcoholic fatty liver disease. Nat Genet. 2014;46:352–6.
31. Struben VM, Hespenheide EE, Caldwell SH. Nonalcoholic steatohepatitis and cryptogenic cirrhosis within kindreds. Am J Med. 2000;108:9–13.
32. Schwimmer JB, Celedon MA, Lavine JE, et al. Heritability of nonalcoholic fatty liver disease. Gastroenterology. 2009;136:1585–92.
33. Loomba R, Schork N, Chen CH, et al. Heritability of hepatic fibrosis and steatosis based on a prospective twin study. Gastroenterology. 2015;149:1784–93.
34. Colicchio P, Tarantino G, del Genio F, et al. Non-alcoholic fatty liver disease in young adult severely obese non-diabetic patients in South Italy. Ann Nutr Metab. 2005;49:289–95.
35. Machado M, Marques-Vidal P, Cortez-Pinto H. Hepatic histology in obese patients undergoing bariatric surgery. J Hepatol. 2006;45:600–6.
36. Pang Q, Zhang JY, Song SI, et al. Central obesity and nonalcoholic fatty liver disease risk after adjusting for body mass index. World J Gastroenterol. 2015;21:1650–62.
37. Liu CJ. Prevalence and risk factors for non-alcoholic fatty liver disease in Asian people who are not obese. J Gastroenterol Hepatol. 2012;27:1555–60.
38. Leite NC, Salles GF, Araujo AL, Villela-Nogueira CA, Cardoso CR. Prevalence and associated factors of non-alcoholic fatty liver disease in patients with type-2 diabetes mellitus. Liver Int. 2009;29:113–9.
39. Prashanth M, Ganesh HK, Vima MV, et al. Prevalence of nonalcoholic fatty liver disease in patients with type 2 diabetes mellitus. J Assoc Physicians India. 2009;57:205–10.

40. Kwok R, Choi KC, Wong GL, et al. Screening diabetic patients for non-alcoholic fatty liver disease with controlled attenuation parameter and liver stiffness measurements: a prospective cohort study. Gut. 2016;65:1359–68.
41. Assy N, Kaita K, Mymin D, Levy C, Rosser B, Minuk G. Fatty infiltration of liver in hyperlipidemic patients. Dig Dis Sci. 2000;45:1929–34.
42. European Association for the Study of the Liver (EASL), European Association for the Study of Diabetes (EASD) and European Association for the Study of Obesity (EASO). EASL–EASD–EASO clinical practice guidelines for the management of non-alcoholic fatty liver disease. J Hepatol. 2016;64:1388–402.
43. Singh S, Allen AM, Wang Z, Prokop LJ, Murad MH, Loomba R. Fibrosis progression in nonalcoholic fatty liver vs nonalcoholic steatohepatitis: a systematic review and meta-analysis of paired-biopsy studies. Clin Gastroenterol Hepatol. 2015;13:643–54.
44. Ekstedt M, Franzén LE, Mathiesen UL, et al. Long-term follow-up of patients with NAFLD and elevated liver enzymes. Hepatology. 2006;44:865–73.
45. Noureddin M, Yates KP, Vaughn IA, et al. Clinical and histological determinants of nonalcoholic steatohepatitis and advanced fibrosis in elderly patients. Hepatology. 2013;58:1644–54.
46. Bazick J, Donithan M, Neuschwander-Tetri BA, et al. Clinical model for NASH and advanced fibrosis in adult patients with diabetes and NAFLD: guidelines for referral in NAFLD. Diabetes Care. 2015;38:1347–55.
47. Ong JP, Elariny H, Collantes R, et al. Predictors of nonalcoholic steatohepatitis and advanced fibrosis in morbidly obese patients. Obes Surg. 2005;15:310–5.
48. Wong VW, Wong GL, Choi PC, et al. Disease progression of non-alcoholic fatty liver disease: a prospective study with paired liver biopsies at 3 years. Gut. 2010;59:969–74.
49. Adams LA, Sanderson S, Lindor KD, Angulo P. The histological course of nonalcoholic fatty liver disease: a longitudinal study of 103 patients with sequential liver biopsies. J Hepatol. 2005;42:132–8.
50. Castera L, Vilgrain V, Angulo P. Noninvasive evaluation of NAFLD. Nat Rev Gastroenterol Hepatol. 2013;10:666–75.
51. Valenti L, Al-Serri A, Daly AK, et al. Homozygosity for the patatin-like phospholipase-3/adiponutrin I148M polymorphism influences liver fibrosis in patients with nonalcoholic fatty liver disease. Hepatology. 2010;51:1209–17.
52. Ferlay J, Soerjomataram I, Ervik M, et al. GLOBOCAN 2012 v1.0, Cancer incidence and mortality worldwide: IARC CancerBase No. 11 [Internet]. Lyon: International Agency for Research on Cancer; 2013.
53. A new prognostic system for hepatocellular carcinoma: a retrospective study of 435 patients: the Cancer of the Liver Italian Program (CLIP) investigators. Hepatology 1998;28:751–5.
54. Okuda K, Ohtsuki T, Obata H, et al. Natural history of hepatocellular carcinoma and prognosis in relation to treatment. Study of 850 patients. Cancer. 1985;56:918–28.
55. Powell EE, Cooksley WG, Hanson R, Searle J, Halliday JW, Powell LW. The natural history of nonalcoholic steatohepatitis: a follow-up study of forty-two patients for up to 21 years. Hepatology. 1990;11:74–80.
56. Younossi ZM, Otgonsuren M, Henry L, et al. Association of nonalcoholic fatty liver disease (NAFLD) with hepatocellular carcinoma (HCC) in the United States from 2004 to 2009. Hepatology. 2015;62:1723–30.
57. Rinella M, Charlton M. The globalization of nonalcoholic fatty liver disease: prevalence and impact on world health. Hepatology. 2016;64:19–22.
58. Ertle J, Dechêne A, Sowa JP, et al. Non-alcoholic fatty liver disease progresses to hepatocellular carcinoma in the absence of apparent cirrhosis. Int J Cancer. 2011;128:2436–43.
59. Dyson J, Jaques B, Chattopadyhay D, et al. Hepatocellular cancer: the impact of obesity, type 2 diabetes and a multidisciplinary team. J Hepatol. 2014;60:110–7.
60. Wallace MC, Preen D, Jeffrey GP, Adams LA. The evolving epidemiology of hepatocellular carcinoma: a global perspective. Expert Rev Gastroenterol Hepatol. 2015;9:765–79.
61. Wang FS, Fan JG, Zhang Z, Gao B, Wang HY. The global burden of liver disease: the major impact of China. Hepatology. 2014;60:2099–108.
62. Zhou M, Wang H, Zhu J, et al. Cause-specific mortality for 240 causes in China during 1990-2013: a systematic subnational analysis for the global burden of disease study 2013. Lancet. 2016;387:251–72.
63. Cho EJ, Kwack MS, Jang ES, et al. Relative etiological role of prior hepatitis B virus infection and non-alcoholic fatty liver disease in the development of non-B non-C hepatocellular carcinoma in a hepatitis B-endemic area. Digestion. 2011;84:17–22.
64. Adams LA, Lymp JF, St Sauver J, et al. The natural history of nonalcoholic fatty liver disease: a population-based cohort study. Gastroenterology. 2005;129:113–21.
65. Kawamura Y, Arase Y, Ikeda K, et al. Large-scale long-term follow-up study of Japanese patients with non-alcoholic fatty liver disease for the onset of hepatocellular carcinoma. Am J Gastroenterol. 2012;107:253–61.
66. Arase Y, Kobayashi M, Suzuki F, et al. Difference in malignancies of chronic liver disease due to non-alcoholic fatty liver disease or hepatitis C in Japanese elderly patients. Hepatol Res. 2012;42:264–72.
67. Hashimoto E, Yatsuji S, Tobari M, et al. Hepatocellular carcinoma in patients with non-alcoholic steatohepatitis. J Gastroenterol. 2009;44:89–95.
68. Sanyal AJ, Banas C, Sargeant C, et al. Similarities and differences in outcomes of cirrhosis due

to nonalcoholic steatohepatitis and hepatitis C. Hepatology. 2006;43:682–9.
69. Kodama K, Tokushige K, Hashimoto E, Taniai M, Shiratori K. Hepatic and extrahepatic malignancies in cirrhosis caused by nonalcoholic steatohepatitis and alcoholic liver disease. Alcohol Clin Exp Res. 2013;37(Suppl 1):E247–52.
70. Ascha MS, Hanouneh IA, Lopez R, Tamimi TA, Feldstein AF, Zein NN. The incidence and risk factors of hepatocellular carcinoma in patients with nonalcoholic steatohepatitis. Hepatology. 2010;51:1972–8.
71. Bhala N, Angulo P, van der Poorten D, et al. The natural history of nonalcoholic fatty liver disease with advanced fibrosis or cirrhosis: an international collaborative study. Hepatology. 2011;54:1208–16.
72. El-Serag HB, Rudolph KL. Hepatocellular carcinoma: epidemiology and molecular carcinogenesis. Gastroenterology. 2007;132:2557–76.
73. Caldwell SH, Oelsner DH, Iezzoni JC, Hespenheide EE, Battle EH, Driscoll CJ. Cryptogenic cirrhosis: clinical characterization and risk factors for underlying disease. Hepatology. 1999;29:664–9.
74. Poonawala A, Nair SP, Thuluvath PJ. Prevalence of obesity and diabetes in patients with cryptogenic cirrhosis: a case-control study. Hepatology. 2000;32:689–92.
75. Paradis V, Zalinski S, Chelbi E, et al. Hepatocellular carcinomas in patients with metabolic syndrome often develop without significant liver fibrosis: a pathological analysis. Hepatology. 2009;49:851–9.
76. Lee SS, Jeong SH, Byoun YS, et al. Clinical features and outcome of cryptogenic hepatocellular carcinoma compared to those of viral and alcoholic hepatocellular carcinoma. BMC Cancer. 2013;13:335.
77. Reddy SK, Steel JL, Chen HW, et al. Outcomes of curative treatment for hepatocellular cancer in nonalcoholic steatohepatitis versus hepatitis C and alcoholic liver disease. Hepatology. 2012;55:1809–19.
78. Marrero JA, Fontana RJ, Su GL, Conjeevaram HS, Emick DM, Lok AS. NAFLD may be a common underlying liver disease in patients with hepatocellular carcinoma in the United States. Hepatology. 2002;36:1349–54.
79. Baffy G, Brunt EM, Caldwell SH. Hepatocellular carcinoma in non-alcoholic fatty liver disease: an emerging menace. J Hepatol. 2012;56:1384–91.
80. Yasui K, Hashimoto E, Komorizono Y, et al. Characteristics of patients with nonalcoholic steatohepatitis who develop hepatocellular carcinoma. Clin Gastroenterol Hepatol. 2011;9:428–33.
81. Guzman G, Brunt EM, Petrovic LM, Chejfec G, Layden TJ, Cotler SJ. Does nonalcoholic fatty liver disease predispose patients to hepatocellular carcinoma in the absence of cirrhosis? Arch Pathol Lab Med. 2008;132:1761–6.
82. Lauby-Secretan B, Scoccianti C, Loomis D, et al. Body fatness and cancer – viewpoint of the IARC Working Group. N Engl J Med. 2016;375(8):794.
83. Larsson SC, Wolk A. Overweight, obesity and risk of liver cancer: a meta-analysis of cohort studies. Br J Cancer. 2007;97:1005–8.
84. Chen Y, Wang X, Wang J, Yan Z, Luo J. Excess body weight and the risk of primary liver cancer: an updated meta-analysis of prospective studies. Eur J Cancer. 2012;48:2137–45.
85. Schlesinger S, Aleksandrova K, Pischon T, et al. Abdominal obesity, weight gain during adulthood and risk of liver and biliary tract cancer in a European cohort. Int J Cancer. 2013;132:645–57.
86. Calle EE, Rodriguez C, Walker-Thurmond K, Thun MJ. Overweight, obesity,and mortality from cancer in a prospectively studied cohort of U.S. adults. N Engl J Med. 2003;348:1625–38.
87. Margini C, Dufour JF. The story of HCC in NAFLD: from epidemiology, across pathogenesis, to prevention and treatment. Liver Int. 2016;36:317–24.
88. Yoshimoto S, Loo TM, Atarashi K, et al. Obesity-induced gut microbial metabolite promotes liver cancer through senescence secretome. Nature. 2013;499:97–101.
89. El-Serag HB, Tran T, Everhart JE. Diabetes increases the risk of chronic liver disease and hepatocellular carcinoma. Gastroenterology. 2004;126:460–8.
90. Davila JA, Morgan RO, Shaib Y, McGlynn KA, El-Serag HB. Diabetes increases the risk of hepatocellular carcinoma in the United States: a population based case control study. Gut. 2005;54:533–9.
91. Adami HO, Chow WH, Nyrén O, et al. Excess risk of primary liver cancer in patients with diabetes mellitus. J Natl Cancer Inst. 1996;88:1472–7.
92. Yang WS, Va P, Bray F, et al. The role of pre-existing diabetes mellitus on hepatocellular carcinoma occurrence and prognosis: a meta-analysis of prospective cohort studies. PLoS One. 2011;6:e27326.
93. Wang P, Kang D, Cao W, Wang Y, Liu Z. Diabetes mellitus and risk of hepatocellular carcinoma: a systematic review and meta-analysis. Diabetes Metab Res Rev. 2012;28:109–22.
94. Kawamura Y, Ikeda K, Arase Y, et al. Diabetes mellitus worsens the recurrence rate after potentially curative therapy in patients with hepatocellular carcinoma associated with nonviral hepatitis. J Gastroenterol Hepatol. 2008;23:1739–46.
95. Singh S, Singh PP, Singh AG, Murad MH, Sanchez W. Anti-diabetic medications and the risk of hepatocellular cancer: a systematic review and meta-analysis. Am J Gastroenterol. 2013;108:881–91.
96. Lai SW, Chen PC, Liao KF, Muo CH, Lin CC, Sung FC. Risk of hepatocellular carcinoma in diabetic patients and risk reduction associated with anti-diabetic therapy: a population-based cohort study. Am J Gastroenterol. 2012;107:46–52.
97. Chen CL, Yang HI, Yang WS, et al. Metabolic factors and risk of hepatocellular carcinoma by chronic hepatitis B/C infection: a follow-up study in Taiwan. Gastroenterology. 2008;135:111–21.

98. Turati F, Talamini R, Pelucchi C, et al. Metabolic syndrome and hepatocellular carcinoma risk. Br J Cancer. 2013;108:222–8.
99. Fargion S, Valenti L, Fracanzani AL. Role of iron in hepatocellular carcinoma. Clin Liver Dis. 2014;3:108–10.
100. George DK, Goldwurm S, MacDonald GA, et al. Increased hepatic iron concentration in nonalcoholic steatohepatitis is associated with increased fibrosis. Gastroenterology. 1998;114:311–8.
101. Fargion S, Mattioli M, Fracanzani AL, et al. Hyperferritinemia, iron overload, and multiple metabolic alterations identify patients at risk for nonalcoholic steatohepatitis. Am J Gastroenterol. 2001;96:2448–55.
102. Hoki T, Miyanishi K, Tanaka S, et al. Increased duodenal iron absorption through up-regulation of divalent metal transporter 1 from enhancement of iron regulatory protein 1 activity in patients with nonalcoholic steatohepatitis. Hepatology. 2015;62:751–61.
103. Sorrentino P, D'Angelo S, Ferbo U, Micheli P, Bracigliano A, Vecchione R. Liver iron excess in patients with hepatocellular carcinoma developed on non-alcoholic steato-hepatitis. J Hepatol. 2009;50:351–7.
104. Kato J, Miyanishi K, Kobune M, et al. Long-term phlebotomy with low-iron diet therapy lowers risk of development of hepatocellular carcinoma from chronic hepatitis C. J Gastroenterol. 2007;42:830–6.
105. Fujita N, Miyachi H, Tanaka H, et al. Iron overload is associated with hepatic oxidative damage to DNA in nonalcoholic steatohepatitis. Cancer Epidemiol Biomark Prev. 2009;18:424–32.
106. Duan XY, Qiao L, Fan JG. Clinical features of nonalcoholic fatty liver disease-associated hepatocellular carcinoma. Hepatobiliary Pancreat Dis Int. 2012;11:18–27.
107. Starley BQ, Calcagno CJ, Harrison SA. Nonalcoholic fatty liver disease and hepatocellular carcinoma: a weighty connection. Hepatology. 2010;51:1820–32.
108. Piscaglia F, Svegliati-Baroni G, Barchetti A, et al. Clinical patterns of hepatocellular carcinoma in nonalcoholic fatty liver disease: a multicenter prospective study. Hepatology. 2016;63:827–38.
109. Tokushige K, Hashimoto E, Horie Y, Taniai M, Higuchi S. Hepatocellular carcinoma in Japanese patients with nonalcoholic fatty liver disease, alcoholic liver disease, and chronic liver disease of unknown etiology: report of the nationwide survey. J Gastroenterol. 2011;46:1230–7.
110. Mittal S, Sada YH, El-Serag HB, et al. Temporal trends of nonalcoholic fatty liver disease-related hepatocellular carcinoma in the veteran affairs population. Clin Gastroenterol Hepatol. 2015;13:594–601.
111. El-Serag HB. Epidemiology of viral hepatitis and hepatocellular carcinoma. Gastroenterology. 2012;142:1264–73.e1
112. Younossi ZM, Blissett D, Blissett R, et al. The economic and clinical burden of nonalcoholic fatty liver disease in the United States and Europe. Hepatology. 2016;64:1577–86.
113. Younossi ZM, Zheng L, Stepanova M, Venkatesan C, Mishra A. Clinical outcomes and resource utilisation in Medicare patients with chronic liver disease: a historical cohort study. BMJ Open. 2014;4:e004318.
114. Martini EM, Garrett N, Lindquist T, Isham GJ. The boomers are coming: a total cost of care model of the impact of population aging on health care costs in the United States by major practice category. Health Serv Res. 2007;42:201–18.
115. Baumeister SE, Völzke H, Marschall P, et al. Impact of fatty liver disease on health care utilization and costs in a general population: a 5-year observation. Gastroenterology. 2008;134:85–94.
116. Younossi ZM, Henry L. Economic and quality-of-life implications of non-alcoholic fatty liver disease. Pharmacoeconomics. 2015;33:1245–53.
117. Newton JL, Jones DE, Henderson E, et al. Fatigue in non-alcoholic fatty liver disease (NAFLD) is significant and associates with inactivity and excessive daytime sleepiness but not with liver disease severity or insulin resistance. Gut. 2008;57:807–13.
118. Thein HH, Isaranuwatchai W, Campitelli MA, et al. Health care costs associated with hepatocellular carcinoma: a population-based study. Hepatology. 2013;58:1375–84.
119. Lang K, Danchenko N, Gondek K, Shah S, Thompson D. The burden of illness associated with hepatocellular carcinoma in the United States. J Hepatol. 2009;50:89–99.
120. Ong JP, Pitts A, Younossi ZM. Increased overall mortality and liver-related mortality in non-alcoholic fatty liver disease. J Hepatol. 2008;49:608–12.
121. Kim D, Kim WR, Kim HJ, Therneau TM. Association between noninvasive fibrosis markers and mortality among adults with nonalcoholic fatty liver disease in the United States. Hepatology. 2013;57:1357–65.
122. Rafiq N, Bai C, Fang Y, et al. Long-term follow-up of patients with nonalcoholic fatty liver. Clin Gastroenterol Hepatol. 2009;7:234–8.
123. Söderberg C, Stål P, Askling J, et al. Decreased survival of subjects with elevated liver function tests during a 28-year follow-up. Hepatology. 2010;51:595–602.

Pathogenesis of NASH: How Metabolic Complications of Overnutrition Favour Lipotoxicity and Pro-Inflammatory Fatty Liver Disease

3

Geoffrey C. Farrell, Fahrettin Haczeyni, and Shivakumar Chitturi

Abstract

Overnutrition, usually with obesity and genetic predisposition, lead to insulin resistance, which is an invariable accompaniment of nonalcoholic fatty liver disease (NAFLD). The associated metabolic abnormalities, pre- or established diabetes, hypertension and atherogenic dyslipidemia (clustered as metabolic syndrome) tend to be worse for nonalcoholic steatohepatitis (NASH), revealing it as part of a continuum of metabolic pathogenesis. The origins of hepatocellular injury and lobular inflammation which distinguish NASH from simple steatosis have intrigued investigators, but it is now widely accepted that NASH results from liver lipotoxicity. The key issue is not the quantity of liver fat but the type(s) of lipid molecules that accumulate, and how they are "packaged" to avoid subcellular injury. Possible lipotoxic mediators include free (unesterified) cholesterol, saturated free fatty acids, diacylglycerols, lysophosphatidylcholine, sphingolipids and ceramide. Lipid droplets are intracellular storage organelles for non-structural lipid whose regulation is influenced by genetic polymorphisms, such as PNPLA3. Cells unable to sequester chemically reactive lipid molecules undergo mitochondrial injury, endoplasmic reticulum (ER) stress and autophagy, all processes of interest for NASH pathogenesis. Lipotoxicity kills hepatocytes by apoptosis, a highly regulated, non-inflammatory form of cell death, but also by necrosis, necroptosis and pyroptosis; the latter involve mitochondrial injury, oxidative stress, activation of c-Jun *N*-terminal kinase (JNK) and release of danger-associated molecular patterns (DAMPs). DAMPs stimulate innate immunity by binding pattern recognition receptors, such as Toll-like receptor 4 (TLR4) and the NOD-like receptor protein 3 (NLRP3) inflammasome, which release a cascade of pro-inflammatory chemokines and cytokines. Thus, lipotoxic hepatocellular injury attracts inflammatory cells, particularly activated macrophages which surround ballooned hepatocytes as crown-like structures. In both experimental and human NASH, livers contain cholesterol crystals which are a second signal for NLRP3 activation; this causes interleukin (IL)-1β and IL18 secretion to attract and activate macrophages and neutrophils. Injured hepatocytes also liberate plasma membrane-

G. C. Farrell (✉) · F. Haczeyni · S. Chitturi
Australian National University Medical School, and Gastroenterology and Hepatology Unit, The Canberra Hospital, Woden, ACT, Australia
e-mail: geoff.farrell@anu.edu.au; fahrettin.haczeyni@anu.edu.au; shiv.chitturi@act.gov.au

J. Yu (ed.), *Obesity, Fatty Liver and Liver Cancer*, Advances in Experimental Medicine and Biology 1061, https://doi.org/10.1007/978-981-10-8684-7_3

derived extracellular vesicles; these have been shown to circulate in NASH and to be pro-inflammatory. The way metabolic dysfunction leads to lipotoxicity, innate immune responses and the resultant pattern of cellular inflammation in the liver are likely also relevant to hepatic fibrogenesis and hepatocarcinogenesis. Pinpointing the key molecules involved pharmacologically should eventually lead to effective pharmacotherapy against NASH.

Keywords
Overnutrition · Lipotoxicity · Nonalcoholic fatty liver disease · Inflammation

3.1 Introduction

Nonalcoholic fatty liver disease (NAFLD) is highly prevalent (15–45%) in North and South America, Europe and the Asia-Pacific region, but only 10–25% of cases develop nonalcoholic steatohepatitis (NASH), which can lead to cirrhosis, liver failure and hepatocellular carcinoma (HCC). The pathology of NASH includes steatosis, hepatocellular degeneration/cell death (ballooning, Mallory hyaline, apoptosis), lobular mixed-cell inflammation (macrophages, neutrophils, lymphocytes) and fibrosis. NASH is more likely than simple steatosis to cause liver fibrosis. We and others have previously reviewed the relationship of steatosis to overnutrition [1–7], with resultant insulin resistance, hyperinsulinemia, hyperglycemia, metabolic syndrome and hypoadiponectinemia. Less is known about hepatocyte cell death and inflammatory recruitment in NASH, despite their defining importance for perpetuating liver injury, hepatic fibrogenesis and hepatocarcinogenesis [8]. Here we consider the origins of hepatocyte injury and resultant patterns of cell death and inflammatory recruitment in NASH. Lipotoxicity is central to current understanding of these processes. It is a form of tissue injury associated with inflammation and wound healing, also thought to be central to the pathogenesis of type 2 diabetes [1, 5, 9].

In lipotoxic liver injury, hepatocytes die by apoptosis, necrosis and necroptosis, and possibly pyroptosis, a more recently recognised form of pro-inflammatory cell death related to inflammasomes (discussed later). An additional phenomenon is that some hepatocytes exhibit the unusual appearance of "ballooning", one of the diagnostic criteria for NASH [3]. Ballooning may reflect cytoskeletal injury as a result of caspase 3 activation with inability to complete programmed cell death ("undead cells") or to enter the cell cycle (senescence) [10]. The interactive roles of cell stressors (oxidative, endoplasmic reticulum [ER], altered membrane fluidity resulting from altered lipid content), intracellular signalling pathways (c-Jun *N*-terminal kinase [JNK], nuclear factor kappa-B [NF-κB]) [8], responses to stress (autophagy [discussed in Chap. 10], senescence), and subcellular injury to mitochondria, lipid droplets (the intracellular storage site for potentially toxic lipids) and plasma membrane are all potentially relevant to NASH pathogenesis. How varying patterns of hepatocyte injury/cell death incite an inflammatory response, particularly by liganding pattern recognition receptors that activate innate immunity (sterile inflammation), interacting with "inputs" from gut microbiota [discussed in Chaps. 8 and 9], stressed adipose and immune/inflammatory cells activated by other processes could be central to the pathological dichotomy between NASH and simple steatosis.

The focus of the present chapter will be on connections between lipotoxic injury to hepatocytes and liver inflammation. Several excellent reviews on sterile liver inflammation and hepatocyte cell death, both of central interest to NASH, have been published recently; for more detailed molecular discussion, the reader is referred to them [5, 11–13].

3.2 What Is Lipotoxicity, and How Does It Fit into a Framework for NASH Pathogenesis?

Unger coined the term "lipotoxicity" in 1994 to describe the pattern of lipid molecule-induced cell injury that occurs in pancreatic β-cells in type 2 diabetes (diabetes) and muscle in metabolic syndrome [9]. Since the first lipidomic data from human NAFLD and NASH livers were published in 2007 and 2009 [14, 15], coupled with the development of animal models where metabolic syndrome determines experimental steatohepatitis [16], the concept that NASH could be a form of liver lipotoxicity has gained ground [1–7, 17]. In 2012, Cusi proposed the term "liver lipotoxicity" be used instead of NASH [5]. We agree with this important conceptual reorientation of NASH (versus "not-NASH" NAFLD), but before adopting the term "liver lipotoxicity" to replace "NASH", it would be useful to know which lipid(s) is/are responsible. Effectively lowering their hepatic levels should reverse NASH.

The central issue in NASH pathogenesis is what is different in livers showing NASH, as opposed to the larger proportion of NAFLD patients whose liver pathology, simple steatosis or steatosis with minor non-specific inflammation (often termed "not-NASH" NAFLD), is less commonly associated with fibrosis progression [3, 8]. Two decades ago it was proposed that NASH reflected operation of a second tier of injury and inflammation-inducing pathways, such as oxidative stress and Th1 cytokine responses (e.g. tumor necrosis factor-alpha [TNF-α]) in a liver that was fatty because of overweight and diabetes (the "first hit"). The second hit was presumed to originate from outside the liver, such as from gut-derived endotoxin (demonstrated experimentally by Yang and colleagues from the Diehl group in 1997 [18] or from inflamed adipose tissue in obesity. This 2-hit hypothesis, eloquently articulated by Day and James in 1998 [19], proved useful to focus attention on injury mechanisms in NASH. With hindsight it now seems simplistic because the metabolic milieu leading to steatosis can also lead "directly" to NASH, as we and others discuss elsewhere [2, 5]. The jaded 2-hit concept is still cited [20]. However, writing in the first book on NAFLD (2003), Bass and Merriman articulated the idea that the lipids which accumulate in NASH could themselves (directly) mediate the disease process [1]. Greg Gores' group then showed that free fatty acid (FFA) lipotoxicity could give rise to TNF-α [21], and by 2007 the concept of "good fat/bad fat" was editorialised in *Hepatology* [22]. Most working in the field now agree that Bass and Merriman were correct. There are multiple responses to lipotoxicity, and these descend through a web of interactions and reactions, a "multiple hit" concept as conceived by Tilg [23], to result in NASH.

3.3 Which Lipid Molecules Accumulate in NASH?

If analogy is drawn with Koch's postulates for determining the infectious aetiology of a disease, similar lines of evidence (or "**rules**") could apply for implicating endogenous toxic molecules as the cause of a pattern of tissue injury. These are encapsulated in Box 3.1.

Box 3.1: Rules for Pathogenicity of Lipotoxic Molecules in NASH

Rule 1 *Phenotypic association.* By phenotypic association, it is reasoned that the causative lipotoxin will be present in human livers showing NASH but not in simple steatosis.

Rule 2 *Congruent explanation.* The reasons why this lipotoxin accumulates will be consistent with a metabolic pathogenesis and/or be explained by genetic predisposition.

Rule 3 *Therapy proves causation.* Ideally, removal of the lipotoxic lipid should reverse NASH pathology, noting that the outcome is likely to be simple steatosis, not a lean liver.

Rule 4 *Direct lipotoxicity.* The putative lipotoxin should be directly toxic to hepatocytes, the cells most conspicuously injured in NASH.

Rule 5 *Lipotoxicity causes NASH.* The way the putative lipotoxin injures hepatocytes must be pro-inflammatory, that is, the injury has an outcome (or form of cell death) that leads to recruitment of macrophages, lymphocytes, and neutrophils to the liver.

3.4 Which Models Should We "Trust" for Interpretation of NASH Pathogenesis Studies?

Before balancing the evidence for and against candidate lipotoxins in NASH, a few words about animal models are salient (animal models are discussed more fully in relation to obesity-related hepatocarcinogenesis by Lau and colleagues in Chap. 11). While the ideal "model" of a human disease is the affected patient, repeated tissue sampling and the challenges (including potential hazards) of experimental interventions generally limit the study of NASH pathogenesis in man to "static measurements", that is, blood or liver samples usually obtained at a single time. The study of Vilar-Gomez et al. [24] is an important rare exception [24]. The next best model might be one that replicates, as faithfully as possible, the preconditions (other than species) for development of human NASH. As reviewed earlier [16], these desirable attributes, and why we think they are prerequisites, are tabulated (Table 3.1).

In addition to the "metabolic determinants" listed in Table 3.1, suitable models should exhibit the pathological spectrum of human NAFLD, which under varying circumstances spans simple steatosis, steatohepatitis (NASH), pericellular fibrosis (noting that rodents are unlikely to develop cirrhosis), and hepatocarcinogenesis (in rats and mice, as well as in an apparently substantial proportion of patients with NASH, HCC does not proceed through advanced liver fibrosis).

While opinions vary widely on the relative merits and weaknesses of numerous NAFLD or steatohepatitis models, we are of the opinion that models whose only virtue is "providing NASH pathology" should not be used uncritically to progress concepts of NASH pathogenesis. For example, rodents with methionine and choline deficiency, the MCD model, was developed by the author's group in 1996 in rats [25] and 2000 in mice [26], as an attempt to provide a model with steatohepatitis, the pathology that is not observed in obese rodents with defects in leptin or the leptin receptor (obesity is associated with simple steatosis) or those fed high fat diet without other nutrient excess. However, Rinella and Green, confirmed by Rizki and Maher, showed that 20–40% weight loss experienced by MCD-fed mice is associated with insulin sensitivity [27, 28], whereas insulin resistance is a *sine qua non* for pathogenesis of NASH [29, 30]. The similar choline-deficient defined L-amino acid (CDAA) diet of Matsumoto et al. [31], popularised by

Table 3.1 Desirable characteristics of animal models of NASH

Characteristic	Importance	Methods to obtain
Overnutrition	Invariable in human NASH	Dietary: High fat
		Mechanical hyperalimentation
		Genetic: Appetite drive
Insulin resistance	Central to metabolic obesity	Genetic predisposition (animal strain)
	Invariable in human NASH	
	Drives hepatic lipotoxicity	Dietary: High fat
Hypoadiponectemia	Found in human NASH	Substantial overnutrition
	Reflects adipose stress	
	Worsens insulin resistance	
Metabolic syndrome (e.g. glucose intolerance, dyslipidemia, hypertension)	85% of patients with NASH	Most dietary models do not achieve metabolic syndrome: Need substantial overnutrition and genetic predisposition
Pathology: Steatosis, ballooned hepatocytes and significant lobular inflammation of mixed cell type	Hallmarks of NASH pathology	Metabolic syndrome-related NASH
		*Methionine and choline deficiency, CDAA, high fat and high cholesterol (atherogenic) diets
Pathological spectrum includes simple steatosis and steatohepatitis with pericellular fibrosis	To understand transition from simple steatosis to NASH: Need model that spans disease phenotypes	An environment determinant of NASH, such as high fat and high cholesterol diet composition, can be modulated to generate steatohepatitis or simple steatosis

*May not cause ballooning

Miura and Brenner [32], appears to be less "nutritionally challenged", but animals still fail to gain excessive weight or develop glucose intolerance; by one biochemical measurement, CDAA-fed mice may have impaired insulin signaling, but physiological insulin resistance has not been demonstrated [31]. Use of the term "NASH" to describe results in MCD or CDAA mice (more than 10 articles in 2014) is curious since, in 2005, the Editor of Gastroenterology specifically instructed the authors to use the more appropriate term "nutritional steatohepatitis" [33].

Other models have provided interesting insights into how "mal-processing" of certain molecules, particularly cholesterol, can lead to steatohepatitis [34–37]. These elegant studies indicate what **can happen** under certain conditions, but do not prove that the same thing **does happen** in humans with NASH. Likewise, diets that promote overnutrition (for example, those rich in simple carbohydrates, particularly fructose or sucrose [38–40], and those that combine excess carbohydrate, fat and cholesterol ("western" or "atherogenic" diets) are most likely to result in NASH [37, 41–43], whereas "unidimensional diets", such as high fat or high sucrose without cholesterol generally cause simple steatosis. On the other hand, for rodents a diet containing 1–2% (wt/wt) cholesterol, which Ginsberg described 10 years ago as the human equivalent of eating >100 big Macs a day [44], is physiologically unrealistic; it is debatable whether such "cholesterol toxicity" is akin to NASH, and the liver histology is not convincing.

Here we draw heavily on studies that have used animal models of overnutrition in which the metabolic determinants of NASH (insulin resistance, hyperglycemia and metabolic syndrome) are present. Such models include rodents and pigs that are deliberately hyper-alimented (e.g. by in-dwelling gastric devices) [45, 46], and rodents with genetically-determined appetite defects, such as melanocortin 4 receptor (*Mc4r*) and *Alms1* mutant mice [42, 47, 48]. The latter is the murine equivalent of Alström syndrome [49], a rare monozygotic form of extreme childhood obesity with diabetes, cardiovascular disease and cirrhosis. Appetite-defective mice are particularly useful as they, like children with monozygotic morbid obesity, "can't stop eating" and soon become quite inactive [50].

3.5 Triglyceride, the Most Abundant Lipid in Fatty Livers, Does Not Injure Hepatocytes

Steatosis is defined by stainable fat in hepatocytes, most of which is triacylglycerol or triglyceride (TG), or by an increase in hepatic TG content (>5.5%) determined, for example, by proton magnetic resonance spectroscopy (MRS). While correlations between hepatic TG content and development of insulin resistance have been derived in human studies [51], these investigations have been based on MRS evidence of steatosis, not on lipid analyses. There is no experimental evidence that TG impairs insulin receptor signalling or has any noxious effect on hepatocytes.

Within hepatocytes, TG is usually stored efficiently in lipid droplets (discussed later). TG is formed by transacylation of diacylglycerols (DG), catalyzed by diacylglyceride acyltransferases (DGAT); DGAT expression protects hepatocytes from palmitic acid-induced lipotoxicity and steatohepatitis caused by MCD diet. Thus, in DGAT2-deficient animals or with DGAT2 knockdown, liver injury (serum alanine aminotransferase [ALT] level) and resultant fibrogenesis were exaggerated, whereas strategies to enhance TG synthesis were protective [52, 53].

3.6 FFAs Are Lipotoxic *in vitro* But Seem Unlikely to Cause NASH

Until recently, FFAs have been the favoured lipotoxin in NASH [54–56], but the evidence for this is based on *in vitro* studies of lipotoxicity (as mentioned above) and the MCD model. FFA, including but not confined to saturated FFA (satFFA), accumulate in all human NAFLD livers, irrespective of disease phenotype [14, 15, 56]. There is no difference in hepatic FFA levels between livers showing NASH and simple steatosis in humans or mice and opossums with metabolic syndrome [37, 57] (Itoh 2012 is an exception [58]).

In vitro, satFFA are more lipotoxic than mono-unsaturated or poly-unsaturated long-chain or very long-chain fatty acids. However, neither the published human nor *foz/foz* mouse analyses indicate important differences in saturation status between NASH and simple steatosis. In mice lacking elongation of long-chain fatty acids family member 6 (Elovl6), which catalyzes formation of stearate (C18:0) from palmitate (C16:0) and oleate (C18:1) from palmitoleate (C16:1), and also promotes expression of sterol-regulatory element-binding protein 1c (SREBP1c), there was no effect on obesity-related liver fat but improved insulin sensitivity attributable to low abundance of DAG [59]; the relevance to human NASH is unclear. An interesting observation has been a relative paucity of polyunsaturated C20-C22 fatty acids in FFA, triacylglycerides and phospholipids in NASH [14, 60]. These reductions include arachidonic (20:4n-6) (the source of eicosanoids), eicosapentanoic (20:5n-3), and docosahexanoic (22:6n-3) acids. This paucity is potentially relevant to liver inflammation because it could change the balance in lipid mediators from antiinflammatory to pro-inflammatory. In mice with forced hepatic overexpression of PNPLA3^{I148M} [61, 62], a polymorphism associated with frequency and severity of human NAFLD [63, 64], relative depletion of polyunsaturated C20-C22 fatty acids was observed among triacylglycerols [65]. Most recently, Chiappini et al. reported the opposite finding, depletion of long-chain fatty acids attributable to decreased activity of the fatty acid desaturase 1 (FADS1) [66]; this particularly altered phospholipid synthesis.

satFFA cytotoxicity to hepatocytes is an experimental paradigm for liver lipotoxicity and resultant inflammation. Some key points are summarised in Box 3.2. satFFA, such as palmitic acid (C16:0) and stearic acid (C18:0), are more toxic than mono-unsaturates, such as palmitoleic (C16:1) and oleic acid (C18:1); the latter *protect* liver cells against saturated FFA lipotoxicity, possibly by promoting their incorporation into TG [54, 67]. Mono-unsaturates also decrease lysophosphatidylcholine (LPC) content [68], which appears to be an essential mediator of FFA lipotoxicity. Lipotoxicity also involves activation of JNK possibly independent of oxidative stress. In turn, JNK activation injures mitochondria leading to oxidative stress, a self-amplifying step in JNK signal transduction.

Box 3.2: Key Points for FFA Toxicity.

1. Saturates are more toxic than unsaturates.
2. Mono-unsaturates confer protective effects.
3. Toxicity proceeds through lysophosphatidylcholine (LPC) formation.
4. Lipotoxicity involves JNK activation.
5. JNK-dependant mitochondrial injury occurs.
6. Secondary oxidative stress causes further damage to the cell.

In studies from Gores' lab using primary murine hepatocytes, which validated key findings in well-differentiated human hepatocytes [69], data confirmed operation of the JNK-mitochondrial cell death pathway in satFFA lipotoxicity via PUMA. They also showed that satFFA lipotoxicity proceeds through the formation of LPC, which had been suggested as the lipotoxic mediator in palmitic acid toxicity studies by Han et al. [68].

3.7 Phospholipids: Lysophosphatidylcholine Is a Candidate Lipotoxin in NASH

Like palmitic acid, LPC produces hepatocyte injury *in vitro*, and it also induces hepatitis *in vivo* [68]. Han and colleagues found increased LPC content in five NASH cases, higher than in seven with simple steatosis or 12 lean livers; few other lipidomic analyses in NAFLD mention LPC. Chiappini et al. recently found decreased phosphatidylcholine-to-phosphatidylethan olamines rates in human NASH livers [66]. They demonstrated experimentally in HCC cell lines and primary human hepatocytes that lipid mixes from NASH patients can strikingly induce cellular toxicity [66].

3.8 Does Ceramide Play a Role?

Ceramide is the prototypic sphingolipid formed in the ER by condensation of palmitoyl CoA (or other fatty acid moiety) with sphingosine. The rate of ceramide synthesis by this pathway depends on availability of satFFA, but, in addition, *de novo* synthesis of ceramide can be rapidly generated from sphingomyelin by sphingomyelinase. Such rapid generation of ceramide has been implicated in apoptosis by the death ligands, TNF-α and Fas ligand (FasL) [70]. Ceramide can also play a role in insulin resistance. A prevailing concept is that satFFA lead to formation of ceramide, accumulation of which kills pancreatic β-cells (and neurons) by death-ligand-induced apoptosis. However, Wei et al. showed that ceramide is not essential for satFFA lipotoxicity in liver cells [71], and Han and colleagues showed that ceramide synthesis inhibitors do not modulate palmitic acid-induced lipoapoptosis to hepatocytes [68]. On the other hand, phospholipase A_2 (PLA_2) inhibitors blocked cell death in these experiments, suggesting a role of PLA_2 or its product LPC. Lipidomic analyses of human or murine NAFLD livers have usually failed to identify ceramide accumulation [72], and bariatric surgery improved NASH without lowering circulating ceramide levels [73]. Sphingosine 1-phosphate (S1P), a derivative of ceramide, contributes to macrophage-related inflammation in some contexts. Mauer and colleagues recently showed that the S1P antagonist, FTY720 reduced inflammation and fibrosis in a high fat, high cholesterol dietary model of steatohepatitis in mice [74].

3.9 Diacylglycerols

DAG activates atypical protein kinase C (PKC) isoforms, which have been implicated in the molecular pathogenesis of insulin resistance. By activating NF-κB, PKCs are also pro-inflammatory. Puri et al. found increased hepatic DAG levels in NAFLD versus lean livers, but no difference between NASH and not-NASH fatty livers [14]. In *foz/foz* mice fed normal rodent chow to cause steatosis or atherogenic diet to cause NASH, hepatic DAG levels increased compared to lean controls, but values were similar in NASH and simple steatosis [75, 76]. Gorden et al.. found increased DAG species, particularly in phospholipids between normal versus NAFLD livers [77, 78], but without specificity to NASH phenotype (see Rule 1, Box 3.1).

3.10 Cholesterol Is a Strong Contender for a Lipotoxin Causing NASH

Three lipidomic analyses found that free cholesterol (FC) is increased in NASH livers but not simple steatosis [60, 76, 77, 79]. Caballero et al used filipin which fluoresces blue upon binding FC but not cholesterol esters [15]. They observed that all 14 NASH livers fluoresced for FC within hepatocytes, versus 4 of 17 with simple steatosis. In *foz/foz* mice, atherogenic dietary intake caused NASH with major increases of hepatic cholesterol ester and FC; chow-fed *foz/foz* mice with simple steatosis showed no such increase [76]. Atherogenic diet-fed *Wt* mice exhibited a transient increase in FC, after which adaptation occurred with return of hepatic FC to normal; this was associated with simple steatosis, not NASH [76].

Epidemiological studies reveal a positive association of dietary cholesterol intake with cirrhosis (irrespective of aetiology) and HCC [80]. Some but not all nutritional studies confirm diets high in saturated fat and cholesterol are associated with NASH [81]. On the other hand, intake of fructose or simple carbohydrates is more consistently identified, and there is a reproducible inverse relationship with micronutrients [82]. Japanese workers showed a strong effect of atherogenic diet (7.5% cocoa butter, 1.25% cholesterol) on NASH in rodents [43], and the co-requirement for cholesterol as well as saturated fat, often with simple carbohydrate, has been found repeatedly [17, 40, 41, 83].

Appetite-defective animals eat more and readily become obese, particularly when fed high fat diet. *Mc4r* mutant mice fed a 60% fat diet (0.04% cholesterol) develop liver and adipose inflammation, with a pattern of crown-like structures (CLSs) of macrophages around hepatocytes that exhibited large lipid droplets [58]. In our studies, modulation of the cholesterol content of atherogenic diet (0, 0.2–2.0% wt/wt) caused a stepwise increase in hepatic FC content, and this was associated with corresponding increases in serum ALT, hepatocyte apoptosis, activated macrophage and neutrophil accumulation, and NASH severity estimated by NAFLD Activity Score (NAS). In *ABCB4* mutant opossums (*ABCB4* encodes a canalicular transporter of bile acids and glutathione conjugates), consumption of a "western diet" (0.7% cholesterol) caused hepatic cholesterol accumulation, atherogenic dyslipidemia and NASH [37]. In low density lipoprotein receptor (LDLR) knockout mice, cholesterol content of the diet was a key determinant of whether liver pathology was steatosis or steatohepatitis [36], and this was associated with increased hepatic cholesterol content [34, 35].

3.11 Dysregulation of Hepatic Cholesterol Homeostasis Occurs in NASH

The liver is the central organ for bodily cholesterol homeostasis. Cholesterol synthesis is regulated in response to "need", as perceived by nuclear receptors such as SREBP2 [84]. SREBP2, the master regulator of cholesterol homeostasis, is upregulated by insulin. Three studies confirm upregulation of hepatic SREBP2 in human NASH [14, 15, 60], and similar changes occur in obese, diabetic *foz/foz* mice with NASH [75, 76]. In the rodent model, HMG-CoA reductase enzyme activity was correspondingly suppressed, as expected by the regulatory role of SREBP2. Min et al. [60] measured circulating metabolites of cholesterol synthesis (desmosterol:cholesterol ratio) and decreased hepatic HMG-CoA phosphoprotein, and concluded that cholesterol synthesis is increased in NASH but not simple steatosis [60]; this finding is counter-intuitive, given the observed upregulation of SREBP2. The different results between the mouse and human studies could reflect species or methodological differences.

Tracer studies indicate that most liver lipid in human NASH arises from peripheral sources, albeit an increase in *de novo* synthesis (hepatic lipogenesis) also occurs [85]. Hepatocytes express three cholesterol uptake pathways: scavenger receptor B1 (SRB1), CD36 (uptake pathway for cholesterol and FFAs) and LDLR. LDLR expression is not increased in human NASH [60], but CD36-enriched extracellular vesicles (EVs) circulate in diabetes and metabolic syndrome, and in patients with NASH (Chen B, Farrell GC, Teoh NC – unpublished data). Further, hepatic CD36 expression is upregulated in obese, diabetic mice with NASH [86].

FC is highly reactive. Thus, cells form fatty acyl esters (CEs) catalyzed by acyl-CoA:cholesterol transferase (ACAT) 2, and also sequester FC into lipid droplets. While hepatic expression of ACAT2 increases in NASH (human and mouse), the reverse pathway of esterolysis, catalyzed by cholesterol ester hydrolase (CEH), is also upregulated [60, 76].

A uniquely important pathway for FC disposition in the liver is biotransformation into bile acids. The rate-limiting steps are cytochromes P450 (CYP) 7A1 and 2B1 in ER, and CYP27A in mitochondria. Profound dysregulation of cholesterol homeostasis occurs in NASH: *CYP7A1* expression (human liver) and *Cyps7a1*, *2b1* and *27a* (mouse liver) are all near-totally suppressed in NASH, but not in simple steatosis [60, 76].

Hepatocytes rid themselves of cholesterol by passage into blood (via basolateral ATP-binding cassette transporter 1 [ABCA1]) or bile, directly via ABCG5/G8 heterodimers, or as bile acids via ABCB11 (bile salt export pump, BSEP) and ABCB4 (mdr2). ABCA1 is downregulated in human NASH [60], and profound suppression of ABCB11, ABCB4 and ABCG5/8 occurs in *foz/foz* mice with NASH [76].

In summary, while details may vary between species, it is clear that cholesterol inputs (uptake or synthesis) are increased in NASH versus simple steatosis. Cholesterol ester hydrolysis is also increased, but biotransformation and egress of cholesterol (directly or as bile acids) is profoundly impaired. The net effect is FC trapping in hepatocytes. Van Rooyen et al. showed that insulin concentrations that circulate in insulin-resistant animals are sufficient to upregulate SREBP2 and LDLR, and to downregulate ABCB11 in murine primary hepatocytes [76].

Recently, it has become apparent that hepatic cholesterol trapping in NASH leads to precipitation of cholesterol crystals. To study the conditions that lead to this change in physical state, Ioannou and colleagues [87] fed mice diet high in fat and with increasing amounts of cholesterol for 6 months [87]. Mice fed diets with 0.5% cholesterol or higher developed NASH with fibrosis whereas those fed lower cholesterol high fat diet showed simple steatosis (Fig. 3.1). It was evident that cholesterol crystal-laden lipid droplet remnants from dead or dying hepatocytes were processed by lysosomal enzymes within Kupffer cells. These Kupffer cells (and presumably also recruited macrophages) formed the centre of CLSs, which stained positive for NLRP3 and active caspase 1 (see later section on inflammasome). This phenomenon could be modelled in culture: thus, HepG2 cells exposed to LDL-cholesterol developed crystals in lipid droplet membranes that upregulated TNF, NLRP3 and IL-1β in co-cultured macrophages, with secretion of IL-1β [87].

Atorvastatin inhibits HMG-CoA reductase but this and other statins have no beneficial effect on NASH pathology [88, 89]; this may be because depletion of hepatic cholesterol upregulates a hepatic cholesterol re-uptake pathway in which Niemann Pick C1-like protein 1 (NPC1L1) transports cholesterol across biliary (and intestinal) epithelium. Conversely, blockade of NPC1L1 by ezetimibe upregulates cholesterol synthesis, and ezetimibe appears ineffective therapy in NASH [90]. We used combination atorvastatin and ezetimibe to return hepatic FC to normal levels in atherogenic diet-fed *foz/foz* mice [57]. There were commensurate reductions in serum ALT, hepatocyte apoptosis, macrophage activation and severity of NASH pathology, including liver fibrosis. Combination atorvastatin and ezetimibe also removed cholesterol crystals [79] (Fig. 3.2). Thus, cholesterol accumulation (with crystal formation) correlates with NASH pathology, and cholesterol removal (FC and crystals) cures NASH.

3.12 Free Cholesterol Is Directly Lipotoxic to Primary Hepatocytes

Caballero and colleagues showed that the mitochondrial cholesterol transporter, steroidogenic acute regulatory protein (StAR) is upregulated in NASH [15], serving as a pathway for mitochondrial cholesterol accumulation. In livers of *foz/foz* mice with NASH, FC partitioned into mitochondria, and to a lesser extent plasma membrane and ER [91]. Ultrastructural studies confirmed mitochondrial damage in this model (swelling, fragmentation of cristae, formation of crystalline material in the matrix), and similar findings have been documented in human NASH since 1999 [92, 93]. Human studies have also found low hepatic ATP levels in NASH [94], which is consistent with mitochondrial injury.

To establish whether FC is directly lipotoxic, we incubated primary murine hepatocytes with unmodified human LDL and showed dose-dependent FC uptake over 24 h [91] (Fig. 3.3). FC loading caused cell injury, apoptosis and necrosis, redox stress, mitochondrial membrane pore transition with cytochrome c leakage into cytosol, and rapid decline in cellular ATP content. These processes were linked mechanistically to JNK1 activation; thus, *Jnk1*$^{-/-}$ hepatocytes were refractory to FC lipotoxicity, and specific JNK inhibitors blocked both apoptosis and necrosis. Mitochondrial protectants (cyclosporine A) and caspase 3/7 inhibitors also rescued hepatocytes from FC lipotoxicity, whereas the ER stress chaperone, 4-phenylbutyric acid, failed to exert any protective effect. The cholesterol loading of HepG2 cells recently reported by Ioannou et al. [87], in which cholesterol crystals were recognised in lipid droplet remnants, also

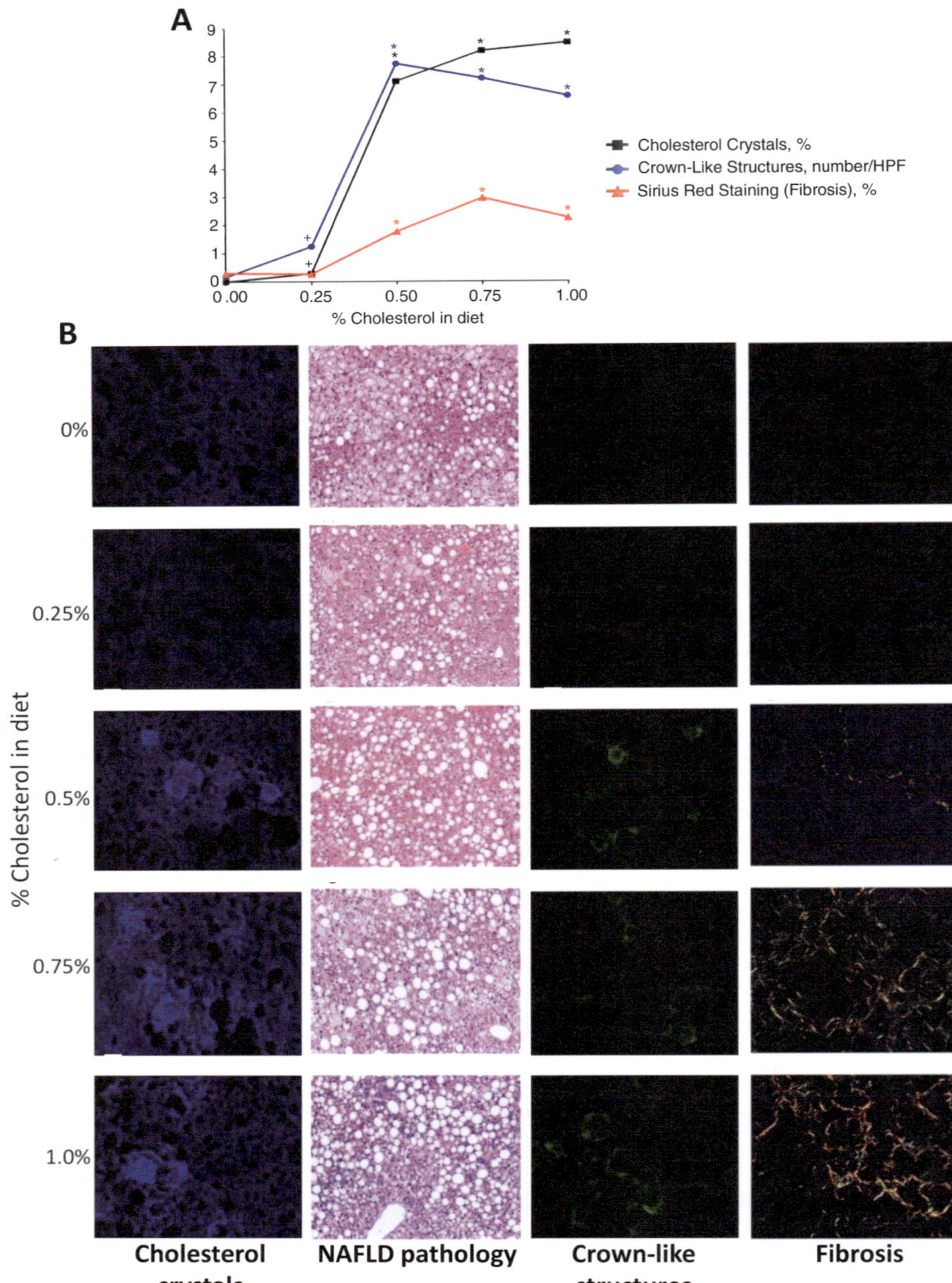

Fig. 3.1 (**A**) Mice were fed high fat (15%) diet with increasing cholesterol content. At 0.5% cholesterol, the number of hepatic cholesterol crystals (black line) increased, associated with macrophage crown-like structures (blue line), and Sirius Red positive area for fibrosis (red line). $^{(*)}P < 0.01$ and $^{(+)}P < 0.05$ compared with 0% cholesterol group. (**B**) Representative mouse liver sections after 6 months on each diet. The first column

support direct toxicity of cholesterol to hepatocyte-like cells.

In summary, among potential lipotoxins causing NASH, FC conforms to the rules of phenotypic association, accumulation by pathways related to metabolic pathogenesis of NASH, is directly toxic to hepatocytes, and its therapeutic removal cures NASH and reverses liver fibrosis (see Box 3.1). Recent data also support a role for selective changes in long-chain fatty acid composition, particularly in selected phospholipid DAGs [66, 95], with alterations in PC:PE ratio that may affect membrane permeability. Whether PNPLA3^{I148M} (discussed later) could underlie such changes requires further study. Meanwhile, it remains possible that fatty acid chain length and accumulation of free cholesterol are both important mechanistically and act synergistically to cause NASH. In order to consider the implications of lipotoxicity for inflammatory recruitment, consideration of the sites of hepatocellular injury in lipotoxic NASH is critical.

3.13 Subcellular Sites of Hepatocyte Injury in NASH

satFFA, LPC and FC lipotoxicity are all associated with mitochondrial membrane pore transition (MPT) that causes disruption of cellular respiration, generation of oxidative stress, and cytochrome c leakage from the matrix into the cytosol where it activates the apoptosome [96]. Provided there is sufficient energy (ATP) required for the final execution steps that involve caspase 3/7-mediated cleavage of the cytoskeleton and cell movement, this causes of apoptosis. When ATP is depleted, programmed cell death is aborted, terminating in necroptosis (caspase 8 is not involved; mixed lineage kinase domain-like pseudokinase [MLKL] is recruited and binds to the receptor-interacting protein 1 [RIP1]/RIP3 complex), or necrosis. Necrosis (sometimes referred to as type 2 necrosis or oncosis) also occurs with more rapid permeabilization of the plasma membrane and dispersion of ion gradients within the cell, a disorganized form of cell death that liberates cell contents. A recent study reported that mitochondrial DNA (mtDNA) was released in mice subjected to a high fat diet, although steatohepatitis was not well-demonstrated in this study model [97]. The authors then showed that mtDNA activated TLR9 (discussed later), and proposed this as a pathway to macrophage recruitment in NASH.

ER is a site of FC deposition in NASH [91], and ER stress is favoured as a pathway to apoptosis (via C/EBP homologous protein [CHOP]-mediated cleavage of Bid) and inflammation (via JNK activation in type 2 diabetes). Triggering of one ER stress response factor but not others, and without CHOP expression, has been described in human NASH [98], and operation of ER stress was reported with MCD steatohepatitis [99]. Legry, Leclercq and colleagues conducted a set of studies in *foz/foz* and *ob/ob* mice, measuring elements of its activation, creating ER stress experimentally, and opposing it pharmacologically [100]. The results provide a strong case against ER stress being conspicuous in steatohepatitis related to obesity, diabetes and metabolic syndrome (NASH) [100, 101]. Likewise, in FC lipotoxicity to hepatocytes there was no increased expression of CHOP, and 4-phenylbutyric acid failed to protect hepatocytes [91]. Finally, in three randomized-controlled clinical trials, ursodeoxycholic acid (which opposes ER stress) was ineffective at improving NASH pathology [102–104].

Ballooned hepatocytes and apoptotic bodies arise from caspase 3/7-mediated lysis of the cytoskeleton. Membrane-bound vesicles are also shed from activated or injured/dying cell types present in NASH livers. Very small vesicles (30–100 mm) are known as exosomes, larger ones (100–

Fig. 3.1 (continued) shows blue-coloured birefringent crystalline material within lipid droplets, which are cholesterol crystals stained by filipin (×200 magnification). Second column is hematoxylin and eosin-stained liver sections. Third column shows TNF-α positive macrophages (within crown-like structures), and the last column exhibits Sirius Red positive areas for fibrosis. (Adopted from Ioannou et al. [87], with permission)

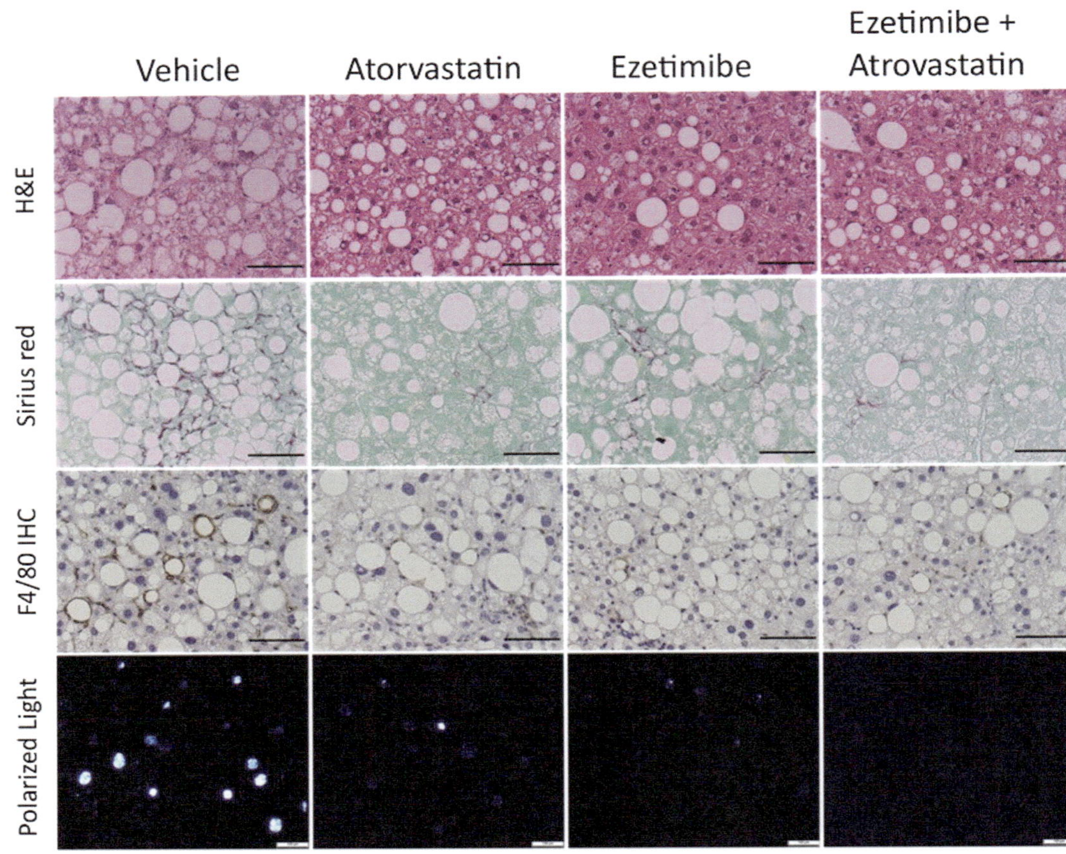

Fig. 3.2 Representative liver sections from *foz/foz* mice fed atherogenic diet (23% fat, 0.2% cholesterol) treated with ezetimibe or atorvastatin, or their combination versus vehicle controls. Liver sections were stained with hematoxylin and eosin, Sirius Red for fibrosis, F4/80 for proinflammatory macrophages (inflammation), and unstained frozen sections viewed with polarized light for birefringent cholesterol crystals. Compared to vehicle controls, there were less cholesterol crystals in the atorvastatin- and ezetimibe-treated groups, and cholesterol crystals were nearly abolished in combination-treated mice. As a result, liver histology improved, and inflammation and fibrosis were less in the drug treatment groups. Black and white scale bars 50 μm and 100 μm, respectively. (Adopted from Ioannou et al. [79], with permission)

1000 nm) are microparticles (MPs); the term extracellular vesicles (EVs) will be used here to encompass both sizes. EVs circulate in hepatic ischemia-reperfusion injury [105], an acute type of sterile liver inflammation, and they have been detected in humans with NAFLD [106]. Povero and colleagues noted that the circulating titre of EVs increases during the transition of steatosis to steatohepatitis in the CDAA model [107]; levels correlated with hepatocyte cell death, fibrosis and angiogenesis. These EVs contained asialoglycoprotein receptor 1 (ASGPR1), a protein unique to hepatocytes, and miR-122 and 192 which are associated with chronic liver disease. Circulating EVs have also been reported to contain mitochondria or mtDNA in experimental fatty and alcoholic liver injury [97, 108]. We recently found that EVs shed from hepatocytes subjected to FC lipotoxicity contain high-mobility group box 1 protein (HMGB1), and activate Kupffer cells via an HMGB1- and TLR4-dependent process (Fig. 3.3, and Gan L, Farrell GC –

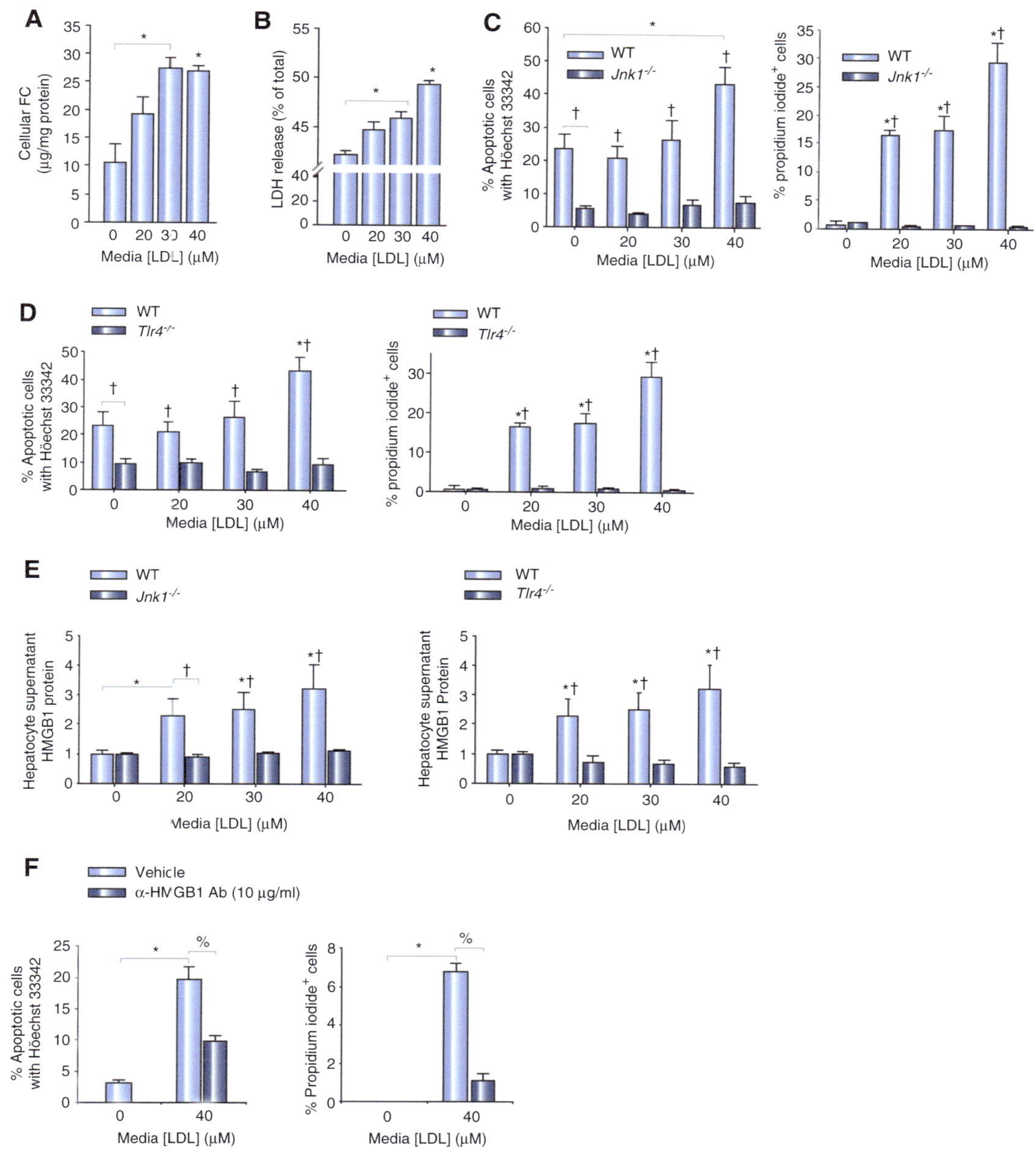

Fig. 3.3 Free cholesterol accumulation causes lipotoxicity in hepatocytes. (**A**) Primary murine hepatocytes incubated with human LDL showed dose-dependent free cholesterol (FC) uptake over 24 h, (**B**) with proportionate LDL release indicating hepatocellular injury with FC loading. Wildtype (WT) hepatocytes showed increased apoptosis (Höechst 33342 positive nuclei) and necrosis (propidium iodide positive cells) with FC-loading; (**C**) JNK1 and (**D**) TLR4 deletion protected cells from both apoptosis and necrosis. (**E**) Hepatocyte release of the danger-associated molecular pattern, high-mobility group box 1 protein (HMGB1), increased with FC-loading of WT hepatocytes, and (**F**) anti-HMGB1 protected cells from both apoptosis and necrosis. $^{(*)}P < 0.05$ compared with 0 μM LDL. $^{(\dagger)}P < 0.05$ compared to WT. $^{(\%)}P < 0.05$ compared to no addition. (Adopted from Gan et al. [91], with permission)

unpublished data). This paracrine process links lipotoxicity to inflammatory cell activation in NASH via the intermediary of EVs and soluble HMGB1. The shedding of EVs from liver cells can also activate hedgehog signalling [109], which has implications for inflammatory recruitment and fibrogenesis [107]. Recently, EVs released from lipotoxic cells were shown to be internalised by both hepatocytes and macrophages; within those cells, NF-κB-mediated upregulation of NLRP3, pro-caspase-1 and pro-interleukin-1 was demonstrated, indicating another link between lipotoxicity and pro-inflammatory pathways in NASH [110].

Using *in vitro* models, it has now been shown that the PNPLA3^{I148M} variant preferentially localises to lipid droplets and is associated with defective remodelling activity, potentially enhancing TG accumulation in lipid droplets [111]. Such lipid droplet "dysfunction" could lead to lipotoxicity indirectly because of "suboptimal storage" of toxic lipids, such as FC [87], and this has now been observed experimentally [66]. Autophagy is another important intracellular pathway, targeting cell constituents to the lysosome for degradation. Mark Czaja and colleagues identified the operation of autophagy for lipid turnover (lipophagy) in fatty liver disease, and the importance of autophagy in opposing apoptosis and influencing insulin sensitivity indicates a possible role in pathogenesis of NASH (elegantly reviewed in Amir and Czaja) [112].

3.14 Hepatocyte Injury and Cell Death in NASH: Relationship to Inflammation

3.14.1 Serum ALT and Ferritin

Circulation of hepatocyte proteins such as ALT and ferritin is evidence of liver injury in NAFLD, but serum ALT level has low sensitivity and specificity for distinguishing NASH from simple steatosis. Maximos et al. found that NAFLD patients with raised ALT had worse adipose insulin resistance, lower plasma adiponectin and higher liver triglyceride (by MRS) than those with normal ALT, but there was no correlation with ballooning, inflammation or fibrosis [51]. Unlike in viral or autoimmune hepatitis, serum ALT values in NASH (and alcoholic hepatitis) rarely exceed tenfold the upper limit of normal (~300 U/L). One reason may be that apoptosis is the predominant form of cell death [113], another is that necrosis tends to be focal rather than zonal or extensive.

3.14.2 Ballooned Hepatocytes

Ballooned hepatocytes are one of three criteria used to calculate the NAS [114], and in global assessment of "NASH vs not NASH" pathology. Further, their number correlates with fibrotic outcome [115]. Ballooned hepatocytes are large, clear cells with "blurred" plasma membrane, possibly reflecting cytoskeletal damage; they lack cytokeratin 8/18 (CK8/18) [116] (suggesting caspase 3 activation) and are ubiquitin positive. They also express hedgehog signalling ligands, which by analogy with *Drosophila melanogaster* may indicate cells have initiated a cell death program but are unable to complete the process (the term "undead" cells has been used) possibly because of deletion of caspase 9 [117]. Hedgehog ligands are chemotactic and could activate stellate cells directly [118]. It is therefore of interest that hedgehog pathway activation correlates with histologic severity of NAFLD, specifically with ballooning, portal inflammation and fibrosis severity [119, 120].

3.14.3 Apoptosis Versus Necrosis and Necroptosis

As reviewed by Luedde and colleagues recently [12], apoptosis is a physiological form of programmed cell death during development and tissue remodelling. It does not release cell contents other than within larger membrane-bound vesicles known as apoptotic bodies. These are typically engulfed by neighbouring cells without an inflammatory response, but often with a "wound healing" response of tissue regeneration and matrix deposition (fibrosis). Feldstein and colleagues showed that hepatocyte apoptosis is prominent in NASH livers [57, 121]. Furthermore, M30, the caspase 3/7-mediated cleavage product of CK8/18, circulates in NASH to a great extent than in simple steatosis [122]. In mice, the number of M30 positive hepatocytes is high in NASH and negligible in simple steatosis [57]. However, while apoptosis is abundant, it is not the only form of cell death that occurs in lipotoxicity or NASH.

In vitro studies of FC lipotoxicity showed a dose-dependent relationship between hepatocyte FC content and necrosis, as well as apoptosis [91]. In addition to release of ALT and ferritin, other evidence suggests that necrosis occurs *in vivo* in NASH, as summarized in Box 3.3. Thus, whole length CK8/18 (among other hepatocyte-specific proteins) circulates [122], and the inflammatory infiltrate that surrounds lipid-laden hepatocytes in NASH contains polymorphonuclear leukocytes (neutrophils) as well as macrophages; these may be a response to lipid peroxidation or to release of neutrophil chemokines. Neutrophils release perforins and other proteolytic enzymes that kill cells by necrosis [123]. Finally, experiments in rodent livers showing NASH have found increased expression of RIP3 (a marker of necrosis) and MLKL (a marker of necroptosis) [124].

3.14.4 Potential Role of Danger-Associated Molecular Patterns (DAMPs)

Release of HMGB1 in FC lipotoxicity experiments is likely a response to oxidative stress or necrosis [91], as has been documented in ischemia-reperfusion injury [125]. HMGB1 is an archetypical DAMP that can activate cell death on neighbouring hepatocytes by binding to TLR4, and it also binds and activates TLR9 and receptor for advanced glycation endproducts (RAGE) [125, 126]. HMGB1 antiserum reduced cell death in FC-loaded hepatocytes, while hepatocytes from *Tlr4*$^{-/-}$ mice, as well as those from *Jnk1*$^{-/-}$ animals, were refractory to FC lipotoxicity [91] (Fig. 3.3). HMGB1 also readily binds TLR4 on Kupffer cells and macrophages, a possible pathway that links hepatocyte necrotic cell death to inflammation in NASH [91]. Ganz and colleagues found hepatic levels of HMGB1 increased during intake of a high fat high cholesterol diet, when steatohepatitis was present at 8 weeks [127]. Consistent with the proposed role of this DAMP in NASH pathogenesis, Li and colleagues documented HMGB1 release and TLR4 involvement in feed-forward hepatocyte injury during the early stages of NAFLD caused by intake of a high fat, 2% cholesterol diet [128].

3.14.5 Sterile Inflammation in NASH

While hepatocytes may generate inflammation in NASH by release of DAMPs that signal through pattern recognition receptors [91, 127], inflammation can kill hepatocytes. In alcoholic hepatitis, the origins of liver inflammation appear to be the gut microbiota [129]. Thus, excessive alcohol compromises intestinal permeability, with resultant absorption of bacterial pathogen-activated molecular patterns (PAMPs) such as endotoxin (lipopolysaccharide). These interact with TLR4 and possibly other TLRs, while bacterial CpG DNA ligands TLR9 to activate NF-κB. We have reviewed the evidence that NF-κB is an essential pro-inflammatory “trigger” in NASH [8]. Its activation results in production and release of chemokines and cytokines that promote a cellular inflammatory response. Normal hepatocytes are not killed by TNF-α. However, under certain conditions, including FC loading of mitochondria

Box 3.3: Evidence that Hepatocyte Necrosis or Necroptosis Occur in NASH.

1. Serum ALT increases.
2. CK8/18 circulates.
3. Neutrophils are present.
4. RIP3 and MLKL expression increase.

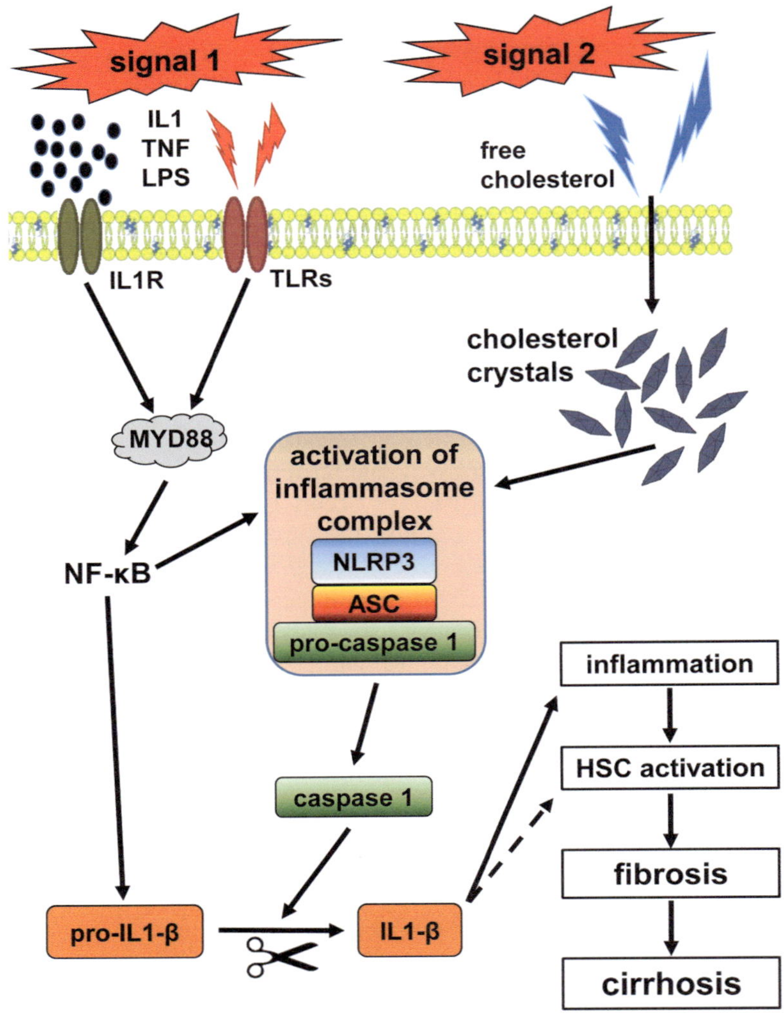

Fig. 3.4 Inflammasomes are intracellular pattern recognition receptors that require a "double trigger" to be assembled. Abbreviations: *ASC* apoptosis-associated speck-like protein containing a card, *HSC* hepatic stellate cell, *IL1* interleukin 1, *LPS* lipopolysaccharide, *MYD88* myeloid differentiation primary response gene 88, *NF-κB* nuclear factor kappa-light-chain-enhancer of activated B cells, *NLRP3* NOD-like receptor protein 3, *ROS* reactive oxygen species, *TLR* toll-like receptor, *TNF* tumour necrosis factor

and glutathione (GSH) depletion caused by oxidative stress, TNF-α can activate hepatocyte apoptosis via caspase 8-mediated death signaling [130]. The evidence that the gut microbiome could play a role in NASH pathogenesis is reviewed in Chaps. 8 and 9.

3.14.6 Role of the NLRP3 Inflammasome

Inflammasomes are intracellular pattern recognition receptors that require a "double trigger" to be assembled (Fig. 3.4). The first signal is MYD88 mediated, and leads to NF-κB-mediated induction of inflammasome components such as NLRP3, pro-caspase 1 and pro-IL-1β. Upon exposure to a second signal, NLRP3 recruits apoptosis-associated speck-like protein containing CARD (ASC) as the scaffold for dimerization of pro-caspase 1, converting it to its active enzyme. Caspase 1 then cleaves pro-IL-1β and pro-IL18 to form the active cytokines. Secreted IL18 attracts and activates macrophages. IL-1β indirectly attracts and then activates neutrophils; it also has direct effects on fibrosis by activating stellate cells.

The MYD88-signaling molecules that could provide a *signal 1* in NASH include RAGE, TLR2, TLR4, TLR9, oxidative stress, and, more controversially, saturated FFAs such as palmitic acid [131]. *Signal 2* can be provided by foreign particulate matter, uric acid crystals (gout) [132], and cholesterol crystals (as in atheroma) [133]. In the presence of a second signal, increased NLRP3 (expressed in hepatocytes as well as kupffer cells) is activated to generate cellular inflammation with macrophages and neutrophils. NLRP3 inflammasome activation also causes pyroptosis, a form of cell death exhibiting features both of apoptosis (DNA fission into ~200 kDa oligonucleotide "ladders") and necrosis (plasma membrane pores). Like necrosis and necroptosis, pyroptosis allows leakage of intracellular contents through such pores to promote inflammation.

Mice defective in inflammasome components (NLRP3, CARD, caspase 1) are protected from MCD steatohepatitis and high fat diet-induced NAFLD. The identification of cholesterol crystals in human NASH and two animal models provides a rationale for NLRP3 activation in the relevant metabolic context [79, 87]. In mice fed a high fat and cholesterol added diet, the number of cholesterol crystals increased from 0.5% cholesterol in the diet, while severity of steatohepatitis and resultant liver fibrosis was proportional to the number of crystals [87] (Fig. 3.1). Conversely, in *foz/foz* mice, the number of cholesterol crystals remaining in livers after treatment with cholesterol-lowering agents correlated with the number of residual F4/80 positive macrophages, neutrophils and extent of liver fibrosis [79]. In both models, active caspase 1 and NLRP3 co-located with cholesterol crystals, and such expression was no longer present when crystals were dissolved as the result of cholesterol-lowering therapy.

If cholesterol crystal-related NLRP3 inflammasome activation is central to the pathogenesis of NASH, NLRP3 inhibitors might provide a new therapeutic opportunity [134], as shown by Szabo and colleagues for the IL-1β receptor inhibitor, anakinra, in alcohol-related fatty liver disease [135]. We used the small molecule NLRP3 inhibitor, MCC950 [134], to test this proposal in atherogenic diet-fed *foz/foz* mice with NASH. We showed that NLRP3 blockade abolishes liver inflammation during development of NASH, with beneficial effects on liver fibrogenesis [136]. Outstanding challenges are to develop NLRP3 inhibitors that can be administered safely to humans with NASH, and to show that they reverse established NASH and fibrosis, as well as arrest its development.

3.14.7 Other Pattern Recognition Receptors

TLR4 is upregulated in human as well as experimental forms of NAFLD [124, 137]. Its likely importance for NASH is reviewed elsewhere [138, 139]. A pro-inflammatory role has also been suggested for TLR3 [131, 138], but there do not appear to be data indicating its upregulation in human NASH. We have recently reported that TLR9 is upregulated in human NASH compared to livers showing simple steatosis [124]. Unlike TLRs 2 and 4, which are located on the cell surface, TLR9 is present in the endosome of macrophages and, to a lesser extent hepatocytes [124]. In rodents, TLR9 appears to govern M1 activation of macrophages, but its role on human macrophages is less clear. Mice deficient in TLR9 are protected from the milder forms of fatty liver disease generated by a high fat diet [97, 124], and also from CDAA-induced steatohepatitis [32]. Neither is associated with obesity, and it is entirely possible that this apparent protection is because *Tlr9*$^{-/-}$ mice are smaller in body weight (less over-nourished). We crossed *Tlr9*$^{-/-}$ with *foz/foz* mice. The resultant obese diabetic mice lacking TLR9 appeared minimally protected against NASH [124]; most critically, resultant liver fibrosis was the same in TLR9-deficient and intact obese animals (Fig. 3.5).

RAGE is another NF-κB-mobilising receptor of potential relevance to *signal 1* for NLRP3 activation. RAGE signals in response to ligation by advanced glycosylation end-products (AGE) that circulate in diabetes and have been linked to diabetic complications. AGE is also found in some charcoal grilled food products. Upregulation of RAGE has been demonstrated in a murine dietary model of NAFLD; its deletion protected mice from exacerbation by a high AGE-containing

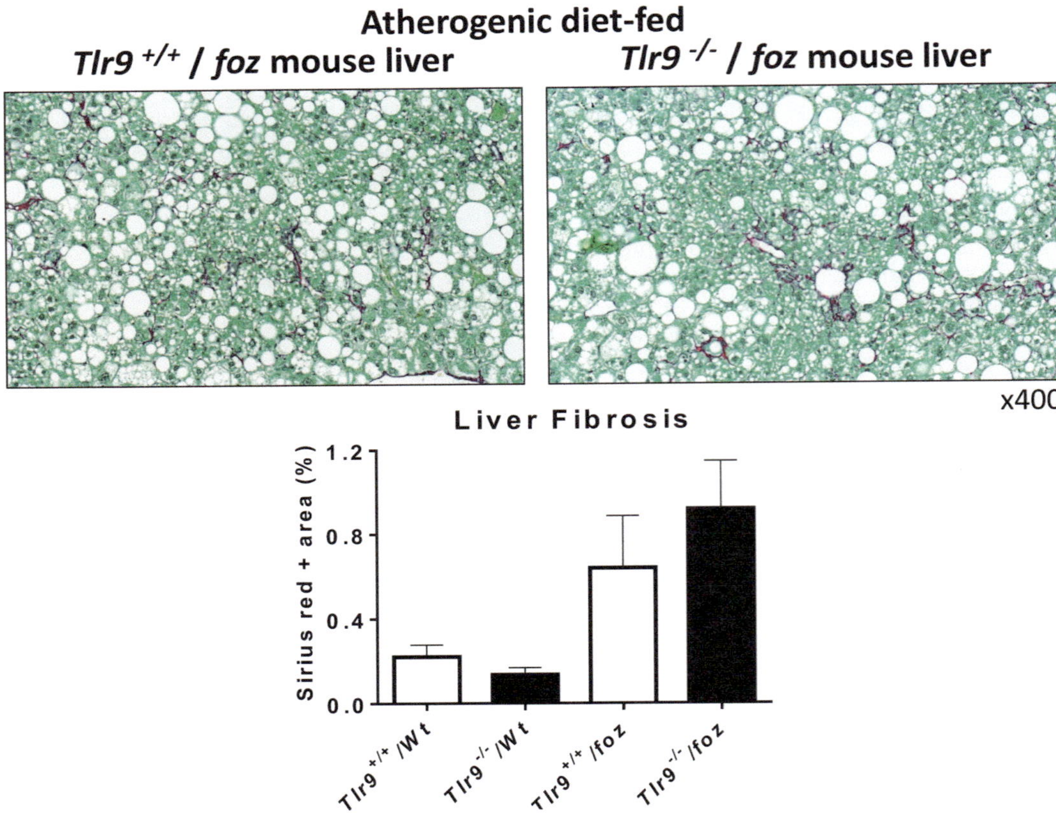

Fig. 3.5 Hepatic Sirius red-positive areas for fibrosis did not change with TLR9 deletion in appetite-defective (hyperphagic) *foz/foz* mice or wildtype (*Wt*) littermates fed an atherogenic diet (23% fat, 0.2% cholesterol)

diet, but not from NASH caused by a HF/HC diet in the absence of AGE [140, 141].

3.14.8 Liver Inflammatory Phenotype

In steatohepatitis, the lobular mixed cell inflammatory infiltrate is comprised of activated (M1) macrophages, lymphocytes and neutrophils. In NASH, macrophages aggregate around ballooned or fat-laden hepatocytes in what are referred to as crown-like structures (CLSs). The same macrophage foci are found in inflamed adipose with type 2 diabetes and metabolic obesity [142, 143]. In NASH, their localization around injured hepatocytes infers signals expressed by or released from those cells are important for their recruitment. Within CLSs, cells exhibit markers of pro-inflammatory (M1) macrophages. Tracking studies suggest most of the expansion in numbers of activated macrophages in NASH is from bone marrow-derived monocytes, and a smaller proportion are derived from resident macrophages (Kupffer cells) [144]. Macrophage chemokines from both the CCL2 and CCL5 families are produced by fatty livers [145]. Such chemokines play an important role in macrophage recruitment and activation in NASH. A CCR2/5 antagonist has recently been shown to improve liver fibrosis in human NASH [146], although it failed to impact NASH pathology.

Among candidate sentinel cell populations responsible for sensing DAMPs in fatty liver injury, Kupffer cells and dendritic cells appear most likely involved. In an experimental system of acute sterile inflammation, CD11b positive cells (likely macrophages) were essential for detection of danger signals [11, 147]. Lymphocytes are among the less well-characterized inflammatory cells that accumulate in NASH livers. In a choline-deficient high fat diet murine model which exhibited insulin resistance and NASH, activated intrahepatic CD8 T cells, natural killer T (NKT) cells and inflammatory cytokines were detected [148]. The authors proposed that CD8 T cells and NKT cells but not myeloid cells promote development of NASH by interactions with hepatocytes (inflammation causes liver injury). In a different murine model (high fat high carbohydrate diet), NKT cells and CD8 T cells were also both required for significant liver injury and hepatic infiltration with macrophages [149].

Neutrophils are a neglected feature of NASH inflammation. By release of reactive oxygen species (ROS) and growth factors, they could augment the effect of M1 macrophages in activating stellate cells to promote fibrosis. The mechanisms that promote neutrophil recruitment and retention in NASH are poorly understood [11, 150]. In acute forms of sterile liver inflammation, such as thermal injury, ATP-induced activation of the P2X7 receptor and the NLRP3 inflammasome are involved (discussed in Kubes and Mehal [11]). In the $LDLR^{-/-}$ model, neutrophil-derived myeloperoxidase contributed importantly to the inflammatory phenotype of fatty liver disease [151].

3.15 Does Inflammation Arise from Other Tissues or from the Liver Itself?

With overnutrition, the essential precondition for NASH, adipose depots are the primary site for energy storage in the body. Adipose stores energy in the form of TG, but is unable to store cholesterol efficiently. By taking up and storing excess glucose and FFAs, adipose counters the potentially toxic effects of these circulating nutrients. The tissue response to chronic energy surplus include adipocyte hypertrophy and hyperplasia. However, there is a limit for adipocyte enlargement, adipose expansion and lipid storage (Haczeyni F review in progress). In metabolic obesity associated with NASH, hypertrophic adipocytes exhibit stress signals and start degenerating [152]. The cellular mechanisms of such degeneration and death of stressed adipocytes exhibit similarities to those seen in lipotoxic hepatocytes, as discussed earlier. Further, the consequences of emission of stress signals and cell degeneration/death of lipotoxic adipocytes and hepatocytes are similar, inflammatory recruitment [142]. Thus, both lipid-engorged adipocytes and hepatocytes attract a group of classically-activated, pro-inflammatory macrophages to form CLSs, as discussed earlier for livers with NASH [58, 79] (Fig. 3.6). The properties of macrophage CLSs around degenerating adipocytes or hepatocytes are also similar. The presence of adipose inflammation, and the loss of highly differentiated adipocyte functions, such as secretion of the insulin-sensitizing adipokine, adiponectin, contribute to the development of adipose insulin resistance in NAFLD [153]. A recent human study found that NAFLD patients with raised serum ALT had more severe adipose insulin resistance, lower serum adiponectin and higher hepatic TG levels than those with normal ALT levels, although there was no correlation with the histological indices of NASH [51]. In mice fed HFD 16 weeks, both hepatic and adipose insulin resistance developed with adipose but not liver inflammation [154]. Early (but not late) depletion of Kupffer cells attenuated adiposity and adipose inflammation and insulin resistance. These kind of data indicate links between liver and adipose responses to overnutrition in terms of insulin resistance and inflammation, now termed "metaflammation", but it seems likely that pro-inflammatory pathways operate in each tissue separately rather than simply "spilling over" from adipose to liver [153, 155]. This proposal is supported by our recent observations of separate effects of obeticholic acid on adipose morphometry and inflammation in relation to hepatic steatosis and inflammation in different models of NAFLD and NASH [156].

3.16 Therapeutic Relevance and New Directions

Over the last 20 years, the Holy Grail of research into NASH pathogenesis has been to find a critical juncture at which the pathology and clinical

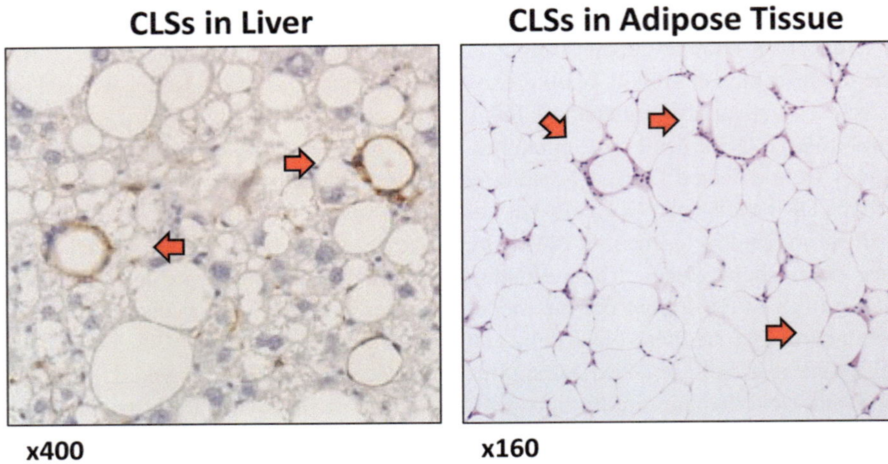

Fig. 3.6 F4/80 positive macrophages in liver and adipose tissue of appetite-defective *foz/foz* mice fed an atherogenic diet (23% fat, 0.2% cholesterol). In both tissues, pro-inflammatory macrophages aggregate around injured hepatocytes and adipocytes in what we termed "crown-like structures", as a feature of NASH and metabolic obesity

course of NASH separate from simple steatosis, the more benign and more common NAFLD phenotype. The rationale is to design mechanism-based and effective drug treatment for NASH because currently there is none. Correction of the metabolic preconditions for NASH, obesity, insulin resistance and metabolic syndrome, does reverse NASH, but the non-pharmacological approaches required for success (lifestyle intervention with 10% reduction in body weight [24]; bariatric surgery [157]) are often not accessed, not achieved or not sustained. To date, empirical approaches or drugs aimed at lipid partitioning are either not effective (metformin) or marginally so (thiazolidinediones) [158]. Similar comments apply to antioxidants (vitamin E), TNF-α release inhibitors (pentoxifylline), FXR agonists (obeticholic acid) and ER stress blockade (ursodeoxycholic acid) [89]. The literature on individual cholesterol-lowering agents has been reviewed [88–90], and is no longer encouraging, but use of combination statin plus ezetimibe does not appear to have been studied in NASH. Recent evidence of the synergistic effect for lowering cardiovascular risk [159], the impressive results of animal studies [57], and recent discovery of cholesterol crystals in NASH [79] indicates that this is a logical approach to NASH therapy worthy of clinical trial.

While it remains possible that the inflammation found in NASH originates from outside the liver [23], in inflamed adipose tissue or is provoked by PAMPs generated by the gut microbiota through a "leaky gut" (Chaps. 8 and 9), the authors' view is that we need look no further than the processes involved with hepatocyte lipotoxicity. If this is the case, preventing accumulation of lipotoxic lipids (like FC) is the logical approach to prevent NASH or to reverse its earliest stages. Unless there is substantial weight reduction, the outcome is likely to be simple steatosis, not a non-fatty liver. We are not convinced that LIGHT from NKT cells [148], or IL-1β [32] are responsible for clinically relevant lipid accumulation in overnourished individuals with NASH (inflammation begets steatosis) [23, 136]. If this is the case, continued use of 2 points improvement of the NAS as the endpoint of NASH drug trials, as recommended by American Association for Liver Disease (AASLD) and mandated by the Federal Drug Authority (FDA) may be inappropriate because 3 of the 7 possible points are allocated to steatosis. Resolution of NASH, preferably with reversal of fibrosis, is more relevant [160].

The sequence of molecular signalling and subcellular injury by which lipotoxicity injures hepatocytes in NASH now presents a more logical "palette" of potential therapeutic opportunities than does the global issue of hepatic lipid partitioning, though it remains possible that newer approaches to improve glycemic control in type 2 diabetes with incretin-based therapies, and agents that improve muscle and adipose insulin sensitivity (PPAR-α/δ [161] or PPAR-δ agonists [162]) could be useful. JNK inhibitors, mitochondrial protectants, antiHMGB1 strategies, TLR4 blockade and NLRP3 inhibitors are all worth exploring. The most appropriate models in which to test such agents are animals with NASH that is attributable to metabolic syndrome.

References

1. Bass NM, Merriman RB. Fatty acid metabolism and lipotoxicity in the pathogenesis of NAFLD/NASH. In: Farrell GC, George J, Hall P de la M, McCullough AJ, editors. Fatty liver disease: NASH and related disorders. Malden: Blackwell Publishing; 2005. p. 109–22.
2. Larter CZ, Chitturi S, Heydet D, Farrell GC. A fresh look at NASH pathogenesis. Part 1: the metabolic movers. J Gastroenterol Hepatol. 2010;25:672–90.
3. Farrell GC, McCullough AJ, Day CP. Non-alcoholic fatty liver disease: A practical guide. Somerset: Wiley; 2013. p. 1–313.
4. Cohen JC, Horton JD, Hobbs HH. Human fatty liver disease: old questions and new insights. Science. 2011;332:1519–23.
5. Cusi K. Role of obesity and lipotoxicity in the development of nonalcoholic steatohepatitis: pathophysiology and clinical implications. Gastroenterology. 2012;142:711–25. e716.
6. Musso G, Cassader M, Rosina F, Gambino R. Impact of current treatments on liver disease, glucose metabolism and cardiovascular risk in non-alcoholic fatty liver disease (NAFLD): a systematic review and meta-analysis of randomised trials. Diabetologia. 2012;55:885–904.
7. Machado MV, Diehl AM. Pathogenesis of nonalcoholic steatohepatitis. Gastroenterology. 2016;150:1769–77.
8. Farrell GC, Van Rooyen D, Gan L, Chitturi S. NASH is an inflammatory disorder: pathogenic, prognostic and therapeutic implications. Gut and Liver. 2012;6:149.
9. Lee Y, Hirose H, Ohneda M, Johnson J, McGarry JD, Unger RH. Beta-cell lipotoxicity in the pathogenesis of non-insulin-dependent diabetes mellitus of obese rats: impairment in adipocyte-beta-cell relationships. Proc Natl Acad Sci (USA). 1994:91:10878–82.
10. Hirsova P, Gores GJ. Death receptor-mediated cell death and proinflammatory signaling in nonalcoholic steatohepatitis. Cell Mol Gastroenterol Hepatol. 2015;1:17–27.
11. Kubes P, Mehal WZ. Sterile inflammation in the liver. Gastroenterology. 2012;143:1158–72.
12. Luedde T, Kaplowitz N, Schwabe RF. Cell death and cell death responses in liver disease: mechanisms and clinical relevance. Gastroenterology. 2014;147:765–83. e764.
13. Zimmermann HW, Tacke F. Modification of chemokine pathways and immune cell infiltration as a novel therapeutic approach in liver inflammation and fibrosis. Inflamm Allergy Drug Targets. 2011;10:509–36.
14. Puri P, Baillie RA, Wiest MM, Mirshahi F, Choudhury J, Cheung O, et al. A lipidomic analysis of nonalcoholic fatty liver disease. Hepatology. 2007;46:1081–90.
15. Caballero F, Fernández A, De Lacy AM, Fernández-Checa JC, Caballería J, García-Ruiz C. Enhanced free cholesterol, SREBP-2 and StAR expression in human NASH. J Hepatol. 2009;50:789–96.
16. Larter CZ, Yeh MM. Animal models of NASH: getting both pathology and metabolic context right. J Gastroenterol Hepatol. 2008;23:1635–48.
17. Neuschwander-Tetri BA. Hepatic lipotoxicity and the pathogenesis of nonalcoholic steatohepatitis: the central role of nontriglyceride fatty acid metabolites. Hepatology. 2010;52:774–88.
18. Yang SQ, Lin HZ, Lane MD, Clemens M, Diehl AM. Obesity increases sensitivity to endotoxin liver injury: implications for the pathogenesis of steatohepatitis. Proc Natl Acad Sci. 1997;94:2557–62.
19. Day CP, James OF. Steatohepatitis: a tale of two "hits"? Gastroenterology. 1998;114:842–5.
20. Henao-Mejia J, Elinav E, Jin C-C, Hao L, Mehal WZ, Strowig T, et al. Inflammasome-mediated dysbiosis regulates progression of NAFLD and obesity. Nature. 2012;482:179.
21. Feldstein AE, Werneburg NW, Canbay A, Guicciardi ME, Bronk SF, Rydzewski R, et al. Free fatty acids promote hepatic lipotoxicity by stimulating TNF-α expression via a lysosomal pathway. Hepatology. 2004;40:185–94.
22. McClain CJ, Barve S, Deaciuc I. Good fat/bad fat. Hepatology. 2007;45:1343–6.
23. Tilg H, Moschen AR. Evolution of inflammation in nonalcoholic fatty liver disease: the multiple parallel hits hypothesis. Hepatology. 2010;52:1836–46.
24. Vilar-Gomez E, Martinez-Perez Y, Calzadilla-Bertot L, Torres-Gonzalez A, Gra-Oramas B, Gonzalez-Fabian L, et al. Weight loss through lifestyle modification significantly reduces features of nonalcoholic steatohepatitis. Gastroenterology. 2015;149:367–8. e365.
25. Weltman MD, Farrell GC, Liddle C. Increased hepatocyte CYP2E1 expression in a rat nutritional model of hepatic steatosis with inflammation. Gastroenterology. 1996;111:1645–53.
26. Leclercq IA, Farrell GC, Field J, Bell DR, Gonzalez FJ, Robertson GR. CYP2E1 and CYP4A as microsomal catalysts of lipid peroxides in murine nonalcoholic steatohepatitis. J Clin Invest. 2000;105:1067.

27. Rizki G, Arnaboldi L, Gabrielli B, Yan J, Lee GS, Ng RK, et al. Mice fed a lipogenic methionine-choline-deficient diet develop hypermetabolism coincident with hepatic suppression of SCD-1. J Lipid Res. 2006;47:2280–90.
28. Rinella ME, Green RM. The methionine-choline deficient dietary model of steatohepatitis does not exhibit insulin resistance. J Hepatol. 2004;40:47–51.
29. Marchesini G, Brizi M, Morselli-Labate AM, Bianchi G, Bugianesi E, McCullough AJ, et al. Association of nonalcoholic fatty liver disease with insulin resistance. Am J Med. 1999;107:450–5.
30. Chitturi S, Abeygunasekera S, Farrell GC, Holmes-Walker J, Hui JM, Fung C, et al. NASH and insulin resistance: insulin hypersecretion and specific association with the insulin resistance syndrome. Hepatology. 2002;35:373–9.
31. Matsumoto M, Hada N, Sakamaki Y, Uno A, Shiga T, Tanaka C, et al. An improved mouse model that rapidly develops fibrosis in non-alcoholic steatohepatitis. Int J Exp Pathol. 2013;94:93–103.
32. Miura K, Kodama Y, Inokuchi S, Schnabl B, Aoyama T, Ohnishi H, et al. Toll-like receptor 9 promotes steatohepatitis by induction of interleukin-1β in mice. Gastroenterology. 2010;139:323–34. e327.
33. dela Peña A, Leclercq I, Field J, George J, Jones B, Farrell G. NF-κB activation, rather than TNF, mediates hepatic inflammation in a murine dietary model of steatohepatitis. Gastroenterology. 2005;129:1663–74.
34. Wouters K, van Gorp PJ, Bieghs V, Gijbels MJ, Duimel H, Lütjohann D, et al. Dietary cholesterol, rather than liver steatosis, leads to hepatic inflammation in hyperlipidemic mouse models of nonalcoholic steatohepatitis. Hepatology. 2008;48:474–86.
35. Wouters K, van Bilsen M, van Gorp PJ, Bieghs V, Lütjohann D, Kerksiek A, et al. Intrahepatic cholesterol influences progression, inhibition and reversal of non-alcoholic steatohepatitis in hyperlipidemic mice. FEBS Lett. 2010;584:1001–5.
36. Bieghs V, Verheyen F, van Gorp PJ, Hendrikx T, Wouters K, Lütjohann D, et al. Internalization of modified lipids by CD36 and SR-A leads to hepatic inflammation and lysosomal cholesterol storage in Kupffer cells. PLoS One. 2012;7:e34378.
37. Chan J, Sharkey FE, Kushwaha RS, VandeBerg JF, VandeBerg JL. Steatohepatitis in laboratory opossums exhibiting a high lipemic response to dietary cholesterol and fat. Am J Physiol Gastrointest Liver Physiol. 2012;303:G12–9.
38. Tetri LH, Basaranoglu M, Brunt EM, Yerian LM, Neuschwander-Tetri BA. Severe NAFLD with hepatic necroinflammatory changes in mice fed trans fats and a high-fructose corn syrup equivalent. Am J Physiol Gastrointest Liver Physiol. 2008;295:G987–95.
39. Pickens MK, Yan JS, Ng RK, Ogata H, Grenert JP, Beysen C, et al. Dietary sucrose is essential to the development of liver injury in the methionine-choline-deficient model of steatohepatitis. J Lipid Res. 2009;50:2072–82.
40. Charlton M, Krishnan A, Viker K, Sanderson S, Cazanave S, McConico A, et al. Fast food diet mouse: novel small animal model of NASH with ballooning, progressive fibrosis, and high physiological fidelity to the human condition. Am J Physiol Gastrointest Liver Physiol. 2011;301:G825–34.
41. Savard C, Tartaglione EV, Kuver R, Haigh WG, Farrell GC, Subramanian S, et al. Synergistic interaction of dietary cholesterol and dietary fat in inducing experimental steatohepatitis. Hepatology. 2013;57:81–92.
42. Itoh M, Suganami T, Nakagawa N, Tanaka M, Yamamoto Y, Kamei Y, et al. Melanocortin 4 receptor–deficient mice as a novel mouse model of nonalcoholic steatohepatitis. Am J Pathol. 2011;179:2454–63.
43. Matsuzawa N, Takamura T, Kurita S, Misu H, Ota T, Ando H, et al. Lipid-induced oxidative stress causes steatohepatitis in mice fed an atherogenic diet. Hepatology. 2007;46:1392–403.
44. Ginsberg HN. Is the slippery slope from steatosis to steatohepatitis paved with triglyceride or cholesterol? Cell Metab. 2006;4:179–81.
45. Qg D, She H, Cheng JH, French SW, Koop DR, Xiong S, et al. Steatohepatitis induced by intragastric overfeeding in mice. Hepatology. 2005;42:905–14.
46. Lee L, Alloosh M, Saxena R, Van Alstine W, Watkins BA, Klaunig JE, et al. Nutritional model of steatohepatitis and metabolic syndrome in the Ossabaw miniature swine. Hepatology. 2009;50:56–67.
47. Arsov T, Larter CZ, Nolan CJ, Petrovsky N, Goodnow CC, Teoh NC, et al. Adaptive failure to high-fat diet characterizes steatohepatitis in Alms1 mutant mice. Biochem Biophys Res Commun. 2006;342:1152–9.
48. Farrell GC, Mridha AR, Yeh MM, Arsov T, Van Rooyen DM, Brooling J, et al. Strain dependence of diet-induced NASH and liver fibrosis in obese mice is linked to diabetes and inflammatory phenotype. Liver Int. 2014;34:1084–93.
49. Arsov T, Silva DG, O'bryan MK, Sainsbury A, Lee NJ, Kennedy C, et al. Fat aussie—a new Alstrom syndrome mouse showing a critical role for ALMS1 in obesity, diabetes, and spermatogenesis. Mol Endocrinol. 2006;20:1610–22.
50. Haczeyni F, Barn V, Mridha AR, Yeh MM, Estevez E, Febbraio MA, et al. Exercise improves adipose function and inflammation and ameliorates fatty liver disease in obese diabetic mice. Obesity. 2015;23:1845–55.
51. Maximos M, Bril F, Portillo Sanchez P, Lomonaco R, Orsak B, Biernacki D, et al. The role of liver fat and insulin resistance as determinants of plasma aminotransferase elevation in nonalcoholic fatty liver disease. Hepatology. 2015;61:153–60.
52. Listenberger LL, Han X, Lewis SE, Cases S, Farese RV, Ory DS, et al. Triglyceride accumulation protects against fatty acid-induced lipotoxicity. Proc Natl Acad Sci (USA). 2003;100:3077–82.
53. Yamaguchi K, Yang L, McCall S, Huang J, Yu XX, Pandey SK, et al. Inhibiting triglyceride synthe-

sis improves hepatic steatosis but exacerbates liver damage and fibrosis in obese mice with nonalcoholic steatohepatitis. Hepatology. 2007;45:1366–74.
54. Alkhouri N, Dixon LJ, Feldstein AE. Lipotoxicity in nonalcoholic fatty liver disease: not all lipids are created equal. Expert Rev Gastroenterol Hepatol. 2009;3:445–51.
55. Cazanave SC, Gores GJ. Mechanisms and clinical implications of hepatocyte lipoapoptosis. Clin Lipidol. 2010;5:71–85.
56. Neuschwander-Tetri BA. Nontriglyceride hepatic lipotoxicity: the new paradigm for the pathogenesis of NASH. Curr Gastroenterol Rep. 2010;12:49–56.
57. Van Rooyen DM, Gan LT, Yeh MM, Haigh WG, Larter CZ, Ioannou G, et al. Pharmacological cholesterol lowering reverses fibrotic NASH in obese, diabetic mice with metabolic syndrome. J Hepatol. 2013;59:144–52.
58. Itoh M, Kato H, Suganami T, Konuma K, Marumoto Y, Terai S, et al. Hepatic crown-like structure: a unique histological feature in non-alcoholic steatohepatitis in mice and humans. PLoS One. 2013;8:e82163.
59. Bruce CR, Febbraio MA. It's what you do with the fat that matters! Nat Med. 2007;13:1137–8.
60. Min H-K, Kapoor A, Fuchs M, Mirshahi F, Zhou H, Maher J, et al. Increased hepatic synthesis and dysregulation of cholesterol metabolism is associated with the severity of nonalcoholic fatty liver disease. Cell Metab. 2012;15:665–74.
61. Boursier J, Diehl AM. Patatin-like phospholipase domain-containing protein 3 and liver disease: opportunities to unravel mechanisms underlying statistical associations. Hepatology. 2015;61:18–20.
62. Smagris E, BasuRay S, Li J, Huang Y, Lai KV, Gromada J, et al. Pnpla3I148M knockin mice accumulate PNPLA3 on lipid droplets and develop hepatic steatosis. Hepatology. 2015;61:108–18.
63. Anstee QM, Day CP. The genetics of NAFLD. Nat Rev Gastroenterol Hepatol. 2013;10:645–55.
64. Zain SM, Mohamed R, Mahadeva S, Cheah PL, Rampal S, Basu RC, et al. A multi-ethnic study of a PNPLA3 gene variant and its association with disease severity in non-alcoholic fatty liver disease. Hum Genet. 2012;131:1145–52.
65. Li JZ, Huang Y, Karaman R, Ivanova PT, Brown HA, Roddy T, et al. Chronic overexpression of PNPLA3I148M in mouse liver causes hepatic steatosis. J Clin Invest. 2012;122:4130.
66. Chiappini F, Coilly A, Kadar H, Gual P, Tran A, Desterke C, et al. Metabolism dysregulation induces a specific lipid signature of nonalcoholic steatohepatitis in patients. Sci Rep. 2017;7:44658.
67. Nolan CJ, Larter CZ. Lipotoxicity: why do saturated fatty acids cause and monounsaturates protect against it? J Gastroenterol Hepatol. 2009;24:703–6.
68. Han MS, Park SY, Shinzawa K, Kim S, Chung KW, Lee J-H, et al. Lysophosphatidylcholine as a death effector in the lipoapoptosis of hepatocytes. J Lipid Res. 2008;49:84–97.
69. Kakisaka K, Cazanave SC, Fingas CD, Guicciardi ME, Bronk SF, Werneburg NW, et al. Mechanisms of lysophosphatidylcholine-induced hepatocyte lipoapoptosis. Am J Physiol Gastrointest Liver Physiol. 2012;302:G77–84.
70. Garcia-Ruiz C, Mari M, Colell A, Morales A, C Fernandez-Checa J. Metabolic therapy: lessons from liver diseases. Curr Pharm Des. 2011;17:3933–44.
71. Wei Y, Wang D, Topczewski F, Pagliassotti MJ. Saturated fatty acids induce endoplasmic reticulum stress and apoptosis independently of ceramide in liver cells. Am J Physiol Endocrinol Metab. 2006;291:E275–81.
72. Kotronen A, Seppänen-Laakso T, Westerbacka J, Kiviluoto T, Arola J, Ruskeepää A-L, et al. Hepatic stearoyl-CoA desaturase (SCD)-1 activity and diacylglycerol but not ceramide concentrations are increased in the nonalcoholic human fatty liver. Diabetes. 2009;58:203–8.
73. Anjani K, Lhomme M, Sokolovska N, Poitou C, Aron-Wisnewsky J, Bouillot J-L, et al. Circulating phospholipid profiling identifies portal contribution to NASH signature in obesity. J Hepatol. 2015;62:905–12.
74. Mauer AS, Hirsova P, Maiers JL, Shah VH, Malhi H. Inhibition of sphingosine 1-phosphate signaling ameliorates murine nonalcoholic steatohepatitis. Am J Physiol Gastrointest Liver Physiol. 2017;312:G300–13.
75. Van Rooyen DM, Farrell GC. SREBP-2: a link between insulin resistance, hepatic cholesterol, and inflammation in NASH. J Gastroenterol Hepatol. 2011;26:789–92.
76. Van Rooyen DM, Larter CZ, Haigh WG, Yeh MM, Ioannou G, Kuver R, et al. Hepatic free cholesterol accumulates in obese, diabetic mice and causes nonalcoholic steatohepatitis. Gastroenterology. 2011;141:1393–403. e1395.
77. Gorden DL, Myers DS, Ivanova PT, Fahy E, Maurya MR, Gupta S, et al. Biomarkers of NAFLD progression: a lipidomics approach to an epidemic. J Lipid Res. 2015;56:722–36.
78. Gorden DL, Ivanova PT, Myers DS, McIntyre JO, VanSaun MN, Wright JK, et al. Increased diacylglycerols characterize hepatic lipid changes in progression of human nonalcoholic fatty liver disease; comparison to a murine model. PLoS One. 2011;6:e22775.
79. Ioannou GN, Van Rooyen DM, Savard C, Haigh WG, Yeh MM, Teoh NC, et al. Cholesterol-lowering drugs cause dissolution of cholesterol crystals and disperse Kupffer cell crown-like structures during resolution of NASH. J Lipid Res. 2015;56:277–85.
80. Yu L, Morishima C, Ioannou GN. Dietary cholesterol intake is associated with progression of liver disease in patients with chronic hepatitis C: analysis of the hepatitis C antiviral long-term treatment against cirrhosis trial. Clin Gastroenterol Hepatol. 2013;11:1661–6. e1663.
81. Marchesini G, Petta S, Dalle Grave R. Diet, weight loss, and liver health in nonalcoholic fatty liver

disease: pathophysiology, evidence, and practice. Hepatology. 2016;63:2032–43.
82. Abdelmalek MF, Suzuki A, Guy C, Unalp-Arida A, Colvin R, Johnson RJ, et al. Increased fructose consumption is associated with fibrosis severity in patients with nonalcoholic fatty liver disease. Hepatology. 2010;51:1961–71.
83. Serviddio G, Bellanti F, Villani R, Tamborra R, Zerbinati C, Blonda M, et al. Effects of dietary fatty acids and cholesterol excess on liver injury: a lipidomic approach. Redox Biol. 2016;9:296–305.
84. Horton JD, Goldstein JL, Brown MS. SREBPs activators of the complete program of cholesterol and fatty acid synthesis in the liver. J Clin Invest. 2002;109:1125.
85. Donnelly KL, Smith CI, Schwarzenberg SJ, Jessurun J, Boldt MD, Parks EJ. Sources of fatty acids stored in liver and secreted via lipoproteins in patients with nonalcoholic fatty liver disease. J Clin Invest. 2005;115:1343.
86. Larter CZ, Yeh MM, Van Rooyen DM, Teoh NC, Brooling J, Hou JY, et al. Roles of adipose restriction and metabolic factors in progression of steatosis to steatohepatitis in obese, diabetic mice. J Gastroenterol Hepatol. 2009;24:1658–68.
87. Ioannou GN, Subramanian S, Chait A, Haigh WG, Yeh MM, Farrell GC, et al. Cholesterol crystallization within hepatocyte lipid droplets and its role in murine NASH. J Lipid Res. 2017;58:1067–79.
88. Musso G, Gambino R, Cassader M. Cholesterol metabolism and the pathogenesis of non-alcoholic steatohepatitis. Prog Lipid Res. 2013;52:175–91.
89. Wong VW-S, Chitturi S, Wong GL-H, Yu J, Chan HL-Y, Farrell GC. Pathogenesis and novel treatment options for non-alcoholic steatohepatitis. Lancet Gastroenterol Hepatol. 2016;1:56–67.
90. Musso G. Ezetimibe in the balance: can cholesterol-lowering drugs alone be an effective therapy for NAFLD? Diabetologia. 2014;57:850–5.
91. Gan LT, Van Rooyen DM, Koina ME, McCuskey RS, Teoh NC, Farrell GC. Hepatocyte free cholesterol lipotoxicity results from JNK1-mediated mitochondrial injury and is HMGB1 and TLR4-dependent. J Hepatol. 2014;61:1376–84.
92. Caldwell SH, Swerdlow RH, Khan EM, Iezzoni JC, Hespenheide EE, Parks JK, et al. Mitochondrial abnormalities in non-alcoholic steatohepatitis. J Hepatol. 1999;31:430–4.
93. Sanyal AJ, Campbell–Sargent C, Mirshahi F, Rizzo WB, Contos MJ, Sterling RK, et al. Nonalcoholic steatohepatitis: association of insulin resistance and mitochondrial abnormalities. Gastroenterology. 2001;120:1183–92.
94. Cortez-Pinto H, Chatham J, Chacko V, Arnold C, Rashid A, Diehl AM. Alterations in liver ATP homeostasis in human nonalcoholic steatohepatitis: a pilot study. JAMA. 1999;282:1659–64.
95. Chiappini F, Desterke C, Bertrand-Michel J, Guettier C, Le Naour F. Hepatic and serum lipid signatures specific to nonalcoholic steatohepatitis in murine models. Sci Rep. 2016;6:31587.
96. Fuchs Y, Steller H. Programmed cell death in animal development and disease. Cell. 2011;147:742–58.
97. Garcia-Martinez I, Santoro N, Chen Y, Hoque R, Ouyang X, Caprio S, et al. Hepatocyte mitochondrial DNA drives nonalcoholic steatohepatitis by activation of TLR9. J Clin Invest. 2016;126:859.
98. Puri P, Mirshahi F, Cheung O, Natarajan R, Maher JW, Kellum JM, et al. Activation and dysregulation of the unfolded protein response in nonalcoholic fatty liver disease. Gastroenterology. 2008;134:568–76.
99. Rahman SM, Schroeder-Gloeckler JM, Janssen RC, Jiang H, Qadri I, Maclean KN, et al. CCAAT/enhancing binding protein β deletion in mice attenuates inflammation, endoplasmic reticulum stress, and lipid accumulation in diet-induced nonalcoholic steatohepatitis. Hepatology. 2007;45:1108–17.
100. Legry V, Van Rooyen DM, Lambert B, Sempoux C, Poekes L, Español-Suñer R, et al. Endoplasmic reticulum stress does not contribute to steatohepatitis in obese and insulin-resistant high-fat-diet-fed foz/foz mice. Clin Sci. 2014;127:507–18.
101. Leclercq IA, Van Rooyen DM, Farrell GC. Hepatic endoplasmic reticulum stress in obesity: deeper insights into processes, but are they relevant to nonalcoholic steatohepatitis? Hepatology. 2011;54:2261–6.
102. Laurin J, Lindor KD, Crippin JS, Gossard A, Gores GJ, Ludwig J, et al. Ursodeoxycholic acid or clofibrate in the treatment of non-alcohol-induced steatohepatitis: a pilot study. Hepatology. 1996;23:1464–7.
103. Leuschner UF, Lindenthal B, Herrmann G, Arnold JC, Rössle M, Cordes HJ, et al. High-dose ursodeoxycholic acid therapy for nonalcoholic steatohepatitis: a double-blind, randomized, placebo-controlled trial. Hepatology. 2010;52:472–9.
104. Ratziu V, De Ledinghen V, Oberti F, Mathurin P, Wartelle-Bladou C, Renou C, et al. A randomized controlled trial of high-dose ursodesoxycholic acid for nonalcoholic steatohepatitis. J Hepatol. 2011;54:1011–9.
105. Teoh NC, Ajamieh H, Wong HJ, Croft K, Mori T, Allison AC, et al. Microparticles mediate hepatic ischemia-reperfusion injury and are the targets of Diannexin (ASP8597). PLoS One. 2014;9:e104376.
106. Kornek M, Lynch M, Mehta SH, Lai M, Exley M, Afdhal NH, et al. Circulating microparticles as disease-specific biomarkers of severity of inflammation in patients with hepatitis C or nonalcoholic steatohepatitis. Gastroenterology. 2012;143:448–58.
107. Povero D, Panera N, Eguchi A, Johnson CD, Papouchado BG, de Araujo Horcel L, et al. Lipid-induced hepatocyte-derived extracellular vesicles regulate hepatic stellate cells via microRNA targeting peroxisome proliferator-activated receptor-γ. Cell Mol Gastroenterol Hepatol. 2015;1:646–63.e644.
108. He Y, Feng D, Li M, Gao Y, Ramirez T, Cao H, et al. Hepatic mitochondrial DNA/Toll-like receptor 9/MicroRNA-223 forms a negative feedback loop to limit neutrophil overactivation and acet-

aminophen hepatotoxicity in mice. Hepatology. 2017;66:220–34.
109. Witek RP, Yang L, Liu R, Jung Y, Omenetti A, Syn WK, et al. Liver cell–derived microparticles activate hedgehog signaling and alter gene expression in hepatic endothelial cells. Gastroenterology. 2009;136:320–30. e322.
110. Cannito S, Morello E, Bocca C, Foglia B, Benetti E, Novo E, et al. Microvesicles released from fat-laden cells promote activation of hepatocellular NLRP3 inflammasome: a pro-inflammatory link between lipotoxicity and non-alcoholic steatohepatitis. PLoS One. 2017;12:e0172575.
111. Ruhanen H, Perttilä J, Hölttä-Vuori M, Zhou Y, Yki-Järvinen H, Ikonen E, et al. PNPLA3 mediates hepatocyte triacylglycerol remodeling. J Lipid Res. 2014;55:739–46.
112. Amir M, Czaja MJ. Autophagy in nonalcoholic steatohepatitis. Expert Rev Gastroenterol Hepatol. 2011;5:159–66.
113. Eguchi A, Feldstein AE. Adipocyte cell death, fatty liver disease and associated metabolic disorders. Dig Dis. 2014;32:579–85.
114. Kleiner DE, Brunt EM, Van Natta M, Behling C, Contos MJ, Cummings OW, et al. Design and validation of a histological scoring system for nonalcoholic fatty liver disease. Hepatology. 2005;41:1313–21.
115. Gramlich T, Kleiner DE, McCullough AJ, Matteoni CA, Boparai N, Younossi ZM. Pathologic features associated with fibrosis in nonalcoholic fatty liver disease. Hum Pathol. 2004;35:196–9.
116. Lackner C, Gogg-Kamerer M, Zatloukal K, Stumptner C, Brunt EM, Denk H. Ballooned hepatocytes in steatohepatitis: the value of keratin immunohistochemistry for diagnosis. J Hepatol. 2008;48:821–8.
117. Kakisaka K, Cazanave SC, Werneburg NW, Razumilava N, Mertens JC, Bronk SF, et al. A hedgehog survival pathway in 'undead' lipotoxic hepatocytes. J Hepatol. 2012;57:844–51.
118. Bijlsma MF, Damhofer H, Roelink H. Hedgehog chemotaxis is mediated by smoothened located outside the primary cilium. Sci Signal. 2012;5:ra60.
119. Guy CD, Suzuki A, Zdanowicz M, Abdelmalek MF, Burchette J, Unalp A, et al. Hedgehog pathway activation parallels histologic severity of injury and fibrosis in human nonalcoholic fatty liver disease. Hepatology. 2012;55:1711–21.
120. Rangwala F, Guy CD, Lu J, Suzuki A, Burchette JL, Abdelmalek MF, et al. Increased production of sonic hedgehog by ballooned hepatocytes. J Pathol. 2011;224:401–10.
121. Castro RE, Ferreira DM, Afonso MB, Borralho PM, Machado MV, Cortez-Pinto H, et al. miR-34a/SIRT1/p53 is suppressed by ursodeoxycholic acid in the rat liver and activated by disease severity in human non-alcoholic fatty liver disease. J Hepatol. 2013;58:119–25.
122. Joka D, Wahl K, Moeller S, Schlue J, Vaske B, Bahr MJ, et al. Prospective biopsy-controlled evaluation of cell death biomarkers for prediction of liver fibrosis and nonalcoholic steatohepatitis. Hepatology. 2012;55:455–64.
123. Ramaiah SK, Jaeschke H. Role of neutrophils in the pathogenesis of acute inflammatory liver injury. Toxicol Pathol. 2007;35:757–66.
124. Mridha AR, Haczeyni F, Yeh MM, Haigh WG, Ioannou GN, Barn V, et al. TLR9 is up-regulated in human and murine NASH: pivotal role in inflammatory recruitment and cell survival. Clin Sci. 2017;131:2145–59.
125. Huebener P, Pradere J-P, Hernandez C, Gwak G-Y, Caviglia JM, Mu X, et al. The HMGB1/RAGE axis triggers neutrophil-mediated injury amplification following necrosis. J Clin Invest. 2015;125:539.
126. Gao B. Innate immunity and steatohepatitis: a critical role of another toll (TLR-9). Gastroenterology. 2010;139:27.
127. Ganz M, Bukong TN, Csak T, Saha B, Park J-K, Ambade A, et al. Progression of non-alcoholic steatosis to steatohepatitis and fibrosis parallels cumulative accumulation of danger signals that promote inflammation and liver tumors in a high fat–cholesterol–sugar diet model in mice. J Transl Med. 2015;13:193.
128. Li L, Chen L, Hu L, Liu Y, Sun HY, Tang J, et al. Nuclear factor high-mobility group box1 mediating the activation of toll-like receptor 4 signaling in hepatocytes in the early stage of nonalcoholic fatty liver disease in mice. Hepatology. 2011;54:1620–30.
129. Csak T, Ganz M, Pespisa J, Kodys K, Dolganiuc A, Szabo G. Fatty acid and endotoxin activate inflammasomes in mouse hepatocytes that release danger signals to stimulate immune cells. Hepatology. 2011;54:133–44.
130. Marí M, Caballero F, Colell A, Morales A, Caballeria J, Fernandez A, et al. Mitochondrial free cholesterol loading sensitizes to TNF-and Fas-mediated steatohepatitis. Cell Metab. 2006;4:185–98.
131. Miura K, Yang L, van Rooijen N, Brenner DA, Ohnishi H, Seki E. Toll-like receptor 2 and palmitic acid cooperatively contribute to the development of nonalcoholic steatohepatitis through inflammasome activation in mice. Hepatology. 2013;57:577–89.
132. Martinon F, Pétrilli V, Mayor A, Tardivel A, Tschopp J. Gout-associated uric acid crystals activate the NALP3 inflammasome. Nature. 2006;440:237.
133. Duewell P, Kono H, Rayner KJ, Sirois CM, Vladimer G, Bauernfeind FG, et al. NLRP3 inflamasomes are required for atherogenesis and activated by cholesterol crystals that form early in disease. Nature. 2010;464:1357.
134. Coll RC, Robertson AA, Chae JJ, Higgins SC, Muñoz-Planillo R, Inserra MC, et al. A small-molecule inhibitor of the NLRP3 inflammasome for the treatment of inflammatory diseases. Nat Med. 2015;21:248–55.
135. Petrasek J, Bala S, Csak T, Lippai D, Kodys K, Menashy V, et al. IL-1 receptor antagonist ameliorates inflammasome-dependent alcoholic steatohepatitis in mice. J Clin Invest. 2012;122:3476.

136. Mridha AR, Wree A, Robertson AA, Yeh MM, Johnson CD, Van Rooyen DM, et al. NLRP3 inflammasome blockade reduces liver inflammation and fibrosis in experimental NASH in mice. J Hepatol. 2017;66:1037–46.
137. Sharifnia T, Antoun J, Verriere TG, Suarez G, Wattacheril J, Wilson KT, et al. Hepatic TLR4 signaling in obese NAFLD. Am J Physiol Gastrointest Liver Physiol. 2015;309:G270–8.
138. Miura K, Ohnishi H. Role of gut microbiota and toll-like receptors in nonalcoholic fatty liver disease. World J Gastroenterol. 2014;20:7381.
139. Roh YS, Seki E. Toll-like receptors in alcoholic liver disease, non-alcoholic steatohepatitis and carcinogenesis. J Gastroenterol Hepatol. 2013;28:38–42.
140. Leung C, Herath CB, Jia Z, Andrikopoulos S, Brown BE, Davies MJ, et al. Dietary advanced glycation end-products aggravate non-alcoholic fatty liver disease. World J Gastroenterol. 2016;22:8026.
141. Goodwin M, Herath C, Jia Z, Leung C, Coughlan MT, Forbes J, et al. Advanced glycation end products augment experimental hepatic fibrosis. J Gastroenterol Hepatol. 2013;28:369–76.
142. Cinti S, Mitchell G, Barbatelli G, Murano I, Ceresi E, Faloia E, et al. Adipocyte death defines macrophage localization and function in adipose tissue of obese mice and humans. J Lipid Res. 2005;46:2347–55.
143. Murano I, Barbatelli G, Parisani V, Latini C, Muzzonigro G, Castellucci M, et al. Dead adipocytes, detected as crown-like structures, are prevalent in visceral fat depots of genetically obese mice. J Lipid Res. 2008;49:1562–8.
144. Tacke F. Targeting hepatic macrophages to treat liver diseases. J Hepatol. 2017;66:1300.
145. Camps J, Joven J. Chemokine ligand 2 and paraoxonase-1 in non-alcoholic fatty liver disease: the search for alternative causative factors. World J Gastroenterol. 2015;21:2875.
146. Friedman SL, Ratziu V, Harrison SA, Abdelmalek MF, Aithal GP, Caballeria J, et al. A randomized, placebo-controlled trial of cenicriviroc for treatment of nonalcoholic steatohepatitis with fibrosis. Hepatology. 2018;67:1754–67.
147. Kono H, Karmarkar D, Iwakura Y, Rock KL. Identification of the cellular sensor that stimulates the inflammatory response to sterile cell death. J Immunol. 2010;184:4470–8.
148. Wolf MJ, Adili A, Piotrowitz K, Abdullah Z, Boege Y, Stemmer K, et al. Metabolic activation of intrahepatic CD8+ T cells and NKT cells causes nonalcoholic steatohepatitis and liver cancer via cross-talk with hepatocytes. Cancer Cell. 2014;26:549–64.
149. Bhattacharjee J, Kirby M, Softic S, Miles L, Salazar-Gonzalez RM, Shivakumar P, et al. Hepatic natural killer T-cell and CD8+ T-cell signatures in mice with nonalcoholic steatohepatitis. Hepatol Commun. 2017;1:299.
150. Heymann F, Tacke F. Immunology in the liver – from homeostasis to disease. Nat Rev Gastroenterol Hepatol. 2016;13:88.
151. Rensen SS, Bieghs V, Xanthoulea S, Arfianti E, Bakker JA, Shiri-Sverdlov R, et al. Neutrophil-derived myeloperoxidase aggravates non-alcoholic steatohepatitis in low-density lipoprotein receptor-deficient mice. PLoS One. 2012;7:e52411.
152. Giordano A, Murano I, Mondini E, Perugini J, Smorlesi A, Severi I, et al. Obese adipocytes show ultrastructural features of stressed cells and die of pyroptosis. J Lipid Res. 2013;54:2423–36.
153. Caputo T, Gilardi F, Desvergne B. From chronic overnutrition to metaflammation and insulin resistance: adipose tissue and liver contributions. FEBS Lett. 2017;591:3061.
154. Lanthier N, Molendi-Coste O, Cani PD, van Rooijen N, Horsmans Y, Leclercq IA. Kupffer cell depletion prevents but has no therapeutic effect on metabolic and inflammatory changes induced by a high-fat diet. FASEB J. 2011;25:4301–11.
155. Ertunc ME, Hotamisligil GS. Lipid signaling and lipotoxicity in metaflammation: indications for metabolic disease pathogenesis and treatment. J Lipid Res. 2016;57:2099–114.
156. Haczeyni F, Poekes L, Wang H, Mridha AR, Barn V, Geoffrey Haigh W, et al. Obeticholic acid improves adipose morphometry and inflammation and reduces steatosis in dietary but not metabolic obesity in mice. Obesity. 2017;25:155–65.
157. Klebanoff MJ, Corey KE, Chhatwal J, Kaplan LM, Chung RT, Hur C. Bariatric surgery for nonalcoholic steatohepatitis: a clinical and cost-effectiveness analysis. Hepatology. 2017;65:1156–64.
158. Musso G, Cassader M, Paschetta E, Gambino R. Thiazolidinediones and advanced liver fibrosis in nonalcoholic steatohepatitis: a meta-analysis. JAMA Intern Med. 2017;177:633–40.
159. Gryn SE, Hegele RA. Ezetimibe plus simvastatin for the treatment of hypercholesterolemia. Expert Opin Pharmacother. 2015;16:1255–62.
160. Wong VWS, Chan WK, Chitturi S, Chawla Y, Dan YY, Duseja A, et al. The Asia-Pacific working party on nonalcoholic fatty liver disease guidelines 2017 part 1: definition, risk factors and assessment. J Gastroenterol Hepatol. 2017;
161. Ratziu V, Harrison SA, Francque S, Bedossa P, Lehert P, Serfaty L, et al. Elafibranor, an agonist of the peroxisome proliferator- activated receptor- α and- δ, induces resolution of nonalcoholic steatohepatitis without fibrosis worsening. Gastroenterology. 2016;150:1147–59.
162. Haczeyni F, Wang H, Barn V, Mridha AR, Yeh MM, Haigh WG, et al. The selective peroxisome proliferator–activated receptor-delta agonist seladelpar reverses nonalcoholic steatohepatitis pathology by abrogating lipotoxicity in diabetic obese mice. Hepatol Commun. 2017;1:663.

Chemokines and Chemokine Receptors in the Development of NAFLD

4

Yoon-Seok Roh and Ekihiro Seki

Abstract

Chemokines are chemo-attractants for leukocyte trafficking, growth, and activation in injured and inflammatory tissues. The chemokine system is comprised of 50 chemokine ligands and 20 cognate chemokine receptors. In the context of liver diseases, leukocytes, hepatocytes, hepatic stellate cells, endothelial cells, and vascular smooth muscle cells are capable of producing chemokines. Chemokine receptors are typically expressed in various leukocyte subsets. Given that inflammation is a critical factor for the transition from simple steatosis to non-alcoholic steatohepatitis (NASH), and fibrosis, the chemokine system may play a prominent role in the pathogenesis of non-alcoholic fatty liver disease (NAFLD). Indeed, accumulating evidence shows elevated expression of chemokines and their receptors in the livers of obese patients with advanced steatosis and NASH. This chapter will discuss the underlying molecular mechanisms and the therapeutic potential of the chemokine systems in the pathogenesis of NAFLD. Among chemokines, we will highlight CCL2, CCL5, CXCL8-10, CX3CL1, and CXCL16 as pivotal mediators in the development of steatosis, NASH, and fibrosis.

Y.-S. Roh
Department of Pharmacy, Chungbuk National University College of Pharmacy, Cheongju, Chungbuk, South Korea
e-mail: ysroh@cbnu.ac.kr

E. Seki (✉)
Division of Digestive and Liver Diseases, Department of Medicine, Cedars-Sinai Medical Center, Los Angeles, CA, USA
e-mail: Ekihiro.Seki@cshs.org

Keywords

Chemokines · Chemokine receptors · NAFLD · NASH · Fibrosis

4.1 Chemokines and NAFLD

Chemokines are chemotactic cytokines which are small heparin-binding proteins. They act as chemo-attractants for leukocyte trafficking, growth, and activation in inflammatory sites [1, 2]. Approximately 50 chemokines were identified and classified into four subfamilies (C, CC, CXC and CX3C) based on the arrangement of the N-terminal conserved cysteine residues. Twenty cognate chemokine receptors have been identified as relevant in the context of liver diseases (Table 4.1) [3]. Various cell types, including leukocytes, hepatocytes, hepatic stellate cells, liver sinusoidal endothelial cells, and vascular smooth muscle cells, can produce chemokines [4]. Chemokine receptors are typically expressed in various leukocyte subsets and immune cells. Chemokine receptors are seven transmembrane

J. Yu (ed.), *Obesity, Fatty Liver and Liver Cancer*, Advances in Experimental Medicine and Biology 1061, https://doi.org/10.1007/978-981-10-8684-7_4

Table 4.1 Important chemokine and chemokine receptor pathways in NAFLD

Chemokine	Alternative name	Cellular source of chemokine	Chemokine receptor	Target cell	Overall effect in NAFLD
CCL2	MCP-1	Hepatocytes, Kupffer cells, HSCs	CCR2	Monocytes/ macrophages, HSCs	Promition
CCL5	RANTES	HSCs, macrophages, hepatocytes, platelets	CCR1, CCR5	NK, Th1, CD8 T, HSCs	Promotion
CXCL8	IL-8	Hepatocytes, macrophages	CXCR1, CXCR2	Neutrophils, monocyte	Promotion
CXCL9	MIG	Hepatocytes, LSECs, HSCs/MFs	CXCR3	NK, Th1, Th17	Promotion
CXCL10	IP-10	Hepatocytes, LSECs, HSCs/MFs	CXCR3	NK, Th1, Th17, HSCs	Promotion
CX3CL1	Fracktalkine	Hepatocytes, HSCs/MFs, LSECs	CX3CR1	Monocytes/ macrophages	Controversial
CXCL16		LSECs, Kupffer cells	CXCR6	NKT cells	Promotion

HSC hepatic stellate cell, *LSEC* liver sinusoidal endothelial cell, *MF* myofibroblast

G-protein coupled receptors. Upon binding of chemokines to the corresponding chemokine receptors, the downstream intracellular cascades, such as phosphatidylinositol 3-kinase, small Rho guanosine triphosphatase, and cellular calcium influx pathways, are activated, which increases in the avidity of leukocyte integrins that promote leukocyte's interactions with adhesion molecules expressed on sinusoidal endothelial cells, such as intercellular adhesion molecules (ICAMs) and vascular cell adhesion molecules (VCAMs), thereby enabling leukocyte adhesion and subsequent extravasation [5]. Secreted chemokines require an interaction with glycosaminoglycans (GAGs) which are bound to the extracellular matrix and endothelial surface. This interaction locally immobilizes and retains chemokines, creating a concentration gradient that allows a coordinated migration of leukocytes toward inflammatory sites [6]. Infiltrated leukocytes produce inflammatory cytokines that further stimulate hepatic immune cells including liver resident macrophages and recruited circulating monocytes, hepatic stellate cells, and hepatocytes, which enhances liver inflammation (Fig. 4.1). Enhanced liver inflammation contributes to the enhancement of hepatocyte lipid accumulation, the transition from simple steatosis to non-alcoholic steatohepatitis (NASH), and the progression from steatohepatitis to fibrosis. Chemokine systems not only act as chemo-attractants, but also have potential to directly stimulate hepatocytes and hepatic stellate cells to enhance their biological activities, such as lipid accumulation and collagen production, respectively. An Accumulation of data has shown evidence of elevated expression of chemokines and their receptors in the livers of obese patients with advanced steatosis and NASH [7]. Inflammation plays a critical role in the progression of non-alcoholic fatty liver disease (NAFLD). Thus, the chemokine systems may play various prominent roles in the pathogenesis of NAFLD [8].

Obesity or western-style diets lead to insulin resistance, adipokine imbalance, and mobilization of lipotoxic free fatty acids to the liver. In the context of liver, fat accumulation contributes to activation of Kupffer cells, which together with hepatocytes and hepatic stellate cells (HSCs) amplify inflammation via production of various chemokines (CCL2, CCL5, CXCL1, CXCL2, CXCL8, CXCL9, and CXCL10), and recruitment of immune cells (monocytes, activated T cells, NKT cells, neutrophils) into the liver. Chemokines have also been directly implicated in the further accumulation of lipids within hepatocytes and collagen deposition by activated HSCs.

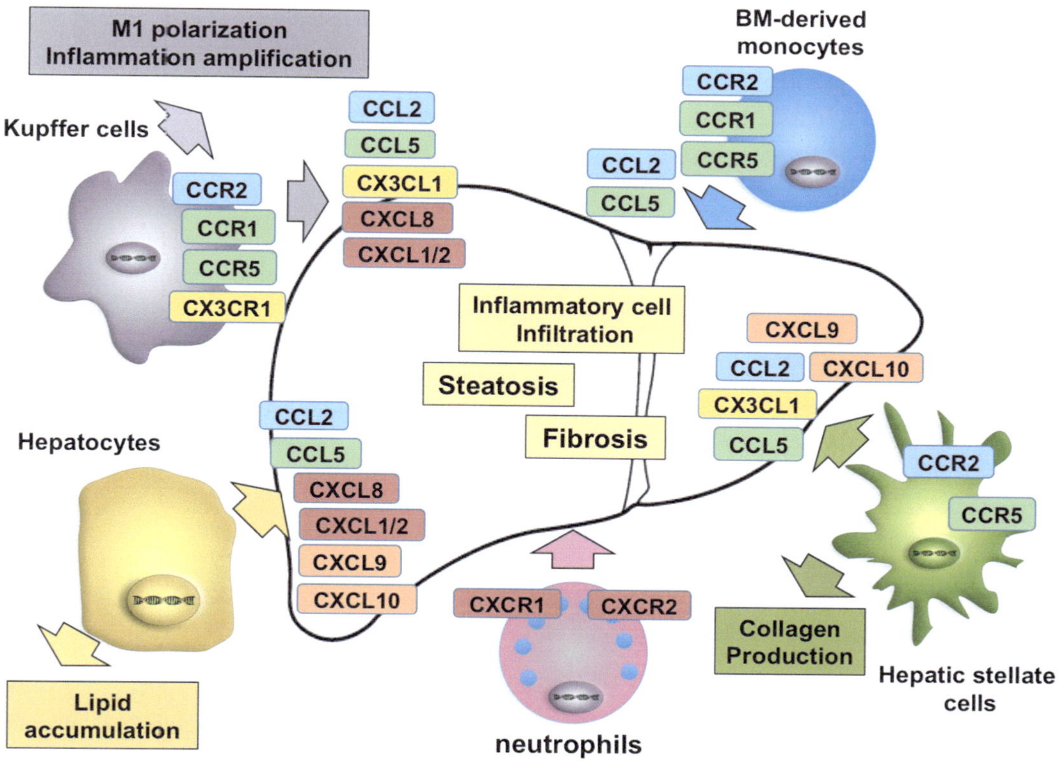

Fig. 4.1 Chemokines in the pathogenesis of nonalcoholic fatty liver disease

4.2 CCL2 (MCP-1) - CCR2

CCL2, also known as Monocyte Chemotactic Protein-1 (MCP-1), is a potent chemoattractant secreted by macrophages, endothelial cells, hepatic stellate cells, and vascular smooth muscle cells in response to inflammatory stimulus, such as interleukin (IL)-1β, tumor necrosis factor (TNF) α, and Toll-like receptor (TLR) ligands (e.g. lipopolysaccharide [LPS]) [9–11]. In pathological settings, hepatocyte CCL2 expression is associated with hepatocyte lipid accumulation in a diet-induced mouse NASH model [12]. In NAFLD, the increases of free fatty acids and activation of TLRs contributes to CCL2 production through NF-κB [13, 14]. In high-fat diet feeding conditions, hepatic CCL2 is upregulated and recruits a subset of myeloid cells, in turn promoting NASH development [15]. Deletion of CCL2 suppresses steatosis and insulin resistance in a diet-induced obese mouse model [16]. Since CCL2 activates the target cells through binding to its receptor CCR2 [17], CCR2 inactivation is expected to show a similar liver phenotype as with CCL2 inactivation. In mice, genetic deletion or pharmacological inhibition of CCR2 has shown the amelioration of inflammation and fibrosis in NASH and insulin resistance by inhibiting the recruitment of CCR2 expressing bone marrow-derived monocytes [14, 18, 19]. In early NAFLD, CCL2 produced from Kupffer cells (liver resident macrophages) is required for recruiting Ly6C positive circulating bone marrow-derived monocytes into the liver, which promotes liver inflammation [14]. Not only do macrophages/monocytes play a role on hepatic stellate cell recruitment and activation through inflammatory and fibrogenic cytokine production, but CCL2 and CCR2 also directly play a role in hepatic stellate cell recruitment and activation that promotes liver fibrosis [20–22]. In NASH progression, adipose tissue macrophages also play an important role. In obesity, macrophages are infiltrated in adipose tissues, in which the CCL2-CCR2 system plays a major role [15]. Infiltration and activation of adipose tissue macrophages release inflammatory cytokines to the systemic circulation, which contributes to liver inflammation progression. In mice, the overexpression of CCL2 in adipose tissue promotes hepatic triglyceride levels and insulin resistance [16]. In human NASH livers, the upregulation of CCL2 was observed [23]. Another study demonstrated that CCL2 production is positively correlated with hepatic fat content in NAFLD patients [24]. These translational studies show additional evidence of the importance of the contribution of the CCL2/CCR2 pathway in the progression of NASH.

4.3 CCL5 (RANTES) – CCR1 and CCR5

CCL5 is also associated with chronic inflammatory diseases, such as NAFLD and liver fibrosis [25]. CCL5 is secreted by various cell types including macrophages, hepatocytes, hepatic stellate cells, and endothelial cells. Excessive lipid accumulation in the liver induces CCL5 production [26]. CCL5 is mainly involved in the migration of T-cells, monocytes, neutrophils, and dendritic cells through binding to its receptors CCR1, CCR3, and CCR5. The association of CCL5 with NAFLD has extensively been discussed in human and mouse studies. Hepatic expression of CCL5 is increased in a murine model of NASH and in obese patients [27, 28]. It should be noted that hepatocytes are a major source of CCL5 in NAFLD [26], suggesting that hepatic lipid accumulation mediates CCL5 release. CCL5 is required for the progression of liver fibrosis through binding to CCR1 and CCR5 [29, 30]. CCR1 is predominantly expressed in liver macrophages while CCR5 is expressed in both liver macrophages and hepatic stellate cells. However, these receptors have not been observed in hepatocytes. In liver fibrosis, CCR5 plays a dominant role in hepatic stellate cells, but not in liver macrophages, for their migration and activation by stimulating with CCL5 [29, 30]. CCR5 also plays a pivotal role in the recruitment of M1-type macrophages and their M1 polarization in adipose tissues, which contributes to insulin resistance and subsequently promotes the development of steatohepatitis [31]. These studies suggest that CCL5/CCR5-mediated signaling contributes to the development of hepatic steatosis, inflammation, fibrosis, and insulin resistance through monocyte/macrophage recruitment and stellate cell activation.

4.4 CXCL8 (IL-8), CXCL1, and CXCL2 – CXCR1 and CXCR2

CXCL8 is a CXC chemokine subfamily secreted by inflammatory cells and endothelial cells, and is also known as IL-8. IL-8 is currently identified only in humans, but not in mice. It is suggested that IL-8 homologues, CXCL1 and CXCL2, substitute the role of IL-8 in mice. These chemokines mainly regulate neutrophil recruitment to inflammatory sites. The serum levels of CXCL8 were significantly higher in NASH patients compared to simple steatosis patients or healthy controls [32]. Moreover, one study demonstrated that serum levels of CXCL8 were higher in subjects with NAFLD as compared to obese and non-obese patients [33]. Conversely, another study also demonstrated no association between serum CXCL8 and NAFLD [34]. More careful and intensive investigations on the function of CXCL8 in the pathogenesis of human NAFLD should be performed in the future. Since CXCL8 was cloned only in humans, the mechanistic analysis is limited. In contrast, the studies of its receptor, CXCR2, that can be activated by its alternative ligands CXCL1, CXCL2, and CXCL5 have been investigated in NAFLD mouse models. In the NAFLD mouse model and in NAFLD patients, circulating and hepatic levels of lipocalin-2 (LCN2), a glycoprotein, are increased.

LCN2 mediates liver injury and inflammation through neutrophil recruitment and CXCR2 in NASH mouse models [35]. We have recently demonstrated that hepatic CXCL1 levels are induced in a TLR4-MyD88-dependent manner and that increased CXCL1 is involved in hepatic neutrophil infiltration, which promotes NASH and liver fibrosis [36]. These studies demonstrate the importance of CXCR1/CXCR2-mediated neutrophil and macrophage recruitment in the development of NAFLD.

4.5 CXCL9/MIG and CXCL10/IP-10 – CXCR3

CXCL9 and CXCL10 bind to CXCR3 as a common receptor, which is highly expressed in macrophages, activated T cells, memory T cells, and natural killer cells [37]. CXCL9 and CXCL10 promote the recruitment of these cell types. However, these chemokines are generally undetectable in most non-lymphoid tissues under physiological conditions. In pathologic conditions, hepatic endothelial cells produce high levels of CXCL9, leading to the migration of the CXCR3-expressing lymphocytes [38]. Moreover, the expression levels of CXCL9 were increased in the livers of NASH patients and mouse NASH models [39, 40]. CXCL10 is produced in macrophages, monocytes, hepatocytes, hepatic stellate cells, and endothelial cells [41]. CXCL10 plays a pivotal role in the pathogenesis of experimental steatohepatitis through induction of inflammation, oxidative stress, and lipogenesis [42]. A recent study reported that extracellular vesicles (EVs) released from lipid-accumulated hepatocytes contain CXCL10 that plays a central role in macrophage recruitment in NAFLD. The production of EVs containing CXCL10 is mediated by MLK3 in hepatocytes [43]. This study provided new evidence that EVs act as vehicles for delivering chemokines as cargos to target organs and cells. Consistently, CXCL10 has been proposed as a potential therapeutic target for the treatment of NASH, progressive liver injury, insulin resistance, and incident diabetes [41, 44].

4.6 CX3CL1/Fractalkine – CX3CR1

CX3CL1, also known as Fractalkine, is a membrane-bound type of chemokine. CX3CL1 is involved in cell recruitment and cell survival through binding to CX3-chemokine receptor 1 (CX3CR1) [45]. In addition, CX3CR1-expressing monocytes circulate in the steady state and differentiate into alternatively activated macrophages [46]. In the liver, CX3CL1 is produced in Kupffer cells/macrophages and hepatic stellate cells [47]. The responsible receptor CX3CR1 is mainly expressed in Kupffer cells/macrophages. The CX3CL1-CX3CR1 interaction induces liver macrophage apoptosis and alternatively acquires anti-inflammatory properties of Kupffer cells/macrophages, which contribute to the negative regulation of liver inflammation and fibrosis [47, 48]. However, the role of CX3CL1/CX3CR1 signaling in NAFLD is still controversial. In an experimental mouse model, CX3CR1 has been reported to protect from excessive hepatic steatosis and inflammation, as well as systemic glucose intolerance through maintaining intestinal homeostasis [49]. Moreover, decreased CX3CL1/CX3CR1 pathway has been suggested to be a mechanism underlying β cell dysfunction in type 2 diabetes [50]. Conversely, CX3CR1+ moDCs (monocyte-derived inflammatory dendritic cells) have a pathologic role in the progression of NASH. The underlying mechanism that the study demonstrated is that the worsening of parenchymal injury was driven by an elevation in hepatic and circulating TNFα levels [51]. This discrepancy might be explained by the different roles of the CX3CL1/CXC3CR1 axis in different cell types.

4.7 CXCL16 – CXCR6

Previous studies demonstrated that the chemokine receptor, CXCR6, and its cognate ligand, CXCL16, control the patrolling of natural killer T (NKT) cells in liver sinusoids to maintain liver homeostasis [52]. In humans, higher CXCR6+ T cells have been detected in the blood of patients with hepatitis C virus infection compared to healthy controls [53]. CXCL16 is expressed in hepatocytes and bile duct epithelial cells of patients with liver disease [53], as well as in murine liver sinusoidal endothelial cells [52]. CXCR6 promotes the infiltration of hepatic NKT cells and inflammatory macrophages, thereby promoting liver inflammation in experimental NAFLD [54, 55]. Indeed, CXCR6 gene expression was positively correlated with the inflammatory activity and ALT levels in patients with NAFLD [55] and injured hepatocytes had increased expression of CXCL16, a ligand of CXCR6, suggesting that the CXCL16-CXCR6 interaction plays a role in the pathogenesis of NAFLD [55].

4.8 Chemokines and Chemokine Receptors As Therapeutic Targets for the Treatment of NAFLD

It has been shown that pharmaceutical inhibition of CCR2 prevents the infiltration of the CCR2-expressing Ly6C-positive monocytes, resulting in an inhibition of NASH-mediated liver inflammation and fibrosis [14]. Consistently, pharmacological blockade of CCL2/CCR2 signaling in several mouse models of metabolic diseases significantly improved steatosis, inflammation, obesity, and insulin resistance [18, 19, 56, 57]. Furthermore, the inhibition of glutaminyl cyclases, an enzyme responsible for the maturation of cytokines to the active form, alleviates CCL2-mediated liver inflammation in an experimental model of NAFLD [58]. CCR5 antagonist, maraviroc, has been shown to be effective in the amelioration of NAFLD, indicating that CCR5 is also a promising therapeutic target for patients with NAFLD [59]. Of note, a CCR2/CCR5 dual antagonist, cenicriviroc, that was originally developed for the treatment of HIV infection is now in a phase 2 clinical trial for NASH-associated liver fibrosis in adult subjects [60]. Since CCR2 and CCR5 are important for the infiltration of both myeloid cells and hepatic stellate cell, we expect that this antagonist can suppress NAFLD development through inhibiting both inflammatory and fibrogenic pathways. Another study showed that pharmacological inhibition of CXCL16 reduced liver macrophage infiltration and steatohepatitis in the NASH mouse model [55]. Moreover, pharmacological inhibition of MLK3 prevented CXCL10 enrichment in hepatocyte-derived EVs and subsequently inhibited macrophage chemotaxis in the pathogenesis of NAFLD [43]. Of note, two recent studies suggest that β-cryptoxanthin protects and reverses NASH in mice through inhibition of lipid accumulation and lipid peroxidation by regulating the M1/M2 polarization of Kupffer cells in the liver. The mechanism of action is partly mediated through a downregulation of the CCL2/CCR2 and CCL5/CCR5 signaling [61, 62]. These previous findings and ongoing clinical trials suggest that targeting chemokines and chemokine receptors on inflammatory cells and hepatic stellate cells to control liver inflammation and fibrogenic response might represent promising therapeutic approaches for NAFLD and its related fibrosis.

4.9 Perspectives and Conclusions

Extensive in vitro and in vivo investigations conducted over the past 20 years have elucidated the pivotal roles played by the inflammation in the pathogenesis of NAFLD and fibrosis. It is becoming increasingly clear that chemokines and chemokine receptors play more important roles than we expected in the NAFLD development. Several chemokine systems may be integrally involved in tissue- and organ-level inflammation caused by interactions among liver, adipose tissue, and macrophages as well as the subsequent development of systemic insulin resistance and metabolic disorders. However, much research remains to be done to elucidate the pathophysiology of NAFLD and to identify specific targets for the treatment. Additionally, the involvement of chemokines and their receptors in the pathogenesis of NAFLD is still only partially understood.

Although the initial studies attempting therapeutic strategies targeting the chemokine system have been reported, further investigations of the underlying molecular mechanisms of NAFLD in which chemokine-chemokine receptor interactions play a role are indeed required. Collectively, all of the evidence supporting the mechanistic link between the chemokine-chemokine receptor system and NAFLD development provides important information for developing new options for the treatment of NAFLD, NASH, and fibrosis. Additional preclinical studies as well as clinical trials targeting chemokines and/or their receptors will provide better understandings of the underlying molecular mechanisms of chemokine system-mediated hepatic inflammation and the pathogenesis of NAFLD, which is crucial for developing novel treatments.

Acknowledgements This work was supported by NIH grant R01DK085252 (E.S) and R21AA025841(E.S), Winnick Research award from Cedars-Sinai Medical Center (E.S), and American Liver Foundation Congressman John Joseph Moakley Postdoctoral Research Fellowship (Y.S.R) and NRF grant 2017R1C1B2004423 (Y.S.R).

References

1. Rollins BJ. Chemokines. Blood. 1997;90:909–28.
2. Gerard C, Rollins BJ. Chemokines and disease. Nat Immunol. 2001;2:108–15.
3. Zlotnik A, Yoshie O. Chemokines: a new classification system and their role in immunity. Immunity. 2000;12:121–7.
4. Saiman Y, Friedman SL. The role of chemokines in acute liver injury. Front Physiol. 2012;3:213.
5. Oo YH, Shetty S, Adams DH. The role of chemokines in the recruitment of lymphocytes to the liver. Dig Dis. 2010;28:31–44.
6. Proudfoot AE, Handel TM, Johnson Z, Lau EK, LiWang P, Clark-Lewis I, et al. Glycosaminoglycan binding and oligomerization are essential for the in vivo activity of certain chemokines. Proc Natl Acad Sci U S A. 2003;100:1885–90.
7. Bertola A, Bonnafous S, Anty R, Patouraux S, Saint-Paul MC, Iannelli A, et al. Hepatic expression patterns of inflammatory and immune response genes associated with obesity and NASH in morbidly obese patients. PLoS One. 2010;5:e13577.
8. Lalor PF, Faint J, Aarbodem Y, Hubscher SG, Adams DH. The role of cytokines and chemokines in the development of steatohepatitis. Semin Liver Dis. 2007;27:173–93.
9. Yla-Herttuala S, Lipton BA, Rosenfeld ME, Sarkioja T, Yoshimura T, Leonard EJ, et al. Expression of monocyte chemoattractant protein 1 in macrophage-rich areas of human and rabbit atherosclerotic lesions. Proc Natl Acad Sci U S A. 1991;88:5252–6.
10. Yu X, Dluz S, Graves DT, Zhang L, Antoniades HN, Hollander W, et al. Elevated expression of monocyte chemoattractant protein 1 by vascular smooth muscle cells in hypercholesterolemic primates. Proc Natl Acad Sci U S A. 1992;89:6953–7.
11. Nelken NA, Coughlin SR, Gordon D, Wilcox JN. Monocyte chemoattractant protein-1 in human atheromatous plaques. J Clin Invest. 1991;88:1121–7.
12. Rull A, Rodriguez F, Aragones G, Marsillach J, Beltran R, Alonso-Villaverde C, et al. Hepatic monocyte chemoattractant protein-1 is upregulated by dietary cholesterol and contributes to liver steatosis. Cytokine. 2009;48:273–9.
13. Luedde T, Schwabe RF. NF-kappaB in the liver--linking injury, fibrosis and hepatocellular carcinoma. Nat Rev Gastroenterol Hepatol. 2011;8:108–18.
14. Miura K, Yang L, van Rooijen N, Ohnishi H, Seki E. Hepatic recruitment of macrophages promotes nonalcoholic steatohepatitis through CCR2. Am J Physiol Gastrointest Liver Physiol. 2012;302:G1310–21.
15. Obstfeld AE, Sugaru E, Thearle M, Francisco AM, Gayet C, Ginsberg HN, et al. C-C chemokine receptor 2 (CCR2) regulates the hepatic recruitment of myeloid cells that promote obesity-induced hepatic steatosis. Diabetes. 2010;59:916–25.
16. Kanda H, Tateya S, Tamori Y, Kotani K, Hiasa K, Kitazawa R, et al. MCP-1 contributes to macrophage infiltration into adipose tissue, insulin resistance, and hepatic steatosis in obesity. J Clin Invest. 2006;116:1494–505.
17. Wobser H, Dorn C, Weiss TS, Amann T, Bollheimer C, Buttner R, et al. Lipid accumulation in hepatocytes induces fibrogenic activation of hepatic stellate cells. Cell Res. 2009;19:996–1005.
18. Tamura Y, Sugimoto M, Murayama T, Minami M, Nishikaze Y, Ariyasu H, et al. C-C chemokine receptor 2 inhibitor improves diet-induced development of insulin resistance and hepatic steatosis in mice. J Atheroscler Thromb. 2010;17:219–28.
19. Baeck C, Wehr A, Karlmark KR, Heymann F, Vucur M, Gassler N, et al. Pharmacological inhibition of the chemokine CCL2 (MCP-1) diminishes liver macrophage infiltration and steatohepatitis in chronic hepatic injury. Gut. 2012;61:416–26.
20. Galastri S, Zamara E, Milani S, Novo E, Provenzano A, Delogu W, et al. Lack of CC chemokine ligand 2 differentially affects inflammation and fibrosis according to the genetic background in a murine model of steatohepatitis. Clin Sci (Lond). 2012;123:459–71.
21. Marra F, Romanelli RG, Giannini C, Failli P, Pastacaldi S, Arrighi MC, et al. Monocyte chemotactic protein-1 as a chemoattractant for human hepatic stellate cells. Hepatology. 1999;29:140–8.
22. Seki E, de Minicis S, Inokuchi S, Taura K, Miyai K, van Rooijen N, et al. CCR2 promotes hepatic fibrosis in mice. Hepatology. 2009;50:185–97.

23. Westerbacka J, Kolak M, Kiviluoto T, Arkkila P, Siren J, Hamsten A, et al. Genes involved in fatty acid partitioning and binding, lipolysis, monocyte/macrophage recruitment, and inflammation are overexpressed in the human fatty liver of insulin-resistant subjects. Diabetes. 2007;56:2759–65.
24. Greco D, Kotronen A, Westerbacka J, Puig O, Arkkila P, Kiviluoto T, et al. Gene expression in human NAFLD. Am J Physiol Gastrointest Liver Physiol. 2008;294:G1281–7.
25. Henao-Mejia J, Elinav E, Jin C, Hao L, Mehal WZ, Strowig T, et al. Inflammasome-mediated dysbiosis regulates progression of NAFLD and obesity. Nature. 2012;482:179–85.
26. Kirovski G, Gabele E, Dorn C, Moleda L, Niessen C, Weiss TS, et al. Hepatic steatosis causes induction of the chemokine RANTES in the absence of significant hepatic inflammation. Int J Clin Exp Pathol. 2010;3:675–80.
27. Desai MS, Mariscalco MM, Tawil A, Vallejo JG, Smith CW. Atherogenic diet-induced hepatitis is partially dependent on murine TLR4. J Leukoc Biol. 2008;83:1336–44.
28. Wu H, Ghosh S, Perrard XD, Feng L, Garcia GE, Perrard JL, et al. T-cell accumulation and regulated on activation, normal T cell expressed and secreted upregulation in adipose tissue in obesity. Circulation. 2007;115:1029–38.
29. Seki E, De Minicis S, Gwak GY, Kluwe J, Inokuchi S, Bursill CA, et al. CCR1 and CCR5 promote hepatic fibrosis in mice. J Clin Invest. 2009;119:1858–70.
30. Berres ML, Koenen RR, Rueland A, Zaldivar MM, Heinrichs D, Sahin H, et al. Antagonism of the chemokine Ccl5 ameliorates experimental liver fibrosis in mice. J Clin Invest. 2010;120:4129–40.
31. Kitade H, Sawamoto K, Nagashimada M, Inoue H, Yamamoto Y, Sai Y, et al. CCR5 plays a critical role in obesity-induced adipose tissue inflammation and insulin resistance by regulating both macrophage recruitment and M1/M2 status. Diabetes. 2012;61:1680–90.
32. Bahcecioglu IH, Yalniz M, Ataseven H, Ilhan N, Ozercan IH, Seckin D, et al. Levels of serum hyaluronic acid, TNF-alpha and IL-8 in patients with nonalcoholic steatohepatitis. Hepato-Gastroenterology. 2005;52:1549–53.
33. Jarrar MH, Baranova A, Collantes R, Ranard B, Stepanova M, Bennett C, et al. Adipokines and cytokines in non-alcoholic fatty liver disease. Aliment Pharmacol Ther. 2008;27:412–21.
34. Abiru S, Migita K, Maeda Y, Daikoku M, Ito M, Ohata K, et al. Serum cytokine and soluble cytokine receptor levels in patients with non-alcoholic steatohepatitis. Liver Int. 2006;26:39–45.
35. Ye D, Yang K, Zang S, Lin Z, Chau HT, Wang Y, et al. Lipocalin-2 mediates non-alcoholic steatohepatitis by promoting neutrophil-macrophage crosstalk via the induction of CXCR2. J Hepatol. 2016;65:988–97.
36. Yang L, Miura K, Zhang B, Matsushita H, Yang YM, Liang S, et al. TRIF differentially regulates hepatic steatosis and inflammation/fibrosis in mice. Cell Mol Gastroenterol Hepatol. 2017;3:469–83.
37. Braunersreuther V, Viviani GL, Mach F, Montecucco F. Role of cytokines and chemokines in non-alcoholic fatty liver disease. World J Gastroenterol. 2012;18:727–35.
38. Schrage A, Wechsung K, Neumann K, Schumann M, Schulzke JD, Engelhardt B, et al. Enhanced T cell transmigration across the murine liver sinusoidal endothelium is mediated by transcytosis and surface presentation of chemokines. Hepatology. 2008;48:1262–72.
39. Wasmuth HE, Lammert F, Zaldivar MM, Weiskirchen R, Hellerbrand C, Scholten D, et al. Antifibrotic effects of CXCL9 and its receptor CXCR3 in livers of mice and humans. Gastroenterology. 2009;137:309–19, 319 e301–303
40. Semba T, Nishimura M, Nishimura S, Ohara O, Ishige T, Ohno S, et al. The FLS (fatty liver Shionogi) mouse reveals local expressions of lipocalin-2, CXCL1 and CXCL9 in the liver with non-alcoholic steatohepatitis. BMC Gastroenterol. 2013;13:120.
41. Xu Z, Zhang X, Lau J, Yu J. C-X-C motif chemokine 10 in non-alcoholic steatohepatitis: role as a pro-inflammatory factor and clinical implication. Expert Rev Mol Med. 2016;18:e16.
42. Zhang X, Shen J, Man K, Chu ES, Yau TO, Sung JC, et al. CXCL10 plays a key role as an inflammatory mediator and a non-invasive biomarker of non-alcoholic steatohepatitis. J Hepatol. 2014;61:1365–75.
43. Ibrahim SH, Hirsova P, Tomita K, Bronk SF, Werneburg NW, Harrison SA, et al. Mixed lineage kinase 3 mediates release of C-X-C motif ligand 10-bearing chemotactic extracellular vesicles from lipotoxic hepatocytes. Hepatology. 2016;63:731–44.
44. Chang CC, Wu CL, Su WW, Shih KL, Tarng DC, Chou CT, et al. Interferon gamma-induced protein 10 is associated with insulin resistance and incident diabetes in patients with nonalcoholic fatty liver disease. Sci Rep. 2015;5:10096.
45. Landsman L, Bar-On L, Zernecke A, Kim KW, Krauthgamer R, Shagdarsuren E, et al. CX3CR1 is required for monocyte homeostasis and atherogenesis by promoting cell survival. Blood. 2009;113:963–72.
46. Auffray C, Fogg D, Garfa M, Elain G, Join-Lambert O, Kayal S, et al. Monitoring of blood vessels and tissues by a population of monocytes with patrolling behavior. Science. 2007;317:666–70.
47. Aoyama T, Inokuchi S, Brenner DA, Seki E. CX3CL1-CX3CR1 interaction prevents carbon tetrachloride-induced liver inflammation and fibrosis in mice. Hepatology. 2010;52:1390–400.
48. Karlmark KR, Zimmermann HW, Roderburg C, Gassler N, Wasmuth HE, Luedde T, et al. The fractalkine receptor CX(3)CR1 protects against liver fibrosis by controlling differentiation and survival of infiltrating hepatic monocytes. Hepatology. 2010;52:1769–82.
49. Schneider KM, Bieghs V, Heymann F, Hu W, Dreymueller D, Liao L, et al. CX3CR1 is a gatekeeper for intestinal barrier integrity in mice: limiting steatohepatitis by maintaining intestinal homeostasis. Hepatology. 2015;62:1405–16.

50. Lee YS, Morinaga H, Kim JJ, Lagakos W, Taylor S, Keshwani M, et al. The fractalkine/CX3CR1 system regulates beta cell function and insulin secretion. Cell. 2013;153:413–25.
51. Sutti S, Locatelli I, Bruzzi S, Jindal A, Vacchiano M, Bozzola C, et al. CX3CR1-expressing inflammatory dendritic cells contribute to the progression of steatohepatitis. Clin Sci (Lond). 2015;129:797–808.
52. Geissmann F, Cameron TO, Sidobre S, Manlongat N, Kronenberg M, Briskin MJ, et al. Intravascular immune surveillance by CXCR6+ NKT cells patrolling liver sinusoids. PLoS Biol. 2005;3:e113.
53. Heydtmann M, Lalor PF, Eksteen JA, Hubscher SG, Briskin M, Adams DH. CXC chemokine ligand 16 promotes integrin-mediated adhesion of liver-infiltrating lymphocytes to cholangiocytes and hepatocytes within the inflamed human liver. J Immunol. 2005;174:1055–62.
54. Wehr A, Baeck C, Heymann F, Niemietz PM, Hammerich L, Martin C, et al. Chemokine receptor CXCR6-dependent hepatic NK T cell accumulation promotes inflammation and liver fibrosis. J Immunol. 2013;190:5226–36.
55. Wehr A, Baeck C, Ulmer F, Gassler N, Hittatiya K, Luedde T, et al. Pharmacological inhibition of the chemokine CXCL16 diminishes liver macrophage infiltration and steatohepatitis in chronic hepatic injury. PLoS One. 2014;9:e112327.
56. Yang SJ, IglayReger HB, Kadouh HC, Bodary PF. Inhibition of the chemokine (C-C motif) ligand 2/chemokine (C-C motif) receptor 2 pathway attenuates hyperglycaemia and inflammation in a mouse model of hepatic steatosis and lipoatrophy. Diabetologia. 2009;52:972–81.
57. Tamura Y, Sugimoto M, Murayama T, Ueda Y, Kanamori H, Ono K, et al. Inhibition of CCR2 ameliorates insulin resistance and hepatic steatosis in db/db mice. Arterioscler Thromb Vasc Biol. 2008;28:2195–201.
58. Cynis H, Kehlen A, Haegele M, Hoffmann T, Heiser U, Fujii M, et al. Inhibition of Glutaminyl Cyclases alleviates CCL2-mediated inflammation of non-alcoholic fatty liver disease in mice. Int J Exp Pathol. 2013;94:217–25.
59. Perez-Martinez L, Perez-Matute P, Aguilera-Lizarraga J, Rubio-Mediavilla S, Narro J, Recio E, et al. Maraviroc, a CCR5 antagonist, ameliorates the development of hepatic steatosis in a mouse model of non-alcoholic fatty liver disease (NAFLD). J Antimicrob Chemother. 2014;69:1903–10.
60. Friedman S, Sanyal A, Goodman Z, Lefebvre E, Gottwald M, Fischer L, et al. Efficacy and safety study of cenicriviroc for the treatment of non-alcoholic steatohepatitis in adult subjects with liver fibrosis: CENTAUR phase 2b study design. Contemp Clin Trials. 2016;47:356–65.
61. Kobori M, Ni Y, Takahashi Y, Watanabe N, Sugiura M. Ogawa K, et al. beta-Cryptoxanthin alleviates diet-induced nonalcoholic steatohepatitis by suppressing inflammatory gene expression in mice. PLoS One. 2014;9:e98294.
62. Ni Y, Nagashimada M, Zhan L, Nagata N, Kobori M, Sugiura M, et al. Prevention and reversal of lipotoxicity-induced hepatic insulin resistance and steatohepatitis in mice by an antioxidant carotenoid, beta-cryptoxanthin. Endocrinology. 2015;156:987–99.

NAFLD Related-HCC: The Relationship with Metabolic Disorders

5

Xiang Zhang

Abstract

Obesity increases death rates of all cancers including non-alcoholic fatty liver disease (NAFLD)-related hepatocellular carcinoma (NAFLD-HCC). NAFLD is considered as hepatic manifestation of metabolic syndrome and is a multi-system disease. Recent prevalence studies have intensively reported the association of obesity, metabolic risk factors and HCC incidence and mortality. Mechanistic studies suggested that immune response, PI3K/AKT/mTOR/PTEN pathway, mitochondrial dysfunction and genetic alterations are important mediators in the progression of NAFLD-HCC from metabolic disorder. In this book chapter, we attempt to collate current research on NAFLD-HCC that lead to our understandings on how metabolic disorders may intersect with cancer development. We also discussed the prevention options of NAFLD-HCC in view of obesity and metabolic disorder. These studies have extended our knowledge on the complicated mechanism of NAFLD and HCC, and provided the prevention options of NAFLD-HCC in patients with obesity and metabolic diseases.

X. Zhang (✉)
Institute of Digestive Disease and Department of Medicine & Therapeutics, State Key Laboratory of Digestive Disease, LKS Institute of Health Sciences, The Chinese University of Hong Kong, Hong Kong, Hong Kong
e-mail: jenniferzhang@link.cuhk.edu.hk

Keywords

Obesity · Metabolic syndrome · NAFLD-related HCC · Immune response

5.1 Obesity and Metabolic Syndrome

Metabolic disorders encompass obesity and type 2 diabetes. During the last few decades, the prevalence of overweight and obesity has increased globally and dramatically. Overweight is defined as increased body mass index (BMI) (25–29.9 kg/m^2) and waist circumference (94–101.9 cm in men and 80–87.9 cm in women) with moderate central fat accumulation [1]. Obese is defined as high BMI (> = 30 kg/m^2) and waist circumference (> = 102 cm in men and > =88 cm in women) with high central fat accumulation and high risk of co-morbidities [1]. Metabolic syndrome, as a predicator of type 2 diabetes, is a series of disorders including obesity, hyperlipidemia, diabetes, and insulin resistance. The definition of metabolic syndrome by International Diabetes Federation metabolic syndrome is central obesity (high waist circumference) plus two of the features including raised triglyceride (≥1.7 mmol/L), reduced high density lipoprotein (HDL)-cholesterol (<1.03 mmol/L in male and <1.29 mmol/L in female), raised blood pressure (Systolic > = 130 mmHg or Diastolic > = 85 mmHg) and raised fasting glucose

J. Yu (ed.), *Obesity, Fatty Liver and Liver Cancer*, Advances in Experimental Medicine and Biology 1061, https://doi.org/10.1007/978-981-10-8684-7_5

(≥5.6 mmol/L) [2]. High triglyceride levels and low HDL-cholesterol levels are key factors for metabolic syndrome and could increase the levels of low density lipoprotein (LDL)-cholesterol. High blood pressure can be caused by insulin resistance through insulin-mediated renal tubular reabsorption of sodium and high catecholamine activity [1]. Raised fasting glucose can be induced by unresponsiveness to insulin due to changes in receptor binding. Among these parameters, insulin resistance is the main feature for metabolic syndrome and central obesity is the main cause of insulin resistance [3]. Accumulated studies have suggested the close relationship between obesity and metabolic syndrome through inflammation, adipocyte dysfunction, microbiota, and so on. However, one should be noted that healthy obese phenotype also exists in 30% obese subjects with low risk of cardiovascular diseases [4]. On the other hand, non-obese individuals could also have metabolic disorders [5].

5.2 NAFLD

Non-alcoholic fatty liver diseases (NAFLD) is a spectrum of diseases including steatosis, non-alcoholic steatohepatitis (NASH), cirrhosis and hepatocellular carcinoma (HCC). NAFLD is mainly due to over-nutrition and its complications, including obesity, insulin resistance, glucose intolerance and metabolic syndrome [6]. On the other hand, metabolic disorder can be induced in NAFLD patients [7]. Therefore, NAFLD is both the cause and consequence of metabolic syndrome [7] (Fig. 5.1). Patients with obesity and type 2 diabetes are recommended to screening for NAFLD [6]. Although NAFLD is closely related with obesity, it can also be developed in non-obese individuals [8]. However, non-obese NAFLD patients have less severe liver disease compared with their counterparts with obesity due to the lower NAFLD activity scores, fibrosis stage and liver stiffness measurement [8, 9].

The gold standard for NAFLD assessment is liver biopsy. However, it is an invasive method that should only be performed in NAFLD patients whose diagnosis is unclear, or there is a suspected possibility of co-existing chronic liver diseases. Non-invasive test of hepatic steatosis has been widely used in clinical studies [6]. Controlled attenuation parameter (CAP) can be used to diagnose steatosis. Moreover, magnetic resonance imaging (MRI)-based assessment of steatosis is highly reproducible and not affected by obesity. Furthermore, liver fibrosis scores including aspartate aminotransferase-to-platelet ratio index (APRI), fibrosis-4 (FIB-4) score, NAFLD fibrosis score (NFS), and Forns score can be used to predict the outcomes of NAFLD [10].

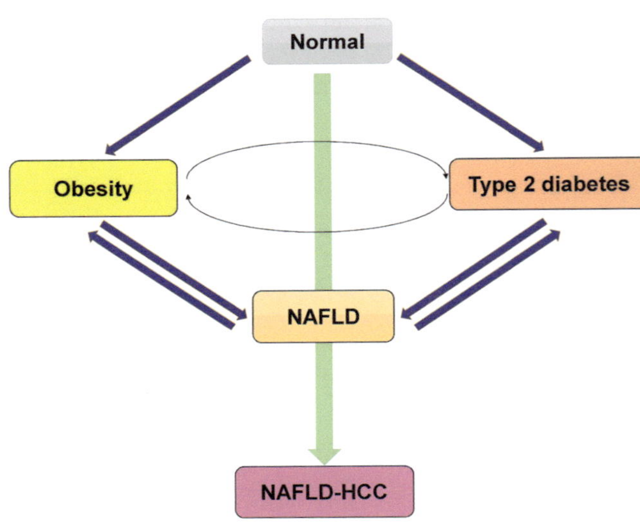

Fig. 5.1 The crosstalk between obesity, type 2 diabetes and NAFLD. Metabolic obesity causes NAFLD. NAFLD is both the cause and consequence of obesity and type 2 diabetes. Obesity and NAFLD can predispose to hepatocellular carcinoma (NAFLD-HCC)

5.3 HCC Prevalence Is Closely Correlated with Obesity and Metabolic Factors

Obesity and diabetes are two major and independent risk factors for NAFLD. NAFLD is considered to be hepatic manifestation of metabolic syndrome and is a multi-system disease, affecting organs besides of liver [11]. Obesity and NAFLD can predispose to hepatocellular carcinoma (NAFLD-HCC), which is more likely to be poorly differentiated than HCC from other etiologies. Accumulating studies have reported that obesity dramatically increases HCC risk [12] and NAFLD has overcome hepatitis C virus (HCV) as the main cause of HCC in the USA. Paris *et al.* investigated the temporal trends, clinical patterns and outcomes of NAFLD-HCC in 323 HCC patients from 1995 to 2004. They stated that the prevalence of NAFLD-HCC increased dramatically over the past 20 years due to the high NAFLD incidence [13]. Patients with NAFLD-HCC have larger tumor size with invasive phenotype compared to HCC patients derived from HCV infection [14]. The association of obesity, metabolic risk factors and HCC incidence and mortality were reported intensively recently. A study involved 5373 male Taiwanese showed that patients with three or more metabolic risk factors had a higher risk of HCC [15]. Consistent with this report, a follow-up study involved more than 34 million person-years in Swedish revealed that obese and overweight men had increased risk of future severe liver diseases, including HCC. Metabolic disorder was related with a further higher risk of severe liver disease [16]. A meta-analysis involved 1,599,453 individuals with 5705 HCC-related deaths showed the direct correlation of obesity with HCC-related mortality [17]. However, in patients with advanced HCC treated with Sorafenib, obesity and metabolic syndrome were not associated with the overall survival of HCC patients [18]. Although recent studies showed that 50% of NAFLD-HCC patients have liver cirrhosis [14], NAFLD-HCC patients with non-cirrhotic liver are less likely to be accompanied with obesity or metabolic syndrome [19]. NAFLD has more than fivefold risk of having HCC in patients without HCC compared to HCV patients.

5.4 Mechanism of Increased NAFLD-HCC Risk by Obesity and Metabolic Disorder

Multiple signaling pathways have been identified to be involved in obesity-associated liver cancer. The link between obesity, metabolic syndrome and NAFLD-HCC are reviewed as follows (Fig. 5.2):

5.4.1 Inflammation and Immune Response

Obesity, metabolic disorder and NAFLD are all inflammatory diseases. Obesity is linked to the activation of inflammatory pathways of adipose tissues. In genetic and dietary obese mouse models, the pro-inflammatory cytokines secreted by the adipocytes and macrophages, including tumor necrosis factor (TNF-α), interleukin (IL)-1, IL-6, and monocyte chemoattractant protein-1 (MCP-1), are up-regulated in the adipose tissues [20]. In obesity, macrophages and adipocytes in the adipose tissues are interrelated. The secreted cytokines by macrophages can damage adipocyte insulin sensitivity, leading to metabolic disorders [20]. On the other hand, the cytokines produced by adipocytes in obese mice could induce adipose macrophage polarization to M1 phenotype [20]. Lipid accumulation and inflammation in the liver can cause NASH development, thereby promoting HCC progression. In obesity, increased TNF-α and IL-6 production could cause hepatic inflammation, leading to HCC development [21]. Gomes *et al.* reported that obesity could lead to DNA damage in hepatocytes, trigger Th17 infiltration, IL-17 production and metabolic disorder-associated insulin resistance, thereby promoting NASH and HCC development [22]. IL-17 blockade could inhibit insulin resistance and prevents NASH and HCC development [22]. In addition, lipid accumulation in obesity and NAFLD induces the loss of

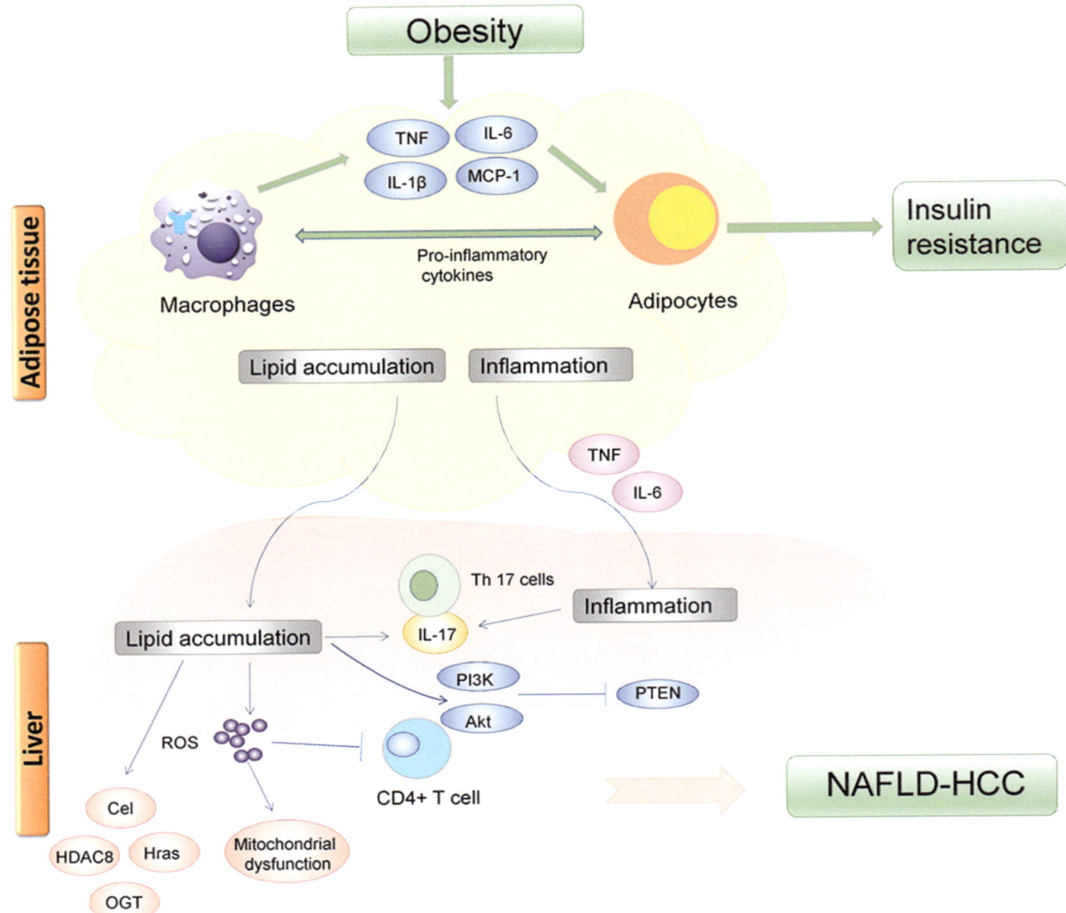

Fig. 5.2 Mechanism of increased NAFLD-HCC risk by obesity and metabolic disorder. Obesity is linked to the activation of inflammatory pathways of adipose tissues through the crosstalk between macrophages and adipocytes. Inflammation, immune response, PI3K/AKT/PTEN pathway, mitochondrial dysfunction and genetic alterations are all involved in the progression of NAFLD-HCC initiated by obesity and insulin resistance

intrahepatic CD4+ T lymphocytes through reactive oxygen species (ROS) production, promoting HCC development [23]. Collectively, inflammation and immune response in obesity and metabolic disorder promote cell proliferation and lead to NAFLD-HCC progression.

5.4.2 PI3K/AKT/mTOR/PTEN Pathway

Hyperinsulinemia in metabolic disorder could induce the activation of phosphatidylinositol 3-kinase (PI3K). Hepatocyte specific overexpression of PI3K in mice leads to steatosis and tumor formation with 94–100% hepatocyte-specific PI3K transgenic mice developed to HCC at 52 weeks age [24]. Lipid accumulation can accelerate tumorigenesis by PI3K activation. Protein kinase Akt is a key factor in glucose output by hepatic insulin. PI3K/Akt deregulation has been implicated in metabolic disorders and tumorigenesis in human [25]. Akt phosphorylation can mediate mammalian target of rapamycin complex 1 (mTORC1) activation. mTOR activation plays an important role in obesity-induced insulin resistance as well as HCC in human and mice [26]. One of the negative regulators of PI3K/Akt/mTOR pathway and insulin signaling pathway is PTEN 10 (phosphatase and tension homologue deleted on chromosome 10). Mice with liver specific PTEN knockout showed NAFLD and insulin hypersensitivity [27]. Further investigation has indicated that PTEN is a crucial mediator of lipogenesis, glucose metabolism, and tumorigenesis in the liver, suggesting PTEN is implicated in the regulation of obesity, metabolic disorders and HCC. 66% of hepatocyte-specific PTEN knockout mice could develop to spontaneous HCC at 74–78 weeks of age [28].

5.4.3 Mitochondrial Dysfunction

Mitochondria, which can generate ATP, play an important role in metabolic process, including oxidative phosphorylation and β-oxidation. Mitochondrial dysfunction is defined as the decreased oxidative phosphorylation, and the reduced mitochondrial oxidation of substrates [29]. In obesity, nutrient excess lead to mitochondrial dysfunction, thereby contribute to the deregulated lipid and glucose metabolism [30]. Moreover, mitochondrial dysfunction has been implicated in insulin resistance, although confounding results generated for the relationship of mitochondria dysfunction and insulin resistance [31]. Overall, mitochondrial dysfunction pathways contribute to the cancer progression through inhibiting apoptosis, ROS production, impaired mitochondrial oxidative phosphorylation and the dysregulation of cancer cell metabolism [32].

5.4.4 Genetic Alteration

Genomic studies of HCC have revealed that gene mutations are frequently present in different chromatin regulators in HCC [33]. Using whole exome sequencing of mice liver tissues from genetic and dietary obese mice and wildtype lean mice, our group has identified that Carboxyl ester lipase (*Cel*) and *4933432B09Rik* are recurrently and specifically mutated in NAFLD-associated HCC [34]. *Cel* is a gene related with lipid metabolism and helps other lipolytic enzymes to lipid nutrients diegestion. *Cel* downregulation could promote HCC cell proliferation through increasing cholesterol level. Besides of *Cel,* the mutation of *Hras*, which is a gene related with Gtase, also plays a crucial role in NAFLD-HCC development. O-GlcNAc transferase (OGT), which is a unique glycosyltransferase involved in metabolic reprogramming, has an oncogeneic role in NAFLD-associated HCC by mediating palmitic acid, endoplasmic reticulum (ER) stress, thereby activating JNK and NF-kB pathway [35]. Histone deacetylase HDAC8, which can be upregulated by the lipogenic factor SREBP-1, can promote insulin resistance and NAFLD-HCC development [36]. Together, these studies indicate that genetic changes are involved in the link between NAFLD-HCC and metabolic disorder.

5.5 Prevention for NAFLD-HCC in View of Obesity and Metabolic Disorder

Drugs to combat obesity and insulin resistance could act as strategies against NAFLD and the prevention of NAFLD-HCC. Lifestyle intervention, insulin sensitizers, anti-inflammatory agents, anti-fibrosis and chemopreventive agents are approaches for NAFLD-HCC prevention.

5.5.1 Weight Loss and Physical Activity

HCC is a disease tightly linked to lifestyle. Lifestyle changes induced weight loss is related with the improvement in NASH histology with highest rate of NASH resolution in patients with body weight losses more than 10% [37]. Fibrosis can also be reversed in patients with more than 10% weight loss. Even without weight loss, exercise could improve liver histology and metabolic disorder. In a study included 139,056 Korean adults, prolonged sitting time and less physical activity were shown to be positively related with the prevalence of NAFLD [38].

Currently, lifestyle intervention is still the gold standard for reversal of NASH and improving fibrosis.

Insulin resistance could also be ameliorated by lifestyle interventions as shown by reduced changes in plasma insulin and insulin-like growth factor-I by physical activity [39]. A parallel group, superiority, randomized controlled trial in Hong Kong showed that a dietitian-led lifestyle modification is effective in remission of NAFLD [40]. Study in rats has showed that physical activity could decrease cancer incidence and cancer multiplicity, strengthening the role of physical activity in cancer inhibition [39]. A randomized single-blind trial showed that weight loss was related with reduced inflammatory markers including IL-6 and C-reactive protein (CRP) as well as insulin resistance [41]. Although weight loss and physical activity could help to prevent NAFLD development, only a few patients can reach and maintain the necessary intervention targets [42].

5.5.2 Insulin Sensitisers

As the incidence of NAFLD-HCC is closely associated with insulin resistance, anti-diabetic drugs may help to reduce the risk of cancer [43]. A widely used anti-diabetic drug, metformin, was reported to reduce cancer risk in patients with type 2 diabetes. Diabetic patients treated with metformin showed significantly reduced cancer incidence compared with patients with other treatments [44].

A randomized, double-blind, placebo-controlled trial showed that long-term pioglitazone with diets improves NAS and reveres NASH pathology in 58% patients with NASH [45]. However, a study involved 19,349 diabetic patients and 77,396 control subjects in Taiwan indicated that metformin or thiazolidinediones (PPAR-r agonists) treatment reduced HCC risks with greater reduction in those taking metformin than those taking thiazolidinediones (51% *v.s.* 44%) [43]. Another study showed that metformin treatment in patients with diabetics decreased the risk of HCC incidence to almost non-diabetic levels in men [46].

Besides, Fibroblast growth factor 21 (FGF21) agonists, which are anti-obesity and anti-diabetic molecules that improve insulin sensitivity, are novel approaches for NAFLD treatment [47]. The dual peroxisome proliferator-activated receptor alpha/delta (PPAR-α/δ) agonist, GFT505, has been demonstrated liver-protective effects on steatosis, inflammation, and fibrosis in mouse models and is a promising liver-targeted drug for treatment of NAFLD [48]. Another PPAR-α/δ agonists Elafibranor, which has been indicated to improve insulin sensitivity, lipid accumulation and inflammation, has entered phase 3 clinical trial for NASH treatment. Although the predefined end point was not met in the intention to treat NASH patients, elafibranor treatment for 1 year resolved NASH without fibrosis worsening [49]. Interestingly, coffee intake, which has inverse relationship with type 2 diabetes, is inversely associated with advanced fibrosis among NAFLD patients with lower insulin resistance [50].

5.6 Conclusion

NAFLD-HCC is always accompanied with obesity and metabolic disorders, which are emerging as a major problem of public health. Inflammation, immune response, PI3K/AKT/mTOR/PTEN pathway, mitochondrial dysfunction and genetic alterations are all involved in the progression of NAFLD-HCC initiated by obesity and metabolic disorders. Lifestyle intervention and insulin sensitisers provide prevention options for NAFLD-HCC. Further studies needed to get more comprehensive mechanism and prevention strategies for NAFLD-HCC.

References

1. Han TS, Lean ME. A clinical perspective of obesity, metabolic syndrome and cardiovascular disease. JRSM Cardiovasc Dis. 2016;5:2048004016633371.
2. Alberti KG, Zimmet P, Shaw J. Metabolic syndrome--a new world-wide definition. A consensus statement from the international diabetes federation. Diabet Med. 2006;23:469–80.

3. Wahba IM, Mak RH. Obesity and obesity-initiated metabolic syndrome: mechanistic links to chronic kidney disease. Clin J Am Soc Nephrol. 2007;2:550–62.
4. Wildman RP. Healthy obesity. Curr Opin Clin Nutr Metab Care. 2009;12:438–43.
5. Lee SC, Hairi NN, Moy FM. Metabolic syndrome among non-obese adults in the teaching profession in Melaka, Malaysia. J Epidemiol. 2017;27:130–4.
6. Wong VW, Chan WK, Chitturi S, Chawla Y, Dan YY, Duseja A, et al. The Asia-Pacific working party on nonalcoholic fatty liver disease guidelines 2017 Part 1: definition, risk factors and assessment. J Gastroenterol Hepatol. 2017;
7. Yki-Jarvinen H. Non-alcoholic fatty liver disease as a cause and a consequence of metabolic syndrome. Lancet Diabetes Endocrinol. 2014;2:901–10.
8. Leake INAFLD. Severity of NAFLD in patients who are not obese. Nat Rev Gastroenterol Hepatol. 2016;13:436.
9. Leung JC, Loong TC, Wei JL, Wong GL, Chan AW, Choi PC, et al. Histological severity and clinical outcomes of nonalcoholic fatty liver disease in nonobese patients. Hepatology. 2017;65:54–64.
10. Unalp-Arida A, Ruhl CE. Liver fibrosis scores predict liver disease mortality in the United States population. Hepatology. 2017;66:84–95.
11. Byrne CD, Targher G. NAFLD: a multisystem disease. J Hepatol. 2015;62:S47–64.
12. Larsson SC, Wolk A. Overweight, obesity and risk of liver cancer: a meta-analysis of cohort studies. Br J Cancer. 2007;97:1005–8.
13. Pais R, Fartoux L, Goumard C, Scatton O, Wendum D, Rosmorduc O, et al. Temporal trends, clinical patterns and outcomes of NAFLD-related HCC in patients undergoing liver resection over a 20-year period. Aliment Pharmacol Ther. 2017;46:856.
14. Piscaglia F, Svegliati-Baroni G, Barchetti A, Pecorelli A, Marinelli S, Tiribelli C, et al. Clinical patterns of hepatocellular carcinoma in nonalcoholic fatty liver disease: a multicenter prospective study. Hepatology. 2016;63:827–38.
15. Yu MW, Lin CL, Liu CJ, Yang SH, Tseng YL, Wu CF. Influence of metabolic risk factors on risk of hepatocellular carcinoma and liver-related death in men with chronic hepatitis B: a large cohort study. Gastroenterology. 2017;153:1006.
16. Hagstrom H, Tynelius P, Rasmussen F. High BMI in late adolescence predicts future severe liver disease and hepatocellular carcinoma: a national, population-based cohort study in 1.2 million men. In: Gut; 2017.
17. Gupta A, Das A, Majumder K, Arora N, Mayo HG, Singh PP, et al. Obesity is independently associated with increased risk of hepatocellular cancer-related mortality: a systematic review and meta-analysis. Am J Clin Oncol. 2017;
18. Labenz C, Prenosil V, Koch S, Huber Y, Marquardt JU, Schattenberg JM, et al. Impact of individual components of the metabolic syndrome on the outcome of patients with advanced hepatocellular carcinoma treated with Sorafenib. Dig Dis. 2017;
19. Mohamad B, Shah V, Onyshchenko M, Elshamy M, Aucejo F, Lopez R, et al. Characterization of hepatocellular carcinoma (HCC) in non-alcoholic fatty liver disease (NAFLD) patients without cirrhosis. Hepatol Int. 2016;10:632–9.
20. Xu H, Barnes GT, Yang Q, Tan G, Yang D, Chou CJ, et al. Chronic inflammation in fat plays a crucial role in the development of obesity-related insulin resistance. J Clin Invest. 2003;112:1821–30.
21. Park EJ, Lee JH, Yu GY, He G, Ali SR, Holzer RG, et al. Dietary and genetic obesity promote liver inflammation and tumorigenesis by enhancing IL-6 and TNF expression. Cell. 2010;140:197–208.
22. Gomes AL, Teijeiro A, Buren S, Tummala KS, Yilmaz M, Waisman A, et al. Metabolic inflammation-associated IL-17A causes non-alcoholic steatohepatitis and hepatocellular carcinoma. Cancer Cell. 2016;30:161–75.
23. Ma C, Kesarwala AH, Eggert T, Medina-Echeverz J, Kleiner DE, Jin P, et al. NAFLD causes selective CD4(+) T lymphocyte loss and promotes hepatocarcinogenesis. Nature. 2016;531:253–7.
24. Kudo Y, Tanaka Y, Tateishi K, Yamamoto K, Yamamoto S, Mohri D, et al. Altered composition of fatty acids exacerbates hepatotumorigenesis during activation of the phosphatidylinositol 3-kinase pathway. J Hepatol. 2011;55:1400–8.
25. Leavens KF, Easton RM, Shulman GI, Previs SF, Birnbaum MJ. Akt2 is required for hepatic lipid accumulation in models of insulin resistance. Cell Metab. 2009;10:405–18.
26. Shaw RJ, Cantley LC. Ras, PI(3)K and mTOR signalling controls tumour cell growth. Nature. 2006;441:424–30.
27. Stiles B, Wang Y, Stahl A, Bassilian S, Lee WP, Kim YJ, et al. Liver-specific deletion of negative regulator Pten results in fatty liver and insulin hypersensitivity [corrected]. Proc Natl Acad Sci U S A. 2004;101:2082–7.
28. Horie Y, Suzuki A, Kataoka E, Sasaki T, Hamada K, Sasaki J, et al. Hepatocyte-specific Pten deficiency results in steatohepatitis and hepatocellular carcinomas. J Clin Invest. 2004;113:1774–83.
29. Montgomery MK, Turner N. Mitochondrial dysfunction and insulin resistance: an update. Endocr Connect. 2015;4:R1–R15.
30. Bournat JC, Brown CW. Mitochondrial dysfunction in obesity. Curr Opin Endocrinol Diabetes Obes. 2010;17:446–52.
31. Kim JA, Wei Y, Sowers JR. Role of mitochondrial dysfunction in insulin resistance. Circ Res. 2008;102:401–14.
32. Ribas V, Garcia-Ruiz C, Fernandez-Checa JC. Mitochondria, cholesterol and cancer cell metabolism. Clin Transl Med. 2016;5:22.
33. Totoki Y, Tatsuno K, Covington KR, Ueda H, Creighton CJ, Kato M, et al. Trans-ancestry mutational landscape of hepatocellular carcinoma genomes. Nat Genet. 2014;46:1267–73.

34. Shen J, Tsoi H, Liang Q, Chu ES, Liu D, Yu AC, et al. Oncogenic mutations and dysregulated pathways in obesity-associated hepatocellular carcinoma. Oncogene. 2016;35:6271–80.
35. Xu W, Zhang X, Wu JL, Fu L, Liu K, Liu D, et al. O-GlcNAc transferase promotes fatty liver-associated liver cancer through inducing palmitic acid and activating endoplasmic reticulum stress. J Hepatol. 2017;67:310–20.
36. Tian Y, Wong VW, Wong GL, Yang W, Sun H, Shen J, et al. Histone deacetylase HDAC8 promotes insulin resistance and beta-catenin activation in NAFLD-associated hepatocellular carcinoma. Cancer Res. 2015;75:4803–16.
37. Vilar-Gomez E, Martinez-Perez Y, Calzadilla-Bertot L, Torres-Gonzalez A, Gra-Oramas B, Gonzalez-Fabian L, et al. Weight loss through lifestyle modification significantly reduces features of nonalcoholic steatohepatitis. Gastroenterology 2015;149:367–78 e365; quiz e314–365.
38. Ryu S, Chang Y, Jung HS, Yun KE, Kwon MJ, Choi Y, et al. Relationship of sitting time and physical activity with non-alcoholic fatty liver disease. J Hepatol. 2015;63:1229–37.
39. Zhu Z, Jiang W, Sells JL, Neil ES, McGinley JN, Thompson HJ. Effect of nonmotorized wheel running on mammary carcinogenesis: circulating biomarkers, cellular processes, and molecular mechanisms in rats. Cancer Epidemiol Biomark Prev. 2008;17:1920–9.
40. Wong VW, Chan RS, Wong GL, Cheung BH, Chu WC, Yeung DK, et al. Community-based lifestyle modification programme for non-alcoholic fatty liver disease: a randomized controlled trial. J Hepatol. 2013;59:536–42.
41. Esposito K, Pontillo A, Di Palo C, Giugliano G, Masella M, Marfella R, et al. Effect of weight loss and lifestyle changes on vascular inflammatory markers in obese women: a randomized trial. JAMA. 2003;289:1799–804.
42. Hannah WN, Jr., Harrison SA. Lifestyle and dietary interventions in the management of nonalcoholic fatty liver disease. Dig Dis Sci 2016;61:1365–1374.
43. Lai SW, Chen PC, Liao KF, Muo CH, Lin CC, Sung FC. Risk of hepatocellular carcinoma in diabetic patients and risk reduction associated with anti-diabetic therapy: a population-based cohort study. Am J Gastroenterol. 2012;107:46–52.
44. Decensi A, Puntoni M, Goodwin P, Cazzaniga M, Gennari A, Bonanni B, et al. Metformin and cancer risk in diabetic patients: a systematic review and meta-analysis. Cancer Prev Res (Phila). 2010;3:1451–61.
45. Cusi K, Orsak B, Bril F, Lomonaco R, Hecht J, Ortiz-Lopez C, et al. Long-term pioglitazone treatment for patients with nonalcoholic steatohepatitis and prediabetes or type 2 diabetes mellitus: a randomized trial. Ann Intern Med. 2016;165:305–15.
46. Lee MS, Hsu CC, Wahlqvist ML, Tsai HN, Chang YH, Huang YC. Type 2 diabetes increases and metformin reduces total, colorectal, liver and pancreatic cancer incidences in Taiwanese: a representative population prospective cohort study of 800,000 individuals. BMC Cancer. 2011;11:20.
47. Sonoda J, Chen MZ, Baruch A. FGF21-receptor agonists: an emerging therapeutic class for obesity-related diseases. Horm Mol Biol Clin Investig. 2017;30
48. Staels B, Rubenstrunk A, Noel B, Rigou G, Delataille P, Millatt LJ, et al. Hepatoprotective effects of the dual peroxisome proliferator-activated receptor alpha/delta agonist, GFT505, in rodent models of nonalcoholic fatty liver disease/nonalcoholic steatohepatitis. Hepatology. 2013;58:1941–52.
49. Ratziu V, Harrison SA, Francque S, Bedossa P, Lehert P, Serfaty L, et al. Elafibranor, an agonist of the peroxisome proliferator-activated receptor-alpha and -delta, induces resolution of nonalcoholic steatohepatitis without fibrosis worsening. Gastroenterology. 2016;150:1147–59. e1145
50. Bambha K, Wilson LA, Unalp A, Loomba R, Neuschwander-Tetri BA, Brunt EM, et al. Coffee consumption in NAFLD patients with lower insulin resistance is associated with lower risk of severe fibrosis. Liver Int. 2014;34:1250–8.

6 Hepatocellular Carcinoma in Obesity: Finding a Needle in the Haystack?

György Baffy

Abstract

Obesity has been implicated in the development of hepatocellular carcinoma (HCC), one of the most common malignancies worldwide with an increasing incidence in the United States. Obesity and associated metabolic disorders such as type II diabetes and the metabolic syndrome are key factors in the development of nonalcoholic fatty liver disease (NAFLD) and promote several molecular mechanisms that may contribute to hepatocarcinogenesis. The vast majority of HCC occur in cirrhotic livers, but a subgroup of patients may develop HCC in non-advanced NAFLD. While the incidence rate for noncirrhotic HCC is low, the population-attributable fraction is still significant due to the extraordinary prevalence of obesity-associated liver disease. This is a challenge since HCC surveillance cannot be provided to the large population of non-advanced NAFLD in a cost-efficient way and requires enhanced risk stratification strategies. Recent advances may offer new clinical, laboratory, and genetic biomarkers and help us meet this important public health need.

G. Baffy (✉)
Department of Medicine, VA Boston Healthcare System and Brigham and Women's Hospital, Harvard Medical School, Boston, MA, USA
e-mail: gbaffy@bwh.harvard.edu

Keywords

Nonalcoholic fatty liver disease · Hepatocarcinogenesis · Oncogenic pathways · Noncirrhotic hepatocellular carcinoma · Biomarkers · Population-attributable fraction

6.1 Introduction

Obesity is recognized as a global epidemic and it has become particularly prevalent in developed countries such as the United States where every third adult and every sixth child is affected [1]. Obesity is a complex disease with a multitude of genetic and environmental factors implicated in highly variable outcomes. The pathophysiological changes associated with increased morbidity and mortality in obesity primarily manifest through the development of cardiovascular disease and type II diabetes, while the liver is almost invariably affected in the form of nonalcoholic fatty liver disease (NAFLD). The spectrum of NAFLD ranges from liver fat accumulation (steatosis) to nonalcoholic steatohepatitis (NASH) featuring a combination of hepatocellular injury, inflammation and fibrosis with a predisposition to progress into end-stage liver disease [2].

Obesity has been implicated in the initiation and progression of several malignancies, including cancer of the breast, endometrium, esophagus, colon, pancreas, kidney and gallbladder [3,

J. Yu (ed.), *Obesity, Fatty Liver and Liver Cancer*, Advances in Experimental Medicine and Biology 1061, https://doi.org/10.1007/978-981-10-8684-7_6

4]. This association is exceptionally strong with primary liver malignancies, mainly in the form of hepatocellular carcinoma (HCC) [5]. This is perhaps not surprising, since cirrhosis multiplies the risk of hepatocarcinogenesis regardless of the original cause of liver disease and advanced NAFLD is no exception. It is quite worrisome, however, that HCC may develop in obesity without frank NAFLD cirrhosis. In fact, among all etiologies linked to chronic liver disease, NAFLD has been associated with the highest rates of noncirrhotic HCC [6, 7]. While a relatively rare event, the specter of noncirrhotic HCC in obesity raises several fundamental questions. What are the major oncogene drivers in NAFLD-associated HCC? Does obesity shift the risk toward developing pre-cirrhotic HCC in viral and alcoholic liver disease? What are the best predictors of HCC in non-advanced NAFLD? Can we define a cost-efficient strategy of risk stratification for pre-cirrhotic HCC in the obese population? In seeking answers to these questions, three M's of obesity-associated HCC are reviewed here: magnitude (disease burden), mechanisms (i.e., oncogene drivers), and markers (risk predictors and early features). Better understanding of these aspects will hopefully improve current strategies of risk stratification and surveillance for HCC in NAFLD.

6.2 Magnitude: The Burden of HCC in Obesity

6.2.1 Obesity and the Risk of HCC

Hepatocellular carcinoma has emerged as the fifth and ninth most common malignancy and the second and sixth leading cause of cancer death worldwide in men and women, respectively [8]. Moreover, HCC is one of a few major malignancies that are becoming increasingly common in the US. Between 1975 and 2000, the age-adjusted incidence of HCC has risen from 1.6 to 4.9 per 100,000 Americans [9]. These values have somewhat slowed with an incidence reaching around 6.7 per 100,000 in 2012 while it shows substantial geographic differences and continues to increase in subgroups such as men aged 55–64 years old and among Caucasians [10]. According to the American Cancer Society, an estimated 42,220 new US cases of primary liver cancer will be diagnosed in 2018, the vast majority being HCC [11]. While chronic hepatitis C remains the dominant cause of HCC among Americans, the spread of obesity has been increasingly implicated in this alarming trend [12]. In fact, it has been predicted that liver disease linked to obesity, diabetes and the metabolic syndrome may soon surpass HCV infection as the primary etiology of HCC in the US and several other industrialized societies [13].

There is substantial literature on the contribution of obesity to the development of HCC from virtually all corners of the world [14]. In a prospective cohort of 18,403 London-based government employees, obesity was associated with a 3.76-fold relative risk for HCC [15]. The Cancer Prevention Study II drawing conclusions from a cohort of 900,000 adult Americans found that the risk of dying from liver cancer was 4.5-fold higher among men with a body mass index (BMI) over 35 kg/m^2 relative to their lean counterparts [16]. According to a meta-analysis of these 2 and 9 additional cohort studies, overweight and obesity increased the risk of liver cancer by 17% and 89%, respectively, when compared to individuals with normal weight [17]. Similar positive association was found between HCC and the metabolic syndrome. A recent meta-analysis of 6 cohort studies found that men having various components of the metabolic syndrome had a relative risk of 1.43 for developing HCC and the risk was comparable among women [18]. An Italian case-control study of 185 HCC cases reported an odds ratio of 1.92 for the metabolic syndrome [19]. Moreover, metabolic syndrome was associated with a twofold risk of HCC in the general US population based on the US Surveillance, Epidemiology and End Results (SEER)-Medicare database reviewed between 1993 and 2005 [20]. When metabolic components were analyzed separately, obesity remained an independent risk factor of HCC [20]. There is also strong association between type II diabetes and the development of HCC. A large prospective cohort study conducted over a 10-year follow-up period in which the risk of HCC was twofold in diabetic vs. non-diabetic US veterans [21]. Subsequent meta-analyses reported pooled odds ratios around 2.5 for the risk of HCC in diabetes without concomitant viral hepatitis or alcoholic liver disease [22, 23]. As expected by the staggering prevalence of obesity, diabetes and the metabolic syndrome, repeated analyses of the SEER-Medicare database confirmed that the population-attributable fraction of metabolic causes for HCC is the highest (32–37%) of all etiologies [24, 25].

6.2.2 Emergence of HCC in NAFLD

When the role of obesity is explored in the development of HCC, it must be noted that some degree of NAFLD, often in the more advanced form of steatohepatitis, is present in the majority of these conditions (Fig. 6.1). Thus, several studies confirmed the presence of biopsy-proven NASH in 16%–43% of obese patients [26–29]. The strong link between obesity and NAFLD is corroborated by a recent meta-analysis encompassing 86 studies and more than 8.5 million cases worldwide to determine long-term outcomes of NAFLD, where obesity affected 51% of individuals with all forms of NAFLD included and it was present in 82% of patients with biopsy-proven NASH [30]. Thus, the liver is almost always affected by NAFLD and obesity-associated HCC is very likely to develop in diseased liver even when cirrhosis is not established.

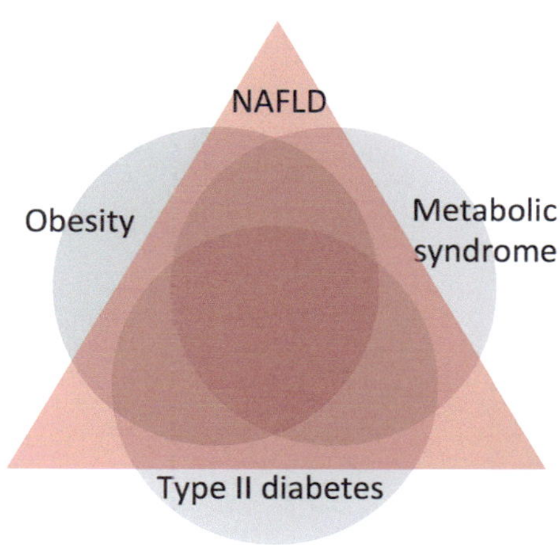

Fig. 6.1 Metabolic disorders and NAFLD. NAFLD mainly occurs at the intersection of obesity, diabetes, and the metabolic syndrome. Multiple overlaps of these disorders are associated with increasing NAFLD severity and their identification and assessment may assist risk stratification for the development of HCC

Based on a recent survey of the SEER registry, the incidence of NAFLD-associated HCC has grown by 9% each year between 2004 and 2009 [31]. NAFLD was linked to 59% of all HCC cases without other apparent etiology identified in a large US health care claims database [32]. Moreover, NAFLD was the single most common cause accounting for 34.8% of all patients diagnosed with HCC in a recent study from Northeastern England, indicating a whopping tenfold increase in this association over a 10-year period [33]. According to a review of the frequency and proportion with which HCC patients have been receiving liver transplant in the US, combined share of HCC associated with NAFLD and cryptogenic cirrhosis (in most cases presumably representing end-stage NAFLD) among recipients has increased fourfold between 2002 and 2012 [34].

Reports from many geographical areas indicate that HCC relatively often develops in noncirrhotic NAFLD [6, 35]. Review of the medical records from 1994 to 2013 at a university hospital in Germany included 714 patients diagnosed with HCC of which 14% occurred in noncirrhotic livers [36]. In a nation-wide cohort of 1500 Americans diagnosed with HCC between 2005 and 2010, detailed chart review found no evidence of cirrhosis in 32.7% of all cases [37]. A Japanese cross-sectional study found that 28% of patients had low-grade fibrosis (less than or equal to F2) at the time of HCC diagnosis [38]. Analysis of the US health care claims database cited above found that 4406 cases of HCC were associated with NAFLD but only 46% carried the ICD code of cirrhosis, while cirrhosis was diagnosed in 78% of all cases with HCV-associated HCC [32].

Incidence estimates of HCC developing in NAFLD greatly differ according to cohort selection and disease severity. In a US single center study of 195 patients referred to liver transplant with NAFLD cirrhosis, the annual cumulative incidence of HCC was 2.6% compared to 4.0% among those with HCV-related cirrhosis in the same analysis [39]. Lower incidence rates of HCC complicating NAFLD cirrhosis have been reported in other studies [40, 41]. The risk of HCC is substantially lower if cirrhosis is not a prerequisite to patient selection. An international study of 247 patients diagnosed with NAFLD and advanced fibrosis (stage F3 or F4) reported a yearly cumulative incidence of 0.34% for HCC (6 cases over an average follow-up of 7.1 years) [42]. A large retrospective study from Japan, analyzing data from 6508 patients with NAFLD diagnosed by ultrasonography and followed for a median period of 5.6 years, found that the annual rate of new HCC was only 0.043% in that cohort [43]. A similar incidence rate of HCC (0.063%) was reported in another retrospective study from Japan that followed 1600 patients aged 60 years or older for 10 years with ultrasonographic evidence of NAFLD [44]. These data have been corroborated by a global meta-analysis that calculated an annual incidence of 0.44 per 1000 person-years (95% CI: 0.29–0.66) for developing HCC among all-comers diagnosed with NAFLD while this figure was 5.29 per 1000 person-years (95% CI: 0.75–37.56) in biopsy-proven NASH [30]. Thus, a diminished yet considerable risk remains present in non-advanced stages of NAFLD (Fig. 6.2).

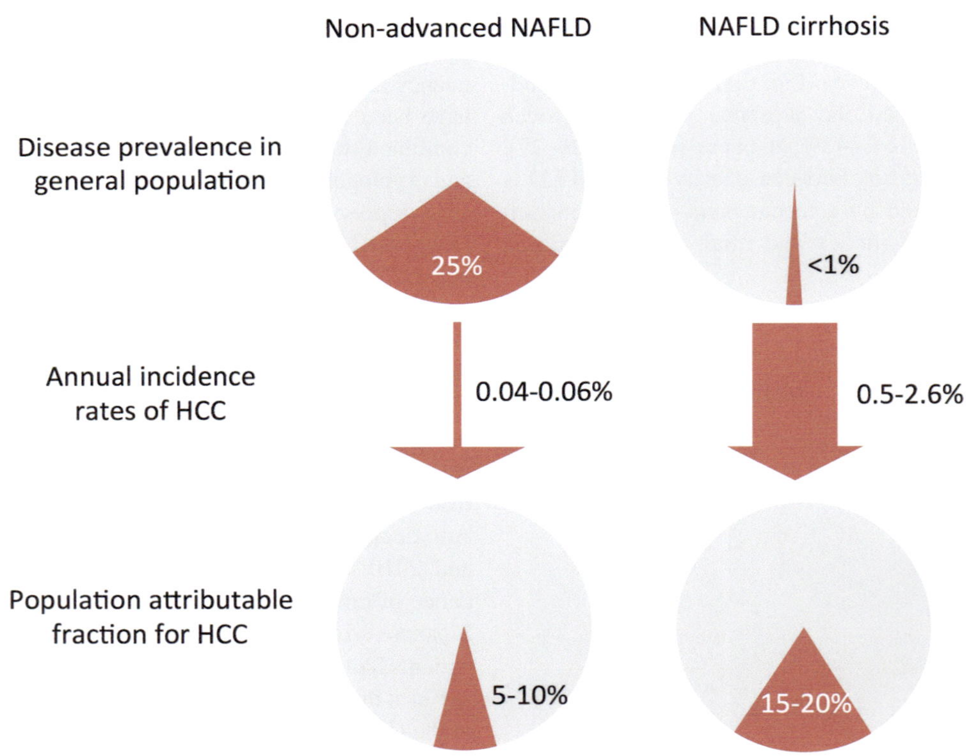

Fig. 6.2 **NAFLD and the burden of HCC** Large-scale follow-up studies indicate highly variable risk of HCC depending on the severity of NAFLD, which correlates with the degree of liver fibrosis. Advanced NAFLD (F3 stage fibrosis or established cirrhosis) is relatively rare with high annual HCC incidence rates and a population-attributable fraction of 15–20%. By contrast, non-advanced NAFLD is extraordinarily prevalent with very low HCC incidence rates and a non-negligible population-attributable fraction of 5–10%, indicating the need for improved risk stratification and cost-efficient surveillance strategies

6.2.3 NAFLD-Associated HCC and Liver Comorbidities

Due to their extraordinarily high prevalence, obesity and NAFLD frequently overlap with chronic liver disease of other etiologies and may boost the risk of HCC in these individuals. Concomitant presence of alcoholic and nonalcoholic liver disease is particularly problematic as excess alcohol consumption is often seen in geographical areas where obesity is prevalent [45, 46]. In a large prospective study from the UK, 48.4% of HCC patients without known chronic liver disease and 51.4% of patient with alcoholic cirrhosis had at least one major (diabetes or obesity) or two minor (hypertension or dyslipidemia) metabolic risk factors [47]. Studies indicate that people in general are less concerned about drinking when diagnosed with NAFLD compared to chronic hepatitis C. This notion was supported by a multicenter Italian study in which the prevalence of social drinkers (not exceeding 30 g alcohol/day) was substantially higher among NAFLD patients than among HCV patients (45.5% versus 8.6%) [48].

Multiple studies confirm the synergistic effects of obesity and alcohol on the severity of liver disease and the risk of HCC. While there is some evidence that some aspects of NAFLD benefit from moderate alcohol consumption [49], the risk of NAFLD-associated HCC was reported to be 3.6-fold higher among Americans who drink small amounts of alcohol compared to teetotalers [39]. Moreover, a retrospective analysis of ~20,000 liver explants in the US found that obesity was an independent predictor of HCC in patients with alcoholic cirrhosis [50]. In A French cohort of 110 patients undergoing liver transplantation for alcoholic cirrhosis, a sixfold higher risk of HCC was linked to a history of overweight or obesity, with an odds ratio further increasing to 9.1 if there also was a history of diabetes [51]. In another French cohort of 771 patients with HCV and alcoholic cirrhosis, simultaneous presence of obesity and diabetes increased the risk of HCC to sixfold [52]. A Swedish study of 616 HCC patients found that the metabolic syndrome was significantly more prevalent among patients with alcoholic liver disease (34%) compared to those with alcoholic liver disease and concomitant HCV infection (10%) or HCV infection alone (13%) [53].

Obesity may also increase the risk of HCC in chronic HBV and HCV infection. A Taiwanese study following 23,820 subjects for 14 years found a total of 291 HCC cases and reported that obesity and central obesity increased the risk of HCC by twofold and fourfold among HCV-seropositive subjects, respectively [54]. A recent analysis of 270 HBV-infected patients from Hong Kong found that fatty liver (present in 39.6% of the cohort) was associated with cirrhosis and independently predicted HCC development with a hazard ratio of 7.27 [55]. Plasma levels of visfatin, an adipokine reflecting the size of visceral fat depots, have been independently associated with an increased risk of HCC (odds ratio = 1.17) diagnosed in chronic HCV and HBV infection [56].

6.3 Mechanisms: Pathogenesis of Obesity-Associated HCC

6.3.1 Hepatocarcinogenesis in Cirrhosis

Cirrhosis represents a fertile soil for oncogenesis due to the repetitive cycles of liver cell death and renewal [57, 58]. The unique microenvironment of liver tissue remodeling may contribute to diverse malfunction among molecular signaling pathways regulating cell growth and proliferation, inflammation and redox balance in addition to altering the expression of oncogenes and tumor suppressors, interfering with epigenetic modifiers and causing mutations that result in genomic instability [59–61]. The panoply of these functional and structural defects in the cirrhotic liver results in highly heterogeneous tumor phenotypes, which explains HCC robustness, treatment resistance and poor overall prognosis [59–61]. Biochemical and genomic analysis has allowed the molecular classification of HCC into subgroups with different genetic signatures and clinical outcomes to correlate with multifocality, therapeutic response and early or late recurrence [62–64]. Emergence of HCC from the accumulation of pathologic changes usually takes several years through a dysplasia-carcinoma sequence seen in other malignancies and may offer a window of early detection [57, 58].

6.3.2 Oncogene Pathways in Noncirrhotic NAFLD

While obesity-associated oncogenesis likely acts in synergy with molecular mechanisms emanating from the destructive/regenerative cycles of cirrhosis, development of HCC in non-advanced NAFLD cannot be attributed to this unique microenvironment. Instead, the pathways promoting HCC in noncirrhotic NAFLD may have more in common with the pathogenesis of obesity-associated malignancies seen in other tissues [65–67]. The occurrence of HCC in a patient with seemingly innocuous steatosis is a relatively rare but highly alarming experience. To understand the oncogenesis that may affect NAFLD at any stage and to allow additional strategies for risk stratification, prevention and early detection, we must consider systemic and local mechanisms unleashed by obesity [14, 35, 65].

Liver-specific and systemic insulin resistance is an essential feature of obesity [3, 68]. Inflammation, oxidative injury, and direct lipotoxicity may impair insulin signaling and result in insulin resistance with compensatory increase in circulating insulin levels [68]. Importantly, insulin resistance is selective and *de novo* lipogenesis in the liver remains responsive to excessive doses of circulating insulin through the action of lipogenic regulators such as steroid response element binding protein (SREBP)-1c and carbohydrate-responsive element-binding protein (ChREBP)-β, liver X receptor α (LXRα), peroxisome proliferator-activated receptor γ (PPARγ), and adipocyte lipid-binding protein 2 (AP2) [69–72]. Sustained hyperinsulinemia also stimulates the production of insulin-like growth factor (IGF)-binding protein, leading to increased bioavailability of liver-derived insulin-like growth factor (IGF) 1 and 2 that may activate additional oncogenic pathways [73–75]. The role of increased insulin levels in hepatocarcinogenesis has been further implicated by studies in which the risk of HCC was several fold higher among diabetic patients taking insulin secretagogues rather than improving peripheral insulin sensitivity [76].

Lipotoxicity is a complex mechanism that links obesity to hepatocarcinogenesis [65]. It has been pointed out that 'pure' or 'simple' steatosis is probably a misnomer as some degree of lobular or portal inflammation is present when hepatocytes store lipids of abnormal sorts and amounts [77]. Indeed, overloading of hepatocytes with lipid molecules may generate sufficient pathology that adversely affects the liver in a number of ways [78]. Excessive lipid breakdown causes mitochondrial dysfunction and oxidative stress, toxic lipid derivatives impair the unfolded protein response in the endoplasmic reticulum, interfere with important homeostatic mechanisms of liver cells such as autophagy and apoptosis, alter the function of many transcription factors and cellular programs, and create a positive feedback loop by suppressing insulin signaling [79–81]. Oxidative damage of DNA and deregulation of gene transcription are major mechanisms by which lipotoxicity may directly contribute to HCC development in the steatotic liver [82–84].

Obesity is defined as excess accumulation of fat due to chronically increased nutrient intake and diminished physical exercise [85]. In response to sustained nutrient excess, adipose tissue expands in order to store surplus energy in the form of lipids. This process involves an elaborate tissue remodeling with multiple cell-cell interactions and recruitment of preadipocytes, endothelial precursors, and macrophages, creating a microenvironment suitable for adipocyte differentiation, connective tissue growth, and angiogenesis [86, 87]. Obesity is accompanied by low-grade, chronic inflammation as a result of adipose tissue remodeling, which results in a profoundly altered pattern of adipokine secretion by adipocytes and recruited macrophages [88, 89]. The growing list of adipose-derived bioactive substances include leptin, adiponectin, resistin, interleukin (IL)-1beta, IL-6, tumor necrosis factor (TNF)-alpha, plasminogen activator inhibitor (PAI)-1, macrophage migration inhibitory factor (MIF), matrix metalloproteinases (e.g., MMP2 and MMP9), vascular endothelial growth factor (VEGF), hypoxia-inducible factor (HIF)-alpha, and various CXC and CC chemokines [87, 90]. In addition, engorged adipocytes serve as a major source of excess sex-steroid hormones (estrogens, progesterone, and androgens) [16].

Adipose tissue remodeling, altered patterns of adipokine secretion and release of pro-inflammatory mediators in obesity provide additional mechanisms of activating potentially oncogenic pathways in the liver [65]. Systemic, low-grade inflammation is maintained under these conditions with increased circulating levels of leptin, a key adipokine with pro-inflammatory and pro-fibrogenic effects facilitating development of HCC [91, 92]. Diminished availability of adiponectin, another adipokine opposing leptin effects through its anti-inflammatory, antiangiogenic and tumor growth-limiting properties, also contributes to activation of oncogenic pathways [93, 94]. Several additional adipokines have been implicated in sustaining a pro-oncogenic environment in the liver tissue and may foster the development of HCC in obesity [95].

There is rapidly growing evidence that obesity affects the composition of the gut microbiota and these changes are related to the pathobiology of NAFLD [96, 97]. Altered gut microbiota may impair the epithelial barrier and cause translocation of intestinal bacteria into the portal circulation, leading to the activation of inflammatory and oncogenic pathways in the liver [98, 99]. A prospective, cross-sectional study comparing gut microbiota profiles of biopsy-proven NAFLD patients found lower percentage of *Bacteroidetes* in patients with NASH compared to steatosis and healthy controls [100]. Recognition of the Gram-negative bacterial cell wall component lipopolysaccharide (LPS) by Toll-like receptor 4 (TLR4) is a key mechanism of this process and has also been implicated in the activation of stellate cells, providing a direct link between the gut microbiota and liver fibrosis [101]. An intriguing link between obesity, gut microbiota, and hepatocarcinogenesis was illustrated by a recent paper in which the growth of chemically induced liver tumors was facilitated by high-fat diet and high serum levels of deoxycholic acid, a secondary bile acid produced by the increasingly dominant intestinal *Clostridia* under these experimental conditions [102]. These and other findings identify the gut microbiota as a key contributor to the risk of HCC in NAFLD. The role of bile acids in the pathogenesis of NAFLD has received increased attention since the recent introduction of obeticholic acid, a synthetic ligand of the farnesoid X receptor (FXR), which limits the conversion of cholesterol into bile acids and inhibits many pro-inflammatory pathways in the liver [103].

Widely applied to the research of complex diseases, an important approach to identify the drivers of HCC development in obesity is to analyze genotype-phenotype associations at various stages of NAFLD. Current advances in systems biology offer powerful methods to search for disease-associated genes that may have a key role in HCC initiation and progression [104]. A recent study used microarray analysis to differentiate mild and severe NAFLD based on a 64-gene profile expressed in human liver biopsy specimens [105]. Functional enrichment analysis indicated significant overlap among the gene expression patterns of severe NAFLD, cardiovascular disease and cancer. A parallel work compared transcriptomic and metabolomic information from human liver tissue representing NAFLD progression (normal, steatosis and steatohepatitis) with published data for HCC [106]. In this study, the majority of changes in gene expression and metabolites occur during the transition from steatosis to steatohepatitis. KEGG pathway analysis associated these changes with the regulation of p53 signaling, cell cycle and apoptosis, suggesting that the transition from steatosis to steatohepatitis is a critical step that may initiate the process of HCC carcinogenesis [106]. These findings suggest that risk stratification for HCC could be most comprehensive and successful if started at the earliest stages of NAFLD.

6.4 Markers: Risk Stratification for HCC in Obesity

6.4.1 Monitoring NAFLD Progression

Since cirrhosis represents by far the highest risk of developing HCC and NAFLD progression is strongly linked to liver fibrosis severity [107, 108], the first task of risk stratification is to detect advanced fibrosis or cirrhosis within the obese population. Unfortunately, cirrhosis often develops insidiously and only comes to attention when liver synthetic functions become impaired or portal hypertension is significant enough to cause complications. Nevertheless, this most vulnerable population can be identified with proper awareness of the clinical practitioner and by increased utilization of noninvasive fibrosis assessment methods. Use of biochemical and imaging-based biomarkers in NAFLD to diagnose advanced liver disease and guide management is the subject of several recent and excellent reviews [109–111].

The next step in HCC risk stratification may involve identification of NAFLD patients who are increasingly prone to develop advanced fibrosis. Histologic and noninvasive follow-up data indicate that fibrosis in NAFLD progresses at highly variable rates. In the global epidemiology review by Younossi et al., the average progression of liver fibrosis among patients with biopsy-proven NASH was 0.09 stage per year (95% CI: 0.06–0.12) [30]. In a Hong Kong study of 52 NAFLD patients followed with paired liver biopsies over 3 years, fibrosis progressed in 27%, remained the same in 48%, and regressed in 25% of the cohort [112]. Surprisingly, fibrosis progressed in 20–30% of all cases independent of the presence of NASH (i.e., it also progressed in steatosis) and in 10% did so by 2 or more fibrosis stages over the follow-up period [112]. These highly variable rates were corroborated in the broader context of a meta-analysis, which found that 36% of all NAFLD patients showed progression of fibrosis, 46% remained stable, and 21% improved [113]. The overall fibrosis progression rates in this study were calculated as 0.07 stage/year in steatosis and 0.14 stage/year in NASH, while a sub-group of patients (7.6% of the total cohort) was identified that may progress rapidly with a baseline fibrosis of F0 changing to ≥F3 over a mean of 5.9 years only and corresponding to a progression of 0.51–0.68 stage per year [113]. There is good evidence that manifest diabetes is strongly associated with higher rates of fibrosis progression in NAFLD [114, 115]. Thus, cohorts of both steatosis and NASH appear to have a sub-group of 'rapid fibrosis progressors', indicating that periodic assessment of liver fibrosis may provide important benefits and timely identification of those in need of HCC surveillance.

Finally, there are the majority of patients with obesity who do not have evidence of advanced NAFLD or rapid fibrosis progression as outlined above. The risk of HCC in this population is quite low and would not justify regular surveillance. However, lifestyle, clinical and laboratory parameters associated with higher risk of HCC may help the identification of subgroups that could benefit from enhanced monitoring in a cost-efficient way. Evidence on novel biomarkers that may assist risk stratification in early stages of NAFLD is summarized below.

6.4.2 Fluid-Based Biomarkers of HCC Development

By far the most studied biomarkers of HCC are serum levels of alpha-fetoprotein (AFP) and des-carboxyprothrombin (DCP). However, these markers have been considered in the detection, rather than risk prediction, of HCC [116–118]. Moreover, the sensitivity of these biomarkers is less than desirable and they do not predict the development of HCC in NAFLD [119, 120]. There is an intense search for novel biomarkers related to the development and progression of HCC. Many of these studies are aimed at further characterization of an already known liver tumor and intend to distinguish multicentric HCC from intrahepatic metastases or predict the risk of HCC recurrence after surgery or loco-regional therapy [106, 121–124]. However, novel biomarkers may reveal genetic predisposition and very early changes in the sequence of hepatocarcinogenesis to help risk stratification and guide surveillance strategies for select individuals among the vast population with non-advanced NAFLD.

Circulating microRNAs (miRNAs) are promising diagnostic markers to monitor NAFLD progression and the risk of HCC development [125]. MicroRNAs (miRNAs) regulate gene-environment interactions and may provide insights into the pathophysiology of complex diseases [126, 127]. Many miRNAs have been associated with the regulation of cell metabolism, redox balance, inflammation and pathways of cell growth and proliferation [128–131]. A number of miRNAs have been associated with the eventual transition of steatosis to NASH to cirrhosis and to HCC [132]. There is increasing evidence that miRNAs can be detected in various bodily fluids including serum and saliva [133, 134]. These circulating miRNAs are remarkably stable, which makes them versatile biomarkers in health and disease [133, 134]. One of the most studied miRNAs in NAFLD pathophysiology is miR-122, which is by far the most abundant miRNA in the liver. Amounts of circulating miR-122 increase in liver injury and may indicate fibrosis severity better than serum cytokeratin-18 or transaminase levels [135, 136]. Genes targeted by miR-122 regulate cholesterol and lipid metabolism, proteasomal protein degradation, cell adhesion and extracellular matrix components [137]. Moreover, miR-122 has tumor suppressor properties and mice deficient in miR-122 rapidly develop steatohepatitis, fibrosis and HCC mice results in rapidly develop steatohepatitis, fibrosis, and HCC [56]. Further studies will hopefully reveal the full predictive and diagnostic potential of miR-122 and many other potentially relevant miRNAs in HCC risk stratification.

An exciting novel direction to explore fluid-based HCC biomarkers is the analysis of saliva for the presence of biomarkers ('salivaomics'). A recent report applied high-throughout RNA sequencing to characterize salivary small non-coding RNAs and found up to 418 and 109 species of miRNA and piRNA, respectively, in cell-free saliva samples of healthy volunteers [138]. Piwi-interacting RNAs or piRNAs are involved, among other biological functions, in the maintenance of genome integrity of germline and stem cells [139]. In a recent work, analysis of liver tissue found an abundance of piRNAs with expression patterns that may differentiate cirrhotic from HCC tissues [140].

Finally, analysis of the urinary 'metabonome' may identify biomarkers for HCC as suggested by several studies in which this approach was able to distinguish patients with HCC associated with HCV-cirrhosis from those with HCV-cirrhosis and healthy controls [141]. Discriminatory metabolites included glycine, trimethylamine-N-oxide, hippurate, citrate, creatinine, creatine and carnitine. Whether similar urinary metabolite profiles have a role and at what disease stage in the risk stratification of NAFLD patients remains to be seen.

6.4.3 Genetic Markers of Predisposition

Several methods have recently become available to analyze genotype-phenotype associations in complex diseases such as obesity and related metabolic disorders [104]. Studies of genome-wide association (GWA) compare frequencies of DNA sequence variants such as single nucleotide polymorphism (SNP) linked to molecular and clinical phenotypes of various disease stages or outcomes [142]. DNA microarrays simultaneously assess the expression of many genes and correlate the data with clinical variables such as tumor progression, recurrence and response to chemotherapeutics [143]. Gene set enrichment analysis ranks genes by their expression relative to a reference microarray or published database to narrow the search for genes most likely to be associated with the disease [144]. These methods may elucidate novel details of the genetic predisposition to HCC developing in obesity.

One of the best characterized genetic variants associated with NAFLD is the rs738409 C>G polymorphism in the PNPLA3 gene leading to I148M substitution in a membrane protein (adiponutrin) implicated in hepatocellular lipid breakdown, lipid droplet remodeling and VLDL secretion [145]. Carriers of the I148M variant were found to have increased risk of cirrhosis and HCC, which was independent from their predisposition to liver fat accumulation [146]. More recently, the rs58542926 C>T polymorphism (E167K) in the transmembrane 6 superfamily 2 (TM6SF2) gene has been associated with the progression of NAFLD [147]. The protein product of this gene may regulate hepatocellular triglyceride and VLDL trafficking and the E167K variant appears to predispose to all components of NASH including advanced fibrosis. Additional SNPs and less frequently observed mutations that may facilitate molecular mechanisms of NAFLD progression and HCC development involve genes regulating hepatic energy metabolism, inflammation, fibrosis and iron homeostasis [148–150]. Futures studies will determine whether screening for these genetic variants can offer a meaningful way to identify patients at higher risk for developing HCC and assist their selection for cancer surveillance.

6.5 Conclusions

Despite substantial advances in our understanding of the pathobiology and management of HCC, it remains a cancer with one of the poorest survival figures. Detection of HCC in its earliest form may multiply the chance of cure or long-term survival. To succeed, we need to optimize our surveillance efforts, which is the best way to reduce mortality from this aggressive cancer. The annual risk of developing HCC in cirrhosis of any etiology ranges between 1% and 6% [151]. Based on cost-effectiveness analyses, surveillance should be offered to patients with cirrhosis of varying etiologies when the annual risk of HCC is 1.5% or greater [152, 153]. Several prospective cohort studies indicate that NAFLD cirrhosis meets these criteria [39–41], and regular HCC surveillance is now recommended by several liver society guidelines for patients with advanced NAFLD [154, 155].

However, timely recognition of HCC that complicates NAFLD remains a challenging goal. Surveillance cannot be initiated if advanced liver disease remains hidden. A recent SEER survey found that patients with NAFLD cirrhosis diagnosed with HCC had higher age, shorter survival time, and increased probability of dying from their primary liver cancer than those who developed HCC from other etiologies, indicating a delay in recognizing the need for surveillance [31]. This problem has been highlighted in a retrospective VA study in which 56.7% of US veterans with NAFLD-associated HCC lacked surveillance in the 3 years preceding the diagnosis of HCC, compared to their counterparts with alcohol-related (40.2%) or HCV-related HCC (13.3%) [156].

The matter is further complicated by the fact that there is no consensus on what surveillance strategy to follow in non-advanced NAFLD, since there are no established guidelines for the detection of noncirrhotic HCC. From a patient's perspective, the risk of HCC in these cases is rather small, since HCC may develop in one out of 2000–3000 cases of non-advanced NAFLD each year [43, 44]. From a public health perspective, however, 14%–54% of all NAFLD-related HCC cases reportedly develop in the absence of advanced fibrosis [32, 36, 37, 48], which is a substantial burden based on the population attributable fraction of NAFLD. Still, regular surveillance of non-advanced NAFLD with biannual liver ultrasonography as it is recommended in cirrhosis is simply not feasible at current incidence rates. Thus, unless the issue becomes more pressing due to worsening trends in the incidence of noncirrhotic HCC, we will continue to search for affordable, simple and safe pre-screening tests and improve our strategies of risk stratification for HCC in obesity, which appears to be more difficult than finding a needle in the haystack.

References

1. Ogden CL, Carroll MD, Kit BK, Flegal KM. Prevalence of childhood and adult obesity in the United States, 2011–2012. JAMA. 2014;311:806–14.
2. Calzadilla Bertot L, Adams LA. The natural course of non-alcoholic fatty liver disease. Int J Mol Sci. 2016;17

3. Calle EE, Kaaks R. Overweight, obesity and cancer: epidemiological evidence and proposed mechanisms. Nat Rev Cancer. 2004;4:579–91.
4. Basen-Engquist K, Chang M. Obesity and cancer risk: recent review and evidence. Curr Oncol Rep. 2011;13:71–6.
5. Vanni E, Bugianesi E. Obesity and liver cancer. Clin Liver Dis. 2014;18:191–203.
6. Baffy G, Brunt EM, Caldwell SH. Hepatocellular carcinoma in nonalcoholic fatty liver disease: an emerging menace. J Hepatol. 2012;56:1384–91.
7. Bellentani S. The epidemiology of non-alcoholic fatty liver disease. Liver Int. 2017;37(Suppl 1):81–4.
8. Torre LA, Bray F, Siegel RL, Ferlay J, Lortet-Tieulent J, Jemal A. Global cancer statistics, 2012. CA Cancer J Clin. 2015;65:87–108.
9. Altekruse SF, McGlynn KA, Reichman ME. Hepatocellular carcinoma incidence, mortality, and survival trends in the United States from 1975 to 2005. J Clin Oncol. 2009;27:1485–91.
10. White DL, Thrift AP, Kanwal F, Davila J, El-Serag HB. Incidence of hepatocellular carcinoma in all 50 United States, from 2000 through 2012. Gastroenterology. 2016
11. American Cancer Society. Cancer Statistics Center. 2018. https://cancerstatisticscenter.cancer.org/#!/cancer-site/Liver%20and%20intrahepatic%20bile%20duct. Accessed 27 Mar 2018.
12. El-Serag HB, Kanwal F. Epidemiology of hepatocellular carcinoma in the United States: where are we? Where do we go? Hepatology. 2014;60:1767–75.
13. Charlton M. Cirrhosis and liver failure in nonalcoholic fatty liver disease: molehill or mountain? Hepatology. 2008;47:1431–3.
14. Marengo A, Rosso C, Bugianesi E. Liver cancer: connections with obesity, fatty liver, and cirrhosis. Annu Rev Med. 2016;67:103–17.
15. Batty GD, Shipley MJ, Jarrett RJ, Breeze E, Marmot MG, Smith GD. Obesity and overweight in relation to organ-specific cancer mortality in London (UK): findings from the original Whitehall study. Int J Obes. 2005;29:1267–74.
16. Calle EE, Rodriguez C, Walker-Thurmond K, Thun MJ. Overweight, obesity, and mortality from cancer in a prospectively studied cohort of U.S. adults. N Engl J Med. 2003;348:1625–38.
17. Larsson SC, Wolk A. Overweight, obesity and risk of liver cancer: a meta-analysis of cohort studies. Br J Cancer. 2007;97:1005–8.
18. Esposito K, Chiodini P, Colao A, Lenzi A, Giugliano D. Metabolic syndrome and risk of cancer: a systematic review and meta-analysis. Diabetes Care. 2012;35:2402–11.
19. Turati F, Talamini R, Pelucchi C, Polesel J, Franceschi S, Crispo A, et al. Metabolic syndrome and hepatocellular carcinoma risk. Br J Cancer. 2013;108:222–08.
20. Welzel TM, Graubard BI, Zeuzem S, El-Serag HB, Davila JA, McGlynn KA. Metabolic syndrome increases the risk of primary liver cancer in the United States: a study in the SEER-Medicare database. Hepatology. 2011;54:463–71.
21. El-Serag HB, Tran T, Everhart JE. Diabetes increases the risk of chronic liver disease and hepatocellular carcinoma. Gastroenterology. 2004;126:460–8.
22. El-Serag HB, Hampel H, Javadi F. The association between diabetes and hepatocellular carcinoma: a systematic review of epidemiologic evidence. Clin Gastroenterol Hepatol. 2006;4:369–80.
23. Wang P, Kang D, Cao W, Wang Y, Liu Z. Diabetes mellitus and risk of hepatocellular carcinoma: a systematic review and meta-analysis. Diabetes Metab Res Rev. 2012;28:109–22.
24. Welzel TM, Graubard BI, Quraishi S, Zeuzem S, Davila JA, El-Serag HB, et al. Population-attributable fractions of risk factors for hepatocellular carcinoma in the United States. Am J Gastroenterol. 2013;108:1314–21.
25. Makarova-Rusher OV, Altekruse SF, McNeel TS, Ulahannan S, Duffy AG, Graubard BI, et al. Population attributable fractions of risk factors for hepatocellular carcinoma in the United States. Cancer. 2016;122:1757–65.
26. Gholam PM, Flancbaum L, Machan JT, Charney DA, Kotler DP. Nonalcoholic fatty liver disease in severely obese subjects. Am J Gastroenterol. 2007;102:399–408.
27. Kallwitz ER, Herdegen J, Madura J, Jakate S, Cotler SJ. Liver enzymes and histology in obese patients with obstructive sleep apnea. J Clin Gastroenterol. 2007;41:918–21.
28. Anty R, Dahman M, Iannelli A, Gual P, Staccini-Myx A, Amor IB, et al. Bariatric surgery can correct iron depletion in morbidly obese women: a link with chronic inflammation. Obes Surg. 2008;18:709–14.
29. Mathurin P, Hollebecque A, Arnalsteen L, Buob D, Leteurtre E, Caiazzo R, et al. Prospective study of the long-term effects of bariatric surgery on liver injury in patients without advanced disease. Gastroenterology. 2009;137:532–40.
30. Younossi ZM, Koenig AB, Abdelatif D, Fazel Y, Henry L, Wymer M. Global epidemiology of nonalcoholic fatty liver disease-meta-analytic assessment of prevalence, incidence, and outcomes. Hepatology. 2016;64:73–84.
31. Younossi ZM, Otgonsuren M, Henry L, Venkatesan C, Mishra A, Erario M, et al. Association of nonalcoholic fatty liver disease (NAFLD) with hepatocellular carcinoma (HCC) in the United States from 2004 to 2009. Hepatology. 2015;62:1723.
32. Sanyal A, Poklepovic A, Moyneur E, Barghout V. Population-based risk factors and resource utilization for HCC: US perspective. Curr Med Res Opin. 2010;26:2183–91.
33. Dyson JK, McPherson S, Anstee QM. Non-alcoholic fatty liver disease: non-invasive investigation and risk stratification. J Clin Pathol. 2013;66:1033–45.
34. Wong RJ, Cheung R, Ahmed A. Nonalcoholic steatohepatitis is the most rapidly growing indication for liver transplantation in patients with

hepatocellular carcinoma in the U.S. Hepatology. 2014;59:2188–95.
35. Hardy T, Oakley F, Anstee QM, Day CP. Nonalcoholic fatty liver disease: pathogenesis and disease spectrum. Annu Rev Pathol. 2016;11:451.
36. Schutte K, Schulz C, Poranzke J, Antweiler K, Bornschein J, Bretschneider T, et al. Characterization and prognosis of patients with hepatocellular carcinoma (HCC) in the non-cirrhotic liver. BMC Gastroenterol. 2014;14:117.
37. Mittal S, El-Serag HB, Sada YH, Kanwal F, Duan Z, Temple S, et al. Hepatocellular carcinoma in the absence of cirrhosis in United States veterans is associated with nonalcoholic fatty liver disease. Clin Gastroenterol Hepatol. 2016;14:124–31. e121
38. Yasui K, Hashimoto E, Komorizono Y, Koike K, Arii S, Imai Y, et al. Characteristics of patients with nonalcoholic steatohepatitis who develop hepatocellular carcinoma. Clin Gastroenterol Hepatol. 2011;9:428–33.
39. Ascha MS, Hanouneh IA, Lopez R, Tamimi TA, Feldstein AF, Zein NN. The incidence and risk factors of hepatocellular carcinoma in patients with nonalcoholic steatohepatitis. Hepatology. 2010;51:1972–8.
40. Hashimoto E, Yatsuji S, Tobari M, Taniai M, Torii N, Tokushige K, et al. Hepatocellular carcinoma in patients with nonalcoholic steatohepatitis. J Gastroenterol. 2009;44(Suppl 19):89–95.
41. Sanyal AJ, Banas C, Sargeant C, Luketic VA, Sterling RK, Stravitz RT, et al. Similarities and differences in outcomes of cirrhosis due to nonalcoholic steatohepatitis and hepatitis C. Hepatology. 2006;43:682–9.
42. Bhala N, Angulo P, van der Poorten D, Lee E, Hui JM, Saracco G, et al. The natural history of nonalcoholic fatty liver disease with advanced fibrosis or cirrhosis: an international collaborative study. Hepatology. 2011;54:1208–16.
43. Kawamura Y, Arase Y, Ikeda K, Seko Y, Imai N, Hosaka T, et al. Large-scale long-term follow-up study of Japanese patients with non-alcoholic fatty liver disease for the onset of hepatocellular carcinoma. Am J Gastroenterol. 2012;107:253–61.
44. Arase Y, Kobayashi M, Suzuki F, Suzuki Y, Kawamura Y, Akuta N, et al. Difference in malignancies of chronic liver disease due to non-alcoholic fatty liver disease or hepatitis C in Japanese elderly patients. Hepatol Res. 2012;42:264–72.
45. Volzke H. Multicausality in fatty liver disease: is there a rationale to distinguish between alcoholic and non-alcoholic origin? World J Gastroenterol. 2012;18:3492–501.
46. Schutte K, Kipper M, Kahl S, Bornschein J, Gotze T, Adolf D, et al. Clinical characteristics and time trends in etiology of hepatocellular cancer in Germany. Digestion. 2013;87:147–59.
47. Dyson J, Jaques B, Chattopadyhay D, Lochan R, Graham J, Das D, et al. Hepatocellular cancer: the impact of obesity, type 2 diabetes and a multidisciplinary team. J Hepatol. 2014;60:110–7.
48. Piscaglia F, Svegliati-Baroni G, Barchetti A, Pecorelli A, Marinelli S, Tiribelli C, et al. Clinical patterns of hepatocellular carcinoma (HCC) in non alcoholic fatty liver disease (NAFLD): a multicenter prospective study. Hepatology. 2015
49. Dunn W, Xu R, Schwimmer JB. Modest wine drinking and decreased prevalence of suspected nonalcoholic fatty liver disease. Hepatology. 2008;47:1947–54.
50. Nair S, Mason A, Eason J, Loss G, Perrillo RP. Is obesity an independent risk factor for hepatocellular carcinoma in cirrhosis? Hepatology. 2002;36:150–5.
51. Pais R, Lebray P, Rousseau G, Charlotte F, Esselma G, Savier E, et al. Nonalcoholic fatty liver disease increases the risk of hepatocellular carcinoma in patients with alcohol-associated cirrhosis awaiting liver transplants. Clin Gastroenterol Hepatol. 2015;13:992–9.
52. N'Kontchou G, Paries J, Htar MT, Ganne-Carrie N, Costentin L, Grando-Lemaire V, et al. Risk factors for hepatocellular carcinoma in patients with alcoholic or viral C cirrhosis. Clin Gastroenterol Hepatol. 2006;4:1062–8.
53. Edenvik P, Davidsdottir L, Oksanen A, Isaksson B, Hultcrantz R, Stal P. Application of hepatocellular carcinoma surveillance in a European setting. What can we learn from clinical practice? Liver Int. 2015;35:1862–71.
54. Chen CL, Yang HI, Yang WS, Liu CJ, Chen PJ, You SL, et al. Metabolic factors and risk of hepatocellular carcinoma by chronic hepatitis B/C infection: a follow-up study in Taiwan. Gastroenterology. 2008;135:111–21.
55. Chan AW, Wong GL, Chan HY, Tong JH, Yu YH, Choi PC, et al. Concurrent fatty liver increases risk of hepatocellular carcinoma among patients with chronic hepatitis B. J Gastroenterol Hepatol. 2016;32(3):667–76.
56. Tsai IT, Wang CP, Yu TH, Lu YC, Lin CW, Lu LF, et al. Circulating visfatin level is associated with hepatocellular carcinoma in chronic hepatitis B or C virus infection. Cytokine. 2017;90:54–9.
57. Thorgeirsson SS, Grisham JW. Molecular pathogenesis of human hepatocellular carcinoma. Nat Genet. 2002;31:339–46.
58. Farazi PA, DePinho RA. Hepatocellular carcinoma pathogenesis: from genes to environment. Nat Rev Cancer. 2006;6:674–87.
59. Aravalli RN, Cressman EN, Steer CJ. Cellular and molecular mechanisms of hepatocellular carcinoma: an update. Arch Toxicol. 2013;87:227–47.
60. Zhang DY, Friedman SL. Fibrosis-dependent mechanisms of hepatocarcinogenesis. Hepatology. 2012;56:769–75.
61. Breuhahn K, Schirmacher P. Signaling networks in human hepatocarcinogenesis – novel aspects and therapeutic options. Prog Mol Biol Transl Sci. 2010;97:251–77.
62. Dufour JF, Johnson P. Liver cancer: from molecular pathogenesis to new therapies summary of

the EASL single topic conference. J Hepatol. 2010;52:296–304.
63. Goossens N, Sun X, Hoshida Y. Molecular classification of hepatocellular carcinoma: potential therapeutic implications. Hepat Oncol. 2015;2:371–9.
64. Zucman-Rossi J, Villanueva A, Nault JC, Llovet JM. Genetic landscape and biomarkers of hepatocellular carcinoma. Gastroenterology. 2015;149:1226–39. e1224
65. Karagozian R, Derdak Z, Baffy G. Obesity-associated mechanisms of hepatocarcinogenesis. Metabolism. 2014;63:607–17.
66. Sanna C, Rosso C, Marietti M, Bugianesi E. Non-alcoholic fatty liver disease and extra-hepatic cancers. Int J Mol Sci. 2016;17(5):717.
67. Tilg H, Moschen AR. Mechanisms behind the link between obesity and gastrointestinal cancers. Best Pract Res Clin Gastroenterol. 2014;28:599–610.
68. Saltiel AR, Kahn CR. Insulin signalling and the regulation of glucose and lipid metabolism. Nature. 2001;414:799–806.
69. Shimomura I, Matsuda M, Hammer RE, Bashmakov Y, Brown MS, Goldstein JL. Decreased IRS-2 and increased SREBP-1c lead to mixed insulin resistance and sensitivity in livers of lipodystrophic and ob/ob mice. Mol Cell. 2000;6:77–86.
70. Brown MS, Goldstein JL. Selective versus total insulin resistance: a pathogenic paradox. Cell Metab. 2008;7:95–6.
71. Eissing L, Scherer T, Todter K, Knippschild U, Greve JW, Buurman WA, et al. De novo lipogenesis in human fat and liver is linked to ChREBP-beta and metabolic health. Nat Commun. 2013;4:1528.
72. Lee JS, Mendez R, Heng HH, Yang ZQ, Zhang K. Pharmacological ER stress promotes hepatic lipogenesis and lipid droplet formation. Am J Transl Res. 2012;4:102–13.
73. Khandekar MJ, Cohen P, Spiegelman BM. Molecular mechanisms of cancer development in obesity. Nat Rev Cancer. 2011;11:886–95.
74. Kim KW, Bae SK, Lee OH, Bae MH, Lee MJ, Park BC. Insulin-like growth factor II induced by hypoxia may contribute to angiogenesis of human hepatocellular carcinoma. Cancer Res. 1998;58:348–51.
75. Tanaka S, Mohr L, Schmidt EV, Sugimachi K, Wands JR. Biological effects of human insulin receptor substrate-1 overexpression in hepatocytes. Hepatology. 1997;26:598–604.
76. Hassan MM, Curley SA, Li D, Kaseb A, Davila M, Abdalla EK, et al. Association of diabetes duration and diabetes treatment with the risk of hepatocellular carcinoma. Cancer. 2010;116:1938–46.
77. Brunt EM. What's in a Name? Hepatology. 2009;50:663–7.
78. Unger RH, Clark GO, Scherer PE, Orci L. Lipid homeostasis, lipotoxicity and the metabolic syndrome. Biochim Biophys Acta. 2010;1801:209–14.
79. Puri P, Mirshahi F, Cheung O, Natarajan R, Maher JW, Kellum JM, et al. Activation and dysregulation of the unfolded protein response in nonalcoholic fatty liver disease. Gastroenterology. 2008;134:568–76.
80. Cazanave SC, Gores GJ. Mechanisms and clinical implications of hepatocyte lipoapoptosis. Clin Lipidol. 2010;5:71–85.
81. Ozcan U, Cao Q, Yilmaz E, Lee AH, Iwakoshi NN, Ozdelen E, et al. Endoplasmic reticulum stress links obesity, insulin action, and type 2 diabetes. Science. 2004;306:457–61.
82. Vinciguerra M, Carrozzino F, Peyrou M, Carlone S, Montesano R, Benelli R, et al. Unsaturated fatty acids promote hepatoma proliferation and progression through downregulation of the tumor suppressor PTEN. J Hepatol. 2009;50:1132–41.
83. Joshi-Barve S, Barve SS, Amancherla K, Gobejishvili L, Hill D, Cave M, et al. Palmitic acid induces production of proinflammatory cytokine interleukin-8 from hepatocytes. Hepatology. 2007;46:823–30.
84. Hussain SP, Hofseth LJ, Harris CC. Radical causes of cancer. Nat Rev Cancer. 2003;3:276–85.
85. Haslam DW, James WP. Obesity. Lancet. 2005;366:1197–209.
86. Virtue S, Vidal-Puig A. Adipose tissue expandability, lipotoxicity and the metabolic syndrome – an allostatic perspective. Biochim Biophys Acta. 2010;1801:338–49.
87. Sun K, Kusminski CM, Scherer PE. Adipose tissue remodeling and obesity. J Clin Invest. 2011;121:2094–101.
88. Shoelson SE, Herrero L, Naaz A. Obesity, inflammation, and insulin resistance. Gastroenterology. 2007;132:2169–80.
89. Hotamisligil GS. Inflammation and metabolic disorders. Nature. 2006;444:860–7.
90. He Q, Gao Z, Yin J, Zhang J, Yun Z, Ye J. Regulation of HIF-1{alpha} activity in adipose tissue by obesity-associated factors: adipogenesis, insulin, and hypoxia. Am J Physiol Endocrinol Metab. 2011;300:E877–85.
91. Marra F, Bertolani C. Adipokines in liver diseases. Hepatology. 2009;50:957–69.
92. Stickel F, Hellerbrand C. Non-alcoholic fatty liver disease as a risk factor for hepatocellular carcinoma: mechanisms and implications. Gut. 2010;59:1303–7.
93. Kadowaki T, Yamauchi T, Kubota N, Hara K, Ueki K, Tobe K. Adiponectin and adiponectin receptors in insulin resistance, diabetes, and the metabolic syndrome. J Clin Investig. 2006;116:1784–92.
94. Dalamaga M, Diakopoulos KN, Mantzoros CS. The role of adiponectin in cancer: a review of current evidence. Endocr Rev. 2012;33:547–94.
95. Duan XF, Tang P, Li Q, Yu ZT. Obesity, adipokines and hepatocellular carcinoma. Int J Cancer. 2013;133:1776–83.
96. Schwabe RF, Jobin C. The microbiome and cancer. Nat Rev Cancer. 2013;13:800–12.
97. Quigley EM, Abu-Shanab A, Murphy EF, Stanton C, Monsour HP Jr. The metabolic role of the microbiome: implications for NAFLD and the metabolic syndrome. Semin Liver Dis. 2016;36:312–6.
98. Schuppan D, Afdhal NH. Liver cirrhosis. Lancet. 2008;371:838–51.

99. Tilg H, Kaser A. Gut microbiome, obesity, and metabolic dysfunction. J Clin Invest. 2011;121:2126–32.
100. Mouzaki M, Comelli EM, Arendt BM, Bonengel J, Fung SK, Fischer SE, et al. Intestinal microbiota in patients with nonalcoholic fatty liver disease. Hepatology. 2013;58:120–7.
101. Dapito DH, Mencin A, Gwak GY, Pradere JP, Jang MK, Mederacke I, et al. Promotion of hepatocellular carcinoma by the intestinal microbiota and TLR4. Cancer Cell. 2012;21:504–16.
102. Yoshimoto S, Loo TM, Atarashi K, Kanda H, Sato S, Oyadomari S, et al. Obesity-induced gut microbial metabolite promotes liver cancer through senescence secretome. Nature. 2013;499:97–101.
103. Fuchs CD, Traussnigg SA, Trauner M. Nuclear receptor modulation for the treatment of nonalcoholic fatty liver disease. Semin Liver Dis. 2016;36:69–86.
104. Baffy G. The impact of network medicine in gastroenterology and hepatology. Clin Gastroenterol Hepatol. 2013;11:1240–4.
105. Moylan CA, Pang H, Dellinger A, Suzuki A, Garrett ME, Guy CD, et al. Hepatic gene expression profiles differentiate presymptomatic patients with mild versus severe nonalcoholic fatty liver disease. Hepatology. 2014;59:471–82.
106. Clarke JD, Novak P, Lake AD, Shipkova P, Aranibar N, Robertson D, et al. Characterization of hepatocellular carcinoma related genes and metabolites in human nonalcoholic fatty liver disease. Dig Dis Sci. 2014;59:365–74.
107. Adams LA, Lymp JF, St Sauver J, Sanderson SO, Lindor KD, Feldstein A, et al. The natural history of nonalcoholic fatty liver disease: a population-based cohort study. Gastroenterology. 2005;129:113–21.
108. Ekstedt M, Franzen LE, Mathiesen UL, Thorelius L, Holmqvist M, Bodemar G, et al. Long-term follow-up of patients with NAFLD and elevated liver enzymes. Hepatology. 2006;44:865–73.
109. Kaswala DH, Lai M, Afdhal NH. Fibrosis assessment in nonalcoholic fatty liver disease (NAFLD) in 2016. Dig Dis Sci. 2016;61:1356–64.
110. Buzzetti E, Lombardi R, De Luca L, Tsochatzis EA. Noninvasive assessment of fibrosis in patients with nonalcoholic fatty liver disease. Int J Endocrinol. 2015;2015:343828.
111. Asrani SK. Incorporation of noninvasive measures of liver fibrosis into clinical practice: diagnosis and prognosis. Clin Gastroenterol Hepatol. 2015;13:2190–204.
112. Wong VW, Wong GL, Choi PC, Chan AW, Li MK, Chan HY, et al. Disease progression of non-alcoholic fatty liver disease: a prospective study with paired liver biopsies at 3 years. Gut. 2010;59:969–74.
113. Singh S, Allen AM, Wang Z, Prokop LJ, Murad MH, Loomba R. Fibrosis progression in nonalcoholic fatty liver vs nonalcoholic steatohepatitis: a systematic review and meta-analysis of paired-biopsy studies. Clin Gastroenterol Hepatol 2015;13:643–654 e641–649; quiz e639–640.
114. McPherson S, Hardy T, Henderson E, Burt AD, Day CP, Anstee QM. Evidence of NAFLD progression from steatosis to fibrosing-steatohepatitis using paired biopsies: implications for prognosis and clinical management. J Hepatol. 2015;62:1148–55.
115. Pais R, Charlotte F, Fedchuk L, Bedossa P, Lebray P, Poynard T, et al. A systematic review of follow-up biopsies reveals disease progression in patients with non-alcoholic fatty liver. J Hepatol. 2013;59:550–6.
116. Davila JA, Morgan RO, Richardson PA, Du XL, McGlynn KA, El-Serag HB. Use of surveillance for hepatocellular carcinoma among patients with cirrhosis in the United States. Hepatology. 2010;52:132–41.
117. Gupta S, Bent S, Kohlwes J. Test characteristics of alpha-fetoprotein for detecting hepatocellular carcinoma in patients with hepatitis C. A systematic review and critical analysis. Ann Intern Med. 2003;139:46–50.
118. Sherman M. Surveillance for hepatocellular carcinoma. Semin Oncol. 2001;28:450–9.
119. Marrero JA, Su GL, Wei W, Emick D, Conjeevaram HS, Fontana RJ, et al. Des-gamma carboxyprothrombin can differentiate hepatocellular carcinoma from nonmalignant chronic liver disease in american patients. Hepatology. 2003;37:1114–21.
120. Voiculescu M, Nanau RM, Neuman MG. Non-invasive biomarkers in non-alcoholic steatohepatitis-induced hepatocellular carcinoma. J Gastrointestin Liver Dis. 2014;23:425–9.
121. Miao R, Luo H, Zhou H, Li G, Bu D, Yang X, et al. Identification of prognostic biomarkers in hepatitis B virus-related hepatocellular carcinoma and stratification by integrative multi-omics analysis. J Hepatol. 2014;61:840–9.
122. Jin GZ, Li Y, Cong WM, Yu H, Dong H, Shu H, et al. iTRAQ-2DLC-ESI-MS/MS based identification of a new set of immunohistochemical biomarkers for classification of dysplastic nodules and small hepatocellular carcinoma. J Proteome Res. 2011;10:3418–28.
123. Nishida N, Kudo M, Nishimura T, Arizumi T, Takita M, Kitai S, et al. Unique association between global DNA hypomethylation and chromosomal alterations in human hepatocellular carcinoma. PLoS One. 2013;8:e72312.
124. Llovet JM, Chen Y, Wurmbach E, Roayaie S, Fiel MI, Schwartz M, et al. A molecular signature to discriminate dysplastic nodules from early hepatocellular carcinoma in HCV cirrhosis. Gastroenterology. 2006;131:1758–67.
125. Gori M, Arciello M, Balsano C. MicroRNAs in nonalcoholic fatty liver disease: novel biomarkers and prognostic tools during the transition from steatosis to hepatocarcinoma. Biomed Res Int. 2014;2014:741465.
126. Bartel DP. MicroRNAs: genomics, biogenesis, mechanism, and function. Cell. 2004;116:281–97.
127. Mohr AM, Mott JL. Overview of microRNA biology. Semin Liver Dis. 2015;35:3–11.

128. Wang XW, Heegaard NH, Orum H. MicroRNAs in liver disease. Gastroenterology. 2012;142:1431–43.
129. Arner P, Kulyte A. MicroRNA regulatory networks in human adipose tissue and obesity. Nat Rev Endocrinol. 2015;11:276–88.
130. Sobolewski C, Calo N, Portius D, Foti M. MicroRNAs in fatty liver disease. Semin Liver Dis. 2015;35:12–25.
131. Finch ML, Marquardt JU, Yeoh GC, Callus BA. Regulation of microRNAs and their role in liver development, regeneration and disease. Int J Biochem Cell Biol. 2014;54:288–303.
132. Afonso MB, Rodrigues PM, Simao AL, Castro RE. Circulating microRNAs as potential biomarkers in non-alcoholic fatty liver disease and hepatocellular carcinoma. J Clin Med. 2016;5(3).
133. Cheng G. Circulating miRNAs: roles in cancer diagnosis, prognosis and therapy. Adv Drug Deliv Rev. 2015;81:75–93.
134. Arrese M, Eguchi A, Feldstein AE. Circulating microRNAs: emerging biomarkers of liver disease. Semin Liver Dis. 2015;35:43–54.
135. Csak T, Bala S, Lippai D, Satishchandran A, Catalano D, Kodys K, et al. microRNA-122 regulates hypoxia-inducible factor-1 and vimentin in hepatocytes and correlates with fibrosis in diet-induced steatohepatitis. Liver Int. 2015;35:532–41.
136. Pirola CJ, Fernandez Gianotti T, Castano GO, Mallardi P, San Martino J. Mora Gonzalez Lopez Ledesma M, et al. circulating microRNA signature in non-alcoholic fatty liver disease: from serum non-coding RNAs to liver histology and disease pathogenesis. Gut. 2015;64:800–12.
137. Ye H, Liu W. Transcriptional networks implicated in human nonalcoholic fatty liver disease. Mol Gen Genomics. 2015; 290:1793–804.
138. Bahn JH, Zhang Q, Li F, Chan TM, Lin X, Kim Y, et al. The landscape of microRNA, Piwi-interacting RNA, and circular RNA in human saliva. Clin Chem. 2015;61:221–30.
139. Iwasaki YW, Siomi MC, Siomi H. PIWI-interacting RNA: its biogenesis and functions. Annu Rev Biochem. 2015;84:405–33.
140. Rizzo F, Rinaldi A, Marchese G, Coviello E, Sellitto A, Cordella A, et al. Specific patterns of PIWI-interacting small noncoding RNA expression in dysplastic liver nodules and hepatocellular carcinoma. Oncotarget. 2016;7:54650–61.
141. Shariff MI, Gomaa AI, Cox IJ, Patel M, Williams HR, Crossey MM, et al. Urinary metabolic biomarkers of hepatocellular carcinoma in an Egyptian population: a validation study. J Proteome Res. 2011;10:1828–36.
142. Pearson TA, Manolio TA. How to interpret a genome-wide association study. JAMA. 2008;299:1335–44.
143. Brown PO, Botstein D. Exploring the new world of the genome with DNA microarrays. Nat Genet. 1999;21:33–7.
144. Subramanian A, Tamayo P, Mootha VK, Mukherjee S, Ebert BL, Gillette MA, et al. Gene set enrichment analysis: a knowledge-based approach for interpreting genome-wide expression profiles. Proc Natl Acad Sci U S A. 2005;102:15545–50.
145. Romeo S, Kozlitina J, Xing C, Pertsemlidis A, Cox D, Pennacchio LA, et al. Genetic variation in PNPLA3 confers susceptibility to nonalcoholic fatty liver disease. Nat Genet. 2008;40:1461–5.
146. Sookoian S, Pirola CJ. Meta-analysis of the influence of I148M variant of patatin-like phospholipase domain containing 3 gene (PNPLA3) on the susceptibility and histological severity of nonalcoholic fatty liver disease. Hepatology. 2011;53:1883–94.
147. Kozlitina J, Smagris E, Stender S, Nordestgaard BG, Zhou HH, Tybjaerg-Hansen A, et al. Exome-wide association study identifies a TM6SF2 variant that confers susceptibility to nonalcoholic fatty liver disease. Nat Genet. 2014;46:352–6.
148. Miele L, Beale G, Patman G, Nobili V, Leathart J, Grieco A, et al. The Kruppel-like factor 6 genotype is associated with fibrosis in nonalcoholic fatty liver disease. Gastroenterology. 2008;135:282–91 e281.
149. Valenti L, Rametta R, Dongiovanni P, Motta BM, Canavesi E, Pelusi S, et al. The A736V TMPRSS6 polymorphism influences hepatic iron overload in nonalcoholic fatty liver disease. PLoS One. 2012;7:e48804.
150. Dongiovanni P, Romeo S, Valenti L. Genetic factors in the pathogenesis of nonalcoholic fatty liver and steatohepatitis. Biomed Res Int. 2015;2015:460190.
151. Sherman M. Hepatocellular carcinoma: epidemiology, surveillance, and diagnosis. Semin Liver Dis. 2010;30:3–16.
152. Arguedas MR, Chen VK, Eloubeidi MA, Fallon MB. Screening for hepatocellular carcinoma in patients with hepatitis C cirrhosis: a cost-utility analysis. Am J Gastroenterol. 2003;98:679–90.
153. Sarasin FP, Giostra E, Hadengue A. Cost-effectiveness of screening for detection of small hepatocellular carcinoma in western patients with child-Pugh class a cirrhosis. Am J Med. 1996;101:422–34.
154. European Association For The Study Of The L, European Organisation For R, Treatment Of C. EASL-EORTC clinical practice guidelines: management of hepatocellular carcinoma. J Hepatol. 2012;56:908–43.
155. Omata M, Lesmana LA, Tateishi R, Chen PJ, Lin SM, Yoshida H, et al. Asian Pacific Association for the study of the liver consensus recommendations on hepatocellular carcinoma. Hepatol Int. 2010;4:439–74.
156. Mittal S, Sada YH, El-Serag HB, Kanwal F, Duan Z, Temple S, et al. Temporal trends of nonalcoholic fatty liver disease-related hepatocellular carcinoma in the veteran affairs population. Clin Gastroenterol Hepatol. 2015;13:594–601 e591.

Dysregulated Epigenetic Modifications in the Pathogenesis of NAFLD-HCC

7

Fung Zhao

Abstract

The pathogenesis of NAFLD is multi-faceted and mechanisms underlying the progression from simple steatosis to NASH have not been fully deciphered. The emerging field of epigenetics, an inheritable phenomenon capable of changing gene expression without altering DNA sequence, unveils a new perspective on the development of NAFLD and subsequent progression to HCC. In fact, numerous studies have highlighted the potential involvement of unhealthy daily habits such as physical inactivity and over-nutrition in the onset and development of NAFLD through epigenetic mechanisms. This chapter will discuss several epigenetic modulations including DNA methylation, histone modifications, functions of non-coding RNAs as well as RNA methylation implicated in the pathogenesis of NAFLD-HCC. On the basis of currently wealthy knowledge of DNA epigenetics, the rapidly growing field of RNA epigenetics will certainly drive forward a new avenue of research direction shedding light on the advancement of better diagnostics, prognostics and therapeutics in the coming era of precision medicine.

F. Zhao (✉)
Institute of Digestive Disease, Department of Medicine and Therapeutics, The Chinese University of Hong Kong, Hong Kong, Hong Kong

Keywords

Non-alcoholic fatty liver disease · Non-alcoholic steatohepatitis · Hepatocellular carcinoma · Epigenetic modifications

7.1 Introduction

As mentioned in previous sections, non-alcoholic fatty liver disease (NAFLD) is defined as the pathological deposition of triglycerides in hepatocytes due to causes other than excessive alcohol consumption. Non-alcoholic steatohepatitis (NASH), the more severe disease entity of NAFLD, represents the most common liver disease in the Western world and has the capacity to progress to cirrhosis and hepatocellular carcinoma (HCC) [1]. Compared to the high prevalence of NAFLD (20–30%) in Western countries, the prevalence in Asian countries is estimated to be around 5–20% [2]. As with other causes of liver disease, only a minor proportion of patients with NASH progress to advanced fibrosis, cirrhosis and/or HCC [3].

The pathogenesis of NAFLD is multi-faceted and mechanisms underlying the progression from simple steatosis to NASH have not been fully deciphered. According to the double-hit theory attempting to explain the development of NAFLD, the first hit is the accumulation of triglycerides in hepatocytes, accompanied by a sec-

J. Yu (ed.), *Obesity, Fatty Liver and Liver Cancer*, Advances in Experimental Medicine and Biology 1061, https://doi.org/10.1007/978-981-10-8684-7_7

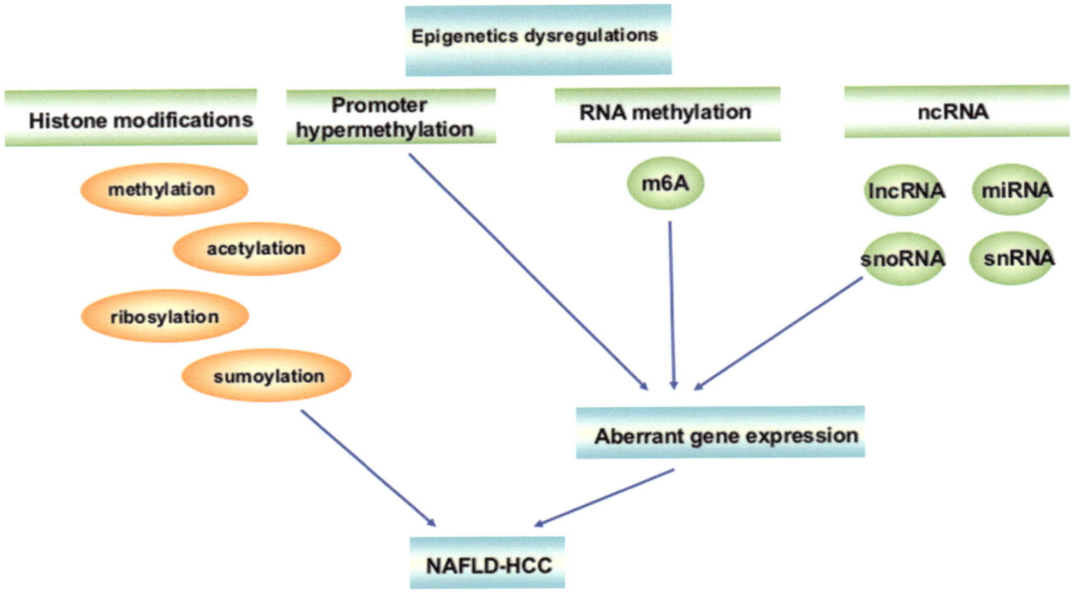

Fig. 7.1 Dysregulated epigenetic modulations including DNA methylation, histone modifications, functions of non-coding RNAs as well as RNA methylation contribute to the pathogenesis of NAFLD-HCC. *m*^{6}*A* N^{6}-methyladenosine, *lncRNA* long non-coding RNA, *snRNA* small nuclear RNA, *snoRNA* small nucleolar RNA

ond hit describing inflammatory cytokine interplay, mitochondrial dysfunction and oxidative stress causing hepatocellular injury, inflammation and fibrosis [4, 5]. Recent studies devised a new model describing multiple parallel hits in the progression of NAFLD. NAFLD pathogenesis is now commonly described as the excessive deposition of fat in hepatocytes, followed by increase in intracellular fat vacuoles, induction of endoplasmic reticulum and oxidative stress eventually leading to apoptosis of hepatocytes [6].

The emerging field of epigenetics, an inheritable phenomenon capable of changing gene expression without altering DNA sequence, unveils a new perspective on the pathogenesis of NAFLD. In fact, numerous studies have highlighted the potential involvement of unhealthy daily habits such as physical inactivity and overnutrition in the onset and development of NAFLD through epigenetic mechanisms [7, 8]. This chapter will discuss several epigenetic modulations including DNA methylation, histone modifications, functions of non-coding RNAs as well as RNA methylation implicated in the pathogenesis of NAFLD-HCC that might serve as novel diagnostic, prognostic and therapeutic options (Fig. 7.1).

7.2 DNA Methylation

The best-known and most intensively studied modification is methylation of cytosine in DNA with a methyl group. DNA methylation is catalyzed by DNA methyltransferases (DNMTs) that transfer a methyl group from S-adenosyl-L-methionine (SAM) to cytosine with guanine as the next nucleotide known as CpG dincleotides, the clustering of which being commonly referred to as CpG islands. Majority of CpG islands are located at the promoter regions of genes and hypermethylation of CpG islands causes gene silencing [9]. On the other hand, the ten-eleven translocation methylcytosine dioxygense (TET) family of enzymes converts the modified DNA base 5-methylcytosine (5-mC) to 5-hydroxymethylcytosine (5-hmC) and this modification has been proposed as the initial step of active demethylation in mammals [10, 11]. Given the central role of DNA methylation in the regulation of gene expression, it comes with no surprise that perturbations to the homeostatic methylation level, due largely to environmental factors, contribute to aberrant gene expressions and trigger various pathological conditions.

7.2.1 DNA Methylation in Fibrosis and Progression of NASH

S-adenosyl-L-methionine (SAM) is the unique methyl donor for DNA methylation and dietary sources include folate, methionine, betaine and choline [12]. Methyl donor deficient diets have been associated with reduced DNA methylation and disturbed lipid metabolism. For example, folate deficiency has been shown to induce hepatic triglyceride accumulation and alter the expression of genes involved in fatty acid synthesis [13]. Likewise, deficiencies in methionine and choline have been correlated with reduced lipoprotein secretion and increased hepatic triglyceride generation accompanied by NAFLD development [14, 15]. Intriguingly, Tryndyak et al. [16] demonstrated *in vivo* that low SAM concentration altered the expressions of a series of genes involved in DNA repair, lipid and glucose metabolisms and hepatic fibrosis. This was consistent with a recent observation reporting a significant decrease in serum betaine levels in NASH patients as compared to those with non-alcoholic fatty liver [17], implicating proper dietary intake and maintenance of homeostatic SAM levels are critical for a harmonious hepatic lipid metabolism.

Liver fibrosis is defined by the excessive accumulation of extracellular matrix and scar formation in the context of chronic liver damage [18]. Activation and trans-differentiation of hepatic stellate cell (HSC) in response to various stimuli such as inflammation, from vitamin A storing pericyte to profibrogenic myofibroblastic phenotype, play a key role in the pathogenesis of liver fibrosis [19]. It has been demonstrated that transforming growth factor- β1 (TGF- β1), an inflammatory cytokine secreted by different types of hepatic cells, represented the main fibrogenic cytokine behind HSC activation [20]. Although the underlying molecular mechanisms driving fibrogenesis await further investigations, DNMTs have recently been implicated in the process. In humans there are three DNMT isoforms: DNMT1, DNMT3a and DNMT3b. While DNMT1 recognizes a hemi-methylated site on a new DNA strand during cell division and regenerates the bi-methylated state thereby safeguarding the faithful propagation of methylation patterns in daughter cells, DNMT3a and DNMT3b are central to the regulation of *de novo* methylation in the absence of cell division [21]. In a mouse model, Pogribny et al. [22] documented a hepatic epigenetic phenotype predetermined individual susceptible to hepatic steatosis in association with altered expressions of DNMT1 and DNMT3a in the liver. DNMT3a has also been shown to enhance HSC activation and liver fibrogenesis via methylation and downregulation of the GTPase Septin-9 [23]. TET enzymes, responsible for catalyzing the stepwise oxidation of methyl groups on DNA leading eventually to the restoration of the unmodified cytosine residue, have been found to fine-tune the *PPARGC1A* transcriptional program in liver. Next-generation sequencing further revealed genetic diversity at *TET* loci was associated with altered 5-hmC levels that might be accountable for the pathogenesis of NAFLD [24]. A recent study elucidating the relationship between methylome and transcriptome in patients with nonalcoholic fatty liver disease revealed differentially methylated genes might distinguish patients with advanced NASH from those with simple steatosis [25]. In the landmark piece of work, 69,247 differentially methylated CpG sites (76% hypomethylated; 24% hypermethylated) were observed in patients with advanced NASH as compared to those with simple steatosis [25]. Aberrant methylation signatures of a plethora of genes have been suggested to predict the progression from NAFLD to NASH. For instance, peroxisome proliferator-activated receptor α (PPAR-α) exhibited significantly higher DNA methylation level in severe NAFLD patients than in mild counterparts [26].

7.2.2 DNA Methylation in the Progression of HCC

Disruption of DNA methylation has long been recognized as one of the key hallmarks of all cancer types [27]. Typical lesions in cancer include loci-specific *de novo* hypermethylation at promoter regions of tumour suppressor genes (TSGs) resulting in transcriptional repression of downstream TSGs. Among the plethora of studies reporting changes in DNA methylation pattern in HCC, Villanueva et al. [28] conducted a comprehensive study profiling the DNA methylation landscape in a cohort of 304 patients with HCC treated with surgical resection. Methylome profiling covering 96% of known CpG islands and 485,000 CpG dinucleotides was performed and a methylation signature generated based on 36 methylation probes accurately predicted survival in patients with HCC. While HCC tissue samples displayed general hypomethylation in the intergenic and body regions as compared with normal liver, hypermethylated probes were mainly located in promoter regions [28]. The authors further demonstrated aberrant methylation in established and candidate epidrivers of disease including well-known tumour suppressors such as Ras association domain family member 1 (*RASSF1*), adenomatous polyposis coli (*APC*), insulin-like growth factor 2 (*IGF2*) and *NOTCH3*, supporting the pivotal role of deregulated DNA methylation in HCC development [28].

The functional relevance of aberrant DNA methylation has been tested in numerous tumour suppressor genes. For instance, sphingomyelin phosphodiesterase 3 (*SMPD3*) and heavy polypeptide (*NEFH*) overexpression could inhibit tumour cell proliferation, whereas stable knockdown of the two enhanced cell migration and invasion *in vitro* and *in vitro* [29]. Noteworthy, persistent Hepatits B virus (HBV) infection has been shown to stimulate the upregulation of DNMTs, leading to hypermethylation and inactivation of p16 and the subsequent progression of HCC [30]. A recent intriguing study uncovered a role of hypoxia in the process of tumour development. Thienpont et al. [31] observed a direct inhibition of the activity of TET enzymes in a series of cancer cell lines (including HCC) and mouse cells in response to a hypoxic environment. The reduction in activity increased hypermethylation at gene promoters resulting in aberrant gene expressions in various signaling pathways and conferring a selective advantage to cancer cells [31]. Taken together, deregulated DNA methylation will continue to be a hot research area as a more thorough understanding of the underlying mechanisms is crucial to formulating novel prognostic markers and therapeutic targets.

7.3 Histone Modifications

Condensation of 2 m of DNA into a human nucleus is achieved through interaction between DNA and specialized histone proteins to form tightly packed chromatin. The basic level of chromatin packing is known as the nucleosome with each core particle comprising of 147 bp of double stranded DNA wrapped around a complex of eight histone proteins (two copies each of H2A, H2B, H3 and H4). The structure is commonly referred to as "beads on string" with linker DNA being the string and the nucleosome core particle representing the beads. In order to allow chromosomal processes such as gene transcription to occur, the chromatin must be packed lightly (euchromatin) or tightly (heterochromatin) in a finely orchestrated fashion. Indeed, each of the core histones harbours an unstructured N-terminal amino acid tail extension that can be subject to a plethora of posttranslational modifications including acetylation, methylation, phosphorylation, ubiquitination, ribosylation and sumoylation which constitute a crucial determinant of chromatin compactness and accessibility [32].

7.3.1 Histone Acetylation in NAFLD-HCC

Among various types of posttranslational modifications, acetylation of lysine residues at the N-terminus of histone tails has been most extensively investigated [33]. While histone acetylation is catalyzed by histone acetyltransferases (HATs), histone deacetylation is mediated by histone deacetylases (HDACs) [34]. Perturbations to the balance between HAT and HDAC have been reported to alter gene expression profiles in NAFLD [35].

7.3.1.1 Histone Acetyltransferases (HATs)

Histone acetyltransferases (HATs) acetylate conserved amino acid residues on histone proteins by transferring an acetyl group from acetyl-CoA to form ε-*N*-acetyllysine enabling enhanced gene expression. HATs can be divided into different classes depending on their subcellular localization [36]. Type A HATs are mainly located in the nucleus including Gcn5-related *N*-acetyltransferases (GNATs), p300/CBP and $TAF_{II}250$, whereas type B HATs function predominantly in the cytoplasm [36]. In particular, p300/CBP has been shown to be involved in NF-κB dependent inflammatory pathways [37]. Inhibition of hepatic p300 was further suggested to be beneficial for treating hepatic steatosis in obesity and type 2 diabetes [38]. On the contrary, a recent report demonstrated p300/CBP-associated factor inhibited the growth of HCC cells by promoting autophagy, suggesting restoration of the specific HAT might prove to be a novel therapeutic strategy of HCC treatment [39].

7.3.1.2 Histone Deacetylases (HDACs)

Histone deacetylases (HDACs) remove acetyl groups from ε-*N*-acetyl lysine residues on histone, a process that is essential for tight wrapping between histones and DNA, as well as subsequent inhibition of gene transcription. HDAC superfamily is sub-divided into four classes: I, II, III (also referred to as Sirtuins or SIRTs) and IV on the basis of varying structure, enzymatic function and subcellular localization. Not surprisingly, dysregulations of HDACs have been implicated in the progression of NAFLD. Disruption of the circadian clock by HDAC3, a member of class I HDACs, resulted in perturbation to hepatic lipid metabolism and obesity [40]. Another member HDAC6 has been documented to function as a tumour suppressor in HCC and suppression of which by induction of miR-221 accompanied by activation of downstream oncogenic pathways contributed to liver tumorigenesis [41].

Silent information regulator 2 proteins (Sirtuins or SIRTs) belong to class III HDACs. Seven members have been identified in human so far (SIRT1-7) with different subcellular localizations. While some are present predominantly in the nucleus, others display cytoplasmic (SIRT1,2) and mitochondrial (SIRT3,4,5) localizations [42]. Research on mammals has been focused on SIRT1, which acts as a potent protector from a wide array of pathological conditions such as diabetes, liver steatosis and various types of cancer [43]. Although overexpression of SIRT1 appeared to offer protection against DNA damage and metabolic derangement induced by high fat diet [44], recent studies highlighted up-regulation of SIRT1 facilitated HCC metastasis and self-renewal of liver cancer stem cells [45, 46]. Similarly, SIRT2 overexpression has also been demonstrated in HCC promoting epithelial-mesenchymal transition and an aggressive phenotype [47]. Another member of the SIRT family of HDACs, SIRT3, represents the primary mitochondrial deacetylase that is indispensable for the maintenance of mitochondrial integrity and metabolism during oxidative stress [48]. In a mouse model fed a high fat diet, Hirschey et al. observed down-regulation of SIRT3 and mice lacking SIRT3 exhibited exacerbated obesity, insulin resistance, hyperlipidemia and steatohepatitis supporting a role of SIRT3 in safeguarding metabolic homeostasis [49]. Studies looking into the potential roles of other SIRT members in the development of liver diseases are expanding.

7.3.2 Histone Methylation in NAFLD-HCC

Though less well studied as compared to DNA methylation, histone methylation can be associated with transcriptional activation or repression. Histone methyltransferases mediate the transfer of methyl groups from S-adenosyl-L-methionine (SAM) to lysine or arginine residues of H3 or H4 histones. Common sites of methylation that have been reported to be involved in gene activation include H3K4, H3K48 and H3K79, whereas H3K9 and H3K27 are associated with gene inactivation [50]. Recent investigations demonstrated participation of histone methyltransferases in the development of diseases. For instance, Fei et al. recently reported the H3K9 methyltransferase SETDB1 was overexpressed in HCC and regulated tumour cell growth via di-methylation of p53 [51].

7.3.3 Histone Ribosylation in NAFLD-HCC

Adenosine diphosphate (ADP)-ribosylation refers to the addition of one or more ADP-ribose moieties from nicotinamide adenine dinucleotide (NAD) to acceptor proteins. The reaction is a reversible posttranslational modification catalyzed by two classes of enzymes: mono-ADP-ribosyltransferases and poly (ADP-ribose) polymerase (PARP) [52]. PARP is involved in a broad range of cellular functions including gene regulation, DNA damage repair, cell signaling as well as apoptosis [53, 54]. As with other types of modifications, aberrant PARP expression has been documented in various types of cancer including HCC. Poly-ADP-ribosylation and PARP expression were found to be significantly upregulated in human HCC when compared to adjacent non-tumour tissues [55]. Since then the potential of PARP as a therapeutic target for cancer has been intensively studied. In combination with DHMEQ (a novel inhibitor of NF-κB), the PARP inhibitor Olaparib has recently been shown to exert synergistic anti-tumour effects on HCC cells [56].

7.3.4 Histone Sumoylation in NAFLD-HCC

Sumoylation describes the covalent attachment of small ubiquitin-related modifier (SUMO) proteins to acceptor proteins. Four SUMO family members, SUMO-1 to SUMO-4, have been identified so far. Though SUMO-1 exhibits 18% sequence identity with ubiquitin and the two share similar three-dimensional structures, sumoylated proteins are not designated for degradation [57]. Indeed, sumoylation is commonly involved in various cellular processes including intracellular trafficking, transcriptional regulation, response to oxidative stress and cell cycle progression [58]. Sumoylation is also a dynamic process catalyzed by SUMO-specific activating (E1), conjugating (E2) and ligating (E3) enzymes [59] and can be reversed by the family of SUMO-specific proteases (SENPs) [60]. In addition to mediating transcriptional repression through recruitment of histone deacetylases and heterochromatin protein 1, sumoylation has been implicated in tumorigenesis [61]. Recently, upregulation of one of the SUMO-specific proteases, SENP5, has been observed in HCC to promote tumorigenesis *in vitro* and *in vivo* via de-sumoylation and regulation of DNA damage response [62]. SUMO1 has also been demonstrated to possess oncogenic properties in HCC by promoting p65 nuclear translocation and regulating NF-κB activity [63].

7.4 Non-coding RNAs (ncRNAs)

Non-coding RNAs (ncRNAs) constitute a significant proportion of the transcribed genome that is not destined to be translated into proteins. ncRNAs comprise highly abundant RNAs including transfer RNAs (tRNAs), ribosomal RNAs (rRNAs), microRNAs (miRNAs), small nuclear RNAs (snRNAs), small nucleolar RNAs (snoRNAs), extracellular RNAs (exRNAs) and long ncRNAs (lncRNAs) [64]. The plethora of ncRNAs play crucial roles in a broad spectrum of biological processes while dysregulations of which contribute to the development of various diseases.

7.4.1 miRNAs

7.4.1.1 Definition

Ever since the discovery of *lin*-4 in the nematode *Caenorhabditis elegans* (*C.elegans*) in 1993, members of the novel class of small non-coding single strand regulatory RNAs, the microRNA (miRNAs) family, have been expanding drawing the attention of research focus [65]. miRNAs are each comprised of approximately 22 nucleotides and are found in a diverse array of organisms ranging from prokaryotes, eukaryotes to viruses. miRNAs can be either encoded by specific genes or located in the introns or exons of protein-coding genes and expressed as a by-product [65]. They play crucial roles in a wide spectrum of cellular and physiological functions, including cell proliferation, cell death, metabolism, haematopoiesis, and chromatin modification by modulating the expression of target genes [66].

7.4.1.2 Biogenesis and Mechanism of Action

Biogenesis of miRNAs in vertebrate initiates with the generation of a long primary miRNA (pri-miRNA) which is transcribed mostly by RNA polymerases type II (Pol-II). Each pri-miRNA is then processed into a hairpin-shaped precursor miRNA (pre-miRNA) of approximately 60–70 nucleotides by Drosha-like RNase III endonucleases. The pre-miRNA is subsequently transported out of nucleus into cytoplasm by Exportin-5 and Ran-GTP, and is then cleaved by Dicer-like RNase III endonuclease to form the mature miRNA duplex. Afterwards, one strand is usually incorporated into the RNA-induced silencing complex (RISC) whereas the other strand is degraded [67]. Regulation of gene expression is mediated through the canonical base pairing of miRNA seed sequence and the complementary sequence of target mRNAs followed by silencing or degradation of target mRNAs [68]. It has been reported an average miRNA has approximately 100 target sites, indicating that miRNAs are capable of regulating a large fraction of protein-coding genes [69]. Given the importance of miRNAs in the regulation of a wide array of cellular functions, it comes with no surprise that deregulating the function of miRNAs could lead to the development of multiple pathological conditions including cancer. Indeed, dysregulated miRNAs have been documented in various cancer types including chronic lymphocytic leukemia [70], breast cancer [71], lung cancer [72], colorectal cancer [73], prostate cancer [74] and ovarian cancer [75].

7.4.1.3 miRNAs in the Progression from NAFLD to HCC

Recent studies have demonstrated aberrant expressions of miRNAs are involved in the acquisition of NAFLD and subsequent progression to NASH. Deregulations of some of the key regulatory miRNAs have been shown to disturb normal glucose, cholesterol and lipid metabolism leading to intra-hepatic excessive accumulation of triglycerides and fatty acids [76]. It has also been demonstrated miRNAs are frequently dysregulated in different phonotypes of NAFLD, from simple steatosis through NASH to cirrhosis and eventually HCC [77].

One of the very first miRNAs associated with lipid metabolism and homeostasis is miR-122, the most abundant miRNA in adult human liver accounting for 70% of the liver's total miRNAs [78]. Using murine models, Krutzfeldt et al. documented antagomirs targeting miR-122 resulted in reduction of plasma cholesterol levels coupled with altered expression of several genes involved in hepatic lipid biosynthesis [79]. A further study demonstrated inhibition of miR-122 significantly increased hepatic fatty acid oxidation and decreased the biosynthesis of hepatic fatty acid and cholesteral *in vivo* [80]. Although specific miRNA signatures responsible for NAFLD progression await further investigations, accumulating evidence has implicated a pivotal role of miR-122 in the process. For instance, mice lacking the gene encoding miR-122a were viable but later developed temporally controlled steatohepatitis, fibrosis and HCC [81]. Reduced expression of miR-122 has also been reported to upregulate modulators of tissue remodeling (including hypoxia-inducible factor 1 and vimentin) contributing to NASH-induced liver fibrosis [82]. A comparison of miR-122 levels in hepatocytes and primary human HCC cells revealed that miR-122 was down-regulated in HCC cells and the tumorigenic properties of cancer cells could be reversed by re-introduction of miR-122 [83]. Consistently, diminished expression of miR-122 has recently been shown to contribute to the acquisition of sorafenib chemoresistance in HCC [84] while miR-122 restoration in human stem-like HCC cells was capable of prompting tumour dormancy via Smad-independent TGF-β pathway [85], implicating that miR-122 might serve as a potential therapeutic target in HCC.

Being one of the firstly identified oncomirs, miR-21 upregulation has been demonstrated in the liver of patients with NAFLD and hepatic miR-21 expression is positively correlated with the severity of NASH [86, 87]. Using different mouse models of NASH, Loyer et al. [88] showed miR-21 was overexpressed in hepatic biliary and inflammatory cells while inhibition of miR-21 diminished liver injury, inflammation and fibrosis via restoration of peroxisome proliferator-activated receptor alpha (PPARα). miR-21 is also involved in the pathogenesis of HCC by suppressing expression of the tumour suppressor gene phosphatase and tensin homolog (PTEN) [89]. A recent study reported that miR-21 acted downstream of the oncogenic signal transducer and activator of transcription 3 (STAT3) mediating the tumorigenic properties of HCC cells, suggesting miR-21 inhibition or suppression might prove to be a novel treatment of HCC [90].

miR-34a represents another key oncomir displaying elevated expression in patients with NAFLD and positive association with the degree of NASH [86]. It has been shown that the miR-34a/SIRT1/p53 pro-apoptotic pathway played a significant role in human NAFLD development which could be suppressed by the inhibitor ursodeoxycholic acid (UDAC) [91]. Administration of pifithrin-α p-nitro (PFT), a p53 inhibitor, was capable of attenuating steatosis and liver injury in a mouse model of NAFLD partially attributed to the resulting transcriptional suppression of miR-34a [92]. In contrast, miR-34a functions as a tumour suppressor in HCC. A small molecule modulator of miR-34a, termed Rubone, has recently been demonstrated to dramatically inhibit tumour growth in a mouse xenograft model via restoration of miR-34a expression and functioning [93].

In an attempt to identify the pattern of altered gene expression at various time points in a high fat diet-induced NAFLD mouse model, Hur et al. [94] found reduced levels of miR-451 in palmitate-exposed HepG2 cells and mouse liver tissue. *In vitro* analysis further showed miR-451 negatively regulated palmitate-induced interleukin-8 (IL-8) and tumour necrosis factor alpha (TNFα) production supporting a role of miR-451 in preventing the progression from simple steatosis to severely advanced liver disease [94]. Concomitantly, miR-451 has also been documented to function as a potential suppressor of tumour angiogenesis in HCC by targeting IL-6R-STAT3-VEGF signaling, thereby implicating a promising therapeutic role of miR-451 in HCC [95]. miR-221/222, which has been intensively studied in the carcinogenesis of breast cancer, has recently been shown to be overexpressed in human liver in a fibrosis progression-dependent manner [96]. miR-221/222 was further established to promote liver tumorigenesis in a mouse transgenic model [97]. Taken together, studies aiming at elucidating the roles of various miRNAs in the progression from NAFLD to HCC are emerging and further investigations are highly anticipated for detailed insights.

7.4.2 lncRNAs

7.4.2.1 Definition and Functions

Long non-coding RNAs (lncRNAs) are another class of non-protein coding transcripts longer than 200 nucleotides in length that can be further divided into three subtypes: (1) antisense lncRNAs overlapping known protein-coding regions; (2) intronic lncRNAs overlapping transcripts and (3) long intergenic RNAs encoded in the intergenic space between protein-coding areas [98]. The majority of lncRNAs display high specificity with respect to cell subtype, tissue and developmental stage. Although lncRNAs are implicated in the fine-tuning of a wide array of biological processes related to liver homeostasis and cancer including cell proliferation, differentiation and migration, in-depth mechanisms by which the majority of lncRNAs mediate their actions remain largely unknown.

LncRNAs are responsible for the regulation of basal transcription machinery, mRNA processing and stability, protein translation and signal transduction [64]. One of the best-characterized lncRNAs functions in X chromosome inactivation in which the 17 kb transcript *Xist* recruits suppressive epigenetic factors to guarantee repression of gene expression and proper gene dosage in females [99]. Since then, research interest has been focusing on the emerging roles of lncRNAs in carcinogenesis with few reports mentioning the potential functions of lncRNAs in NAFLD. Until recently, Chen et al. [100] demonstrated the lncRNA steroid receptor RNA activator (SRA) promoted hepatic steatosis in mouse model via repressing the expression of adipose triglyceride lipase. In contrast, quite a number of studies have documented the roles of various lncRNAs in the development of HCC.

Highly upregulated in liver cancer (HULC), a 500 nt transcript discovered by cDNA microarray sequencing, is overexpressed 33-fold in HCC [101]. Using a transient silencing approach, the authors further reported HULC knockdown altered the expression of several genes related to the proliferation of HCC. HULC might also serve as a novel biomarker since it could be detected in the peripheral blood of HCC patients [101]. HOX transcript antisense intergenic RNA (HOTAIR) is a 2158 nt lncRNA displaying overexpression in HCC that is predictive of tumour recurrence in liver transplant patients [102]. Transient knockdown of HOTAIR has been shown to suppress tumorigenesis through inhibition of tumour cell growth and induction of cell cycle arrest [103]. Another recently identified lncRNA MALAT1 acts as a proto-oncogene via Wnt pathway activation and induction of the oncogenic splicing factor SRSF1 [104]. By and large, future studies using next generation sequencing will certainly shed light on the roles of more lncRNAs in hepatocarcinogenesis.

7.5 RNA Methylation

7.5.1 Introduction

The central dogma of molecular biology coined in the 50's explains the flow of genetic information in living organisms from DNA to RNA and RNA to protein. As such, messenger RNA (mRNA) represents a bridging link faithfully translating the secrets of life encoded in DNA sequences into functional proteins. However, cellular protein levels are not necessarily associated with mRNA levels, suggesting post-transcriptional mRNA modifications are crucial in the regulation of gene expression [105]. In fact, more than 100 different types of chemical modifications have so far been identified in cellular RNA, including mRNA, ribosomal RNA (rRNA), transfer RNA (tRNA), snRNA and lncRNA [106]. The most prevalent modification among all is adenosine methylation, also known as m^6A or N^6-methyladenosine.

Analysis of nucleic acid modifications and the corresponding effects on epigenetic status has been garnering heated research intention. As mentioned in previous sections, much efforts and interests have been focusing on changes in the chemistry of DNA and the actions of histone proteins as well as their subsequent modifications. It was not until the 1970s with the discovery of m^6A in a broad spectrum of eukaryotes-ranging from yeast, *Drosophila*, viruses to mammals-that investigators had realized and added a whole new RNA dimension to the field of epigenetics [107, 108]. Owing to a series of hindrances including the lack of knowledge of m^6A demethylating enzymes, the short life-span of most RNAs, the resulting idea that m^6A modifications are unalterable, coupled with technical limitations in detecting m^6A-containing mRNAs, however, the pace of RNA epigenetic research had slowed down [109]. In 2011, a new surge of interest was sparked by the discovery that the fat mass and obesity associated protein (FTO) was capable of demethylating RNA, implicating m^6A RNA modifications are highly dynamic subject to finely orchestrated regulations [110]. Elucidation of the methylated transcriptome in mammals was further achieved by technical breakthroughs such as m^6A RNA immunoprecipitation followed by high-throughput sequencing (MeRIP-Seq) [111, 112]. Since then studies aiming at deciphering novel functions of the m^6A modification and more members of the methylation/demethylation machinery have been on the rise.

7.5.2 m⁶A Modification and Regulation

Following two independent studies unequivocally demonstrating that m^6A is a widespread phenomenon in mRNA, further investigations revealed m^6A residues are enriched in 5′ untranslated regions (5' UTRs), around stop codons and in 3' UTRs adjacent to stop codons in mammalian mRNAs [111–113]. Bioinformatic analysis of MeRIP-Seq data identified the recognition sequence for m^6A methylation as RRACH (where R = G/A and H = A/C/U). Occurrence of the consensus motif has been estimated at 1 in 2000 bases in human and almost 90% of all m^6A peaks contain at least one of the motif variants [111, 112]. The dynamic regulation of m^6A methylation is mediated by adenosine methyltransferases ("writers") and demethylases ("erasers").

Methyltransferase like 3 (METTL3) is established as the S-adenosyl-L-methionine (SAM)-binding component of a multiprotein methyltransferase complex responsible for catalyzing m^6A mRNA methylation [114, 115]. The catalytic function of METTL3 was then confirmed by *in vitro* studies demonstrating METTL3 knockdown diminished m^6A peaks in mRNAs from various cell lines [112, 113]. Intriguingly, localization of METTL3 in both cytoplasm and nucleus has been reported, implying m^6A mRNA methylation could occur in both cytoplasmic and nuclear compartments [116]. As a close homologue to METTL3, METTL14 has also been shown to mediate methylation reactions and a complex formed by METTL3 and METTL14 possesses much more efficient activity than separated components [117]. As mentioned previously, the discovery of FTO as the first m^6A mRNA demethylase ignited the conception of m^6A as reversible modification and resurged research interest in RNA methylation. Functional investigations documented silencing of FTO increased m^6A peaks while ectopic expression reduced m^6A peaks [110]. AlkB Homolog 5 (ALKBH5), another member of the mRNA demethylase family, was later identified by *in vitro* and *in vivo* analyses [118].

7.5.3 Role of m⁶A Methylation in Disease

Given that m^6A modifications have been demonstrated in many housekeeping genes influencing a wide array of biological processes including transcription splicing, nuclear RNA export, translation, energy production and cell differentiation, it comes with no surprise that dysregulation of the modification inevitably contributes to obesity, brain development abnormality and other pathological conditions [119–121]. In the field of hepatic diseases, FTO was found to be overexpressed in the livers of NASH patients. *In vitro* studies showed FTO knockdown was protective against palmitate-induced oxidative stress, mitochondrial dysfunction, ER stress and apoptosis, suggesting inhibition of FTO might serve as a treatment option for NASH [122].

The year of 2016 witnessed several inspiring studies documenting the involvement of m^6A mRNA modifications in cancer. A hypoxic tumour microenvironment has been reported to stimulate breast cancer stem cell phenotype by increasing NANOG mRNA and protein expression via induction of HIF and ALKBH5 [123]. In lung adenocarcinoma, METTL3 promoted the growth, survival and invasion of cancer cells [124]. Recently, Ma et al. [125] demonstrated a pivotal role of METTL14 in the progression of HCC. Down-regulation of METTL14 accounted for reduced m^6A modifications in HCC, acted as an adverse prognostic factor for disease-free survival and was significantly correlated with tumour metastasis *in vitro* and *in vivo*. The authors further showed METTL14 depletion reduced expression of the tumour suppressor miR-126 by modulating binding of the microprocessor protein DGCR8 to pri-miR-126 in an m^6A-dependent manner [125]. Taken together, while detailed regulations and mechanisms of DNA epigenetics and histone modifications have been thoroughly studied and are already being targeted in various cancer therapies, the emerging RNA epigenetics may represent the next avenue for investigation in the pursuit for novel prognostic and treatment options.

7.6 Concluding Remarks and Future Perspectives

This chapter highlights some of the key epigenetic modulations implicated in the development of NAFLD-HCC. Further in-depth studies would undoubtedly reveal a more comprehensive picture of the role of epigenetics in the development of pathological conditions. On the basis of currently wealthy knowledge of DNA epigenetics, the rapidly growing field of RNA epigenetics will certainly drive forward a new avenue of research direction shedding light on the advancement of better diagnostics, prognostics and therapeutics in the coming era of precision medicine.

References

1. Rinella ME. Nonalcoholic fatty liver disease: a systematic review. JAMA. 2015;313:2263–73.
2. Bellentani S, Scaglioni F, Marino M, Bedogni G. Epidemiology of non-alcoholic fatty liver disease. Dig Dis. 2010;28:155–61.
3. Hardy T, Oakley F, Anstee QM, Day CP. Nonalcoholic fatty liver disease: pathogenesis and disease spectrum. Annu Rev Pathol. 2016;11:451–96.
4. Farrell GC. Larter CZ. Nonalcoholic fatty liver disease: from steatosis to cirrhosis. Hepatology. 2006;43:S99–S112.
5. Sun C, Fan JG, Qiao L. Potential epigenetic mechanism in non-alcoholic fatty liver disease. Int J Mol Sci. 2015;16:5161–79.
6. Berlanga A, Guiu-Jurado E, Porras JA, Auguet T. Molecular pathways in non-alcoholic fatty liver disease. Clin Exp Gastroenterol. 2014;7:221–39.
7. Lee JH, Friso S, Choi SW. Epigenetic mechanisms underlying the link between non-alcoholic fatty liver diseases and nutrition. Forum Nutr. 2014;6:3303–25.
8. Anstee QM, Day CP. The genetics of NAFLD. Nat Rev Gastroenterol Hepatol. 2013;10:645–55.
9. Zilberman D, Henikoff S. Genome-wide analysis of DNA methylation patterns. Development. 2007;134:3959–65.
10. Tahiliani M, Koh KP, Shen Y, Pastor WA, Bandukwala H, Brudno Y, et al. Conversion of 5-methylcytosine to 5-hydroxymethylcytosine in mammalian DNA by MLL partner TET1. Science. 2009;324:930–5.
11. Ito S, Shen L, Dai Q, Wu SC, Collins LB, Swenberg JA, et al. Tet proteins can convert 5-methylcytosine to 5-formylcytosine and 5-carboxylcytosine. Science. 2011;333:1300–3.
12. Park LK, Friso S, Choi SW. Nutritional influences on epigenetics and age-related disease. Proc Nutr Soc. 2012;71:75–83.
13. da Silva RP, Kelly KB, Al Rajabi A, Jacobs RL. Novel insights on interactions between folate and lipid metabolism. Biofactors. 2014;40:277–83.
14. Jacobs RL, Lingrell S, Zhao Y, Francis GA, Vance DE. Hepatic CTP:phosphocholine cytidylyltransferase-alpha is a critical predictor of plasma high density lipoprotein and very low density lipoprotein. J Biol Chem. 2008;283:2147–55.
15. Martinez-Chantar ML, Corrales FJ, Martinez-Cruz LA, Garcia-Trevijano ER, Huang ZZ, Chen L, et al. Spontaneous oxidative stress and liver tumors in mice lacking methionine adenosyltransferase 1A. FASEB J. 2002;16:1292–4.
16. Tryndyak VP, Han T, Muskhelishvili L, Fuscoe JC, Ross SA, Beland FA, et al. Coupling global methylation and gene expression profiles reveal key pathophysiological events in liver injury induced by a methyl-deficient diet. Mol Nutr Food Res. 2011;55:411–8.
17. Sookoian S, Puri P, Castano GO, Scian R, Mirshahi F, Sanyal AJ, et al. Nonalcoholic steatohepatitis is associated with a state of betaine-insufficiency. Liver Int. 2017;37:611–9.
18. Bataller R, Brenner DA. Liver fibrosis. J Clin Invest. 2005;115:209–18.
19. Moreira RK. Hepatic stellate cells and liver fibrosis. Arch Pathol Lab Med. 2007;131:1728–34.
20. Friedman SL. Cytokines and fibrogenesis. Semin Liver Dis. 1999;19:129–40.
21. Law JA, Jacobsen SE. Establishing, maintaining and modifying DNA methylation patterns in plants and animals. Nat Rev Genet. 2010;11:204–20.
22. Pogribny IP, Tryndyak VP, Bagnyukova TV, Melnyk S, Montgomery B, Ross SA, et al. Hepatic epigenetic phenotype predetermines individual susceptibility to hepatic steatosis in mice fed a lipogenic methyl-deficient diet. J Hepatol. 2009;51:176–86.
23. Wu Y, Bu F, Yu H, Li W, Huang C, Meng X, et al. Methylation of Septin9 mediated by DNMT3a enhances hepatic stellate cells activation and liver fibrogenesis. Toxicol Appl Pharmacol. 2016;315:35–49.
24. Pirola CJ, Scian R, Gianotti TF, Dopazo H, Rohr C, Martino JS, et al. Epigenetic modifications in the biology of nonalcoholic fatty liver disease: the role of DNA Hydroxymethylation and TET proteins. Medicine (Baltimore). 2015;94:e1480.
25. Murphy SK, Yang H, Moylan CA, Pang H, Dellinger A, Abdelmalek MF, et al. Relationship between methylome and transcriptome in patients with nonalcoholic fatty liver disease. Gastroenterology. 2013;145:1076–87.
26. Zeybel M, Hardy T, Robinson SM, Fox C, Anstee QM, Ness T, et al. Differential DNA methylation of genes involved in fibrosis progression in non-alcoholic fatty liver disease and alcoholic liver disease. Clin Epigenetics. 2015;7:25.

27. Hanahan D, Weinberg RA. Hallmarks of cancer: the next generation. Cell. 2011;144:646–74.
28. Villanueva A, Portela A, Sayols S, Battiston C, Hoshida Y, Mendez-Gonzalez J, et al. DNA methylation-based prognosis and epidrivers in hepatocellular carcinoma. Hepatology. 2015;61:1945–56.
29. Revill K, Wang T, Lachenmayer A, Kojima K, Harrington A, Li J, et al. Genome-wide methylation analysis and epigenetic unmasking identify tumor suppressor genes in hepatocellular carcinoma. Gastroenterology. 2013;145:1424–1435 e1421–1425.
30. Li H, Yang F, Gao B, Yu Z, Liu X, Xie F, et al. Hepatitis B virus infection in hepatocellular carcinoma tissues upregulates expression of DNA methyltransferases. Int J Clin Exp Med. 2015;8:4175–85.
31. Thienpont B, Steinbacher J, Zhao H, D'Anna F, Kuchnio A, Ploumakis A, et al. Tumour hypoxia causes DNA hypermethylation by reducing TET activity. Nature. 2016;537:63–8.
32. Chen ZJ, Pikaard CS. Epigenetic silencing of RNA polymerase I transcription: a role for DNA methylation and histone modification in nucleolar dominance. Genes Dev. 1997;11:2124–36.
33. Gallego-Duran R, Romero-Gomez M. Epigenetic mechanisms in non-alcoholic fatty liver disease: an emerging field. World J Hepatol. 2015;7:2497–502.
34. Granger A, Abdullah I, Huebner F, Stout A, Wang T, Huebner T, et al. Histone deacetylase inhibition reduces myocardial ischemia-reperfusion injury in mice. FASEB J. 2008;22:3549–60.
35. Tian Y, Wong VW, Chan HL, Cheng AS. Epigenetic regulation of hepatocellular carcinoma in non-alcoholic fatty liver disease. Semin Cancer Biol. 2013;23:471–82.
36. Lee KK, Workman JL. Histone acetyltransferase complexes: one size doesn't fit all. Nat Rev Mol Cell Biol. 2007;8:284–95.
37. Chan HM, La Thangue NB. p300/CBP proteins: HATs for transcriptional bridges and scaffolds. J Cell Sci. 2001;114:2363–73.
38. Bricambert J, Miranda J, Benhamed F, Girard J, Postic C, Dentin R. Salt-inducible kinase 2 links transcriptional coactivator p300 phosphorylation to the prevention of ChREBP-dependent hepatic steatosis in mice. J Clin Invest. 2010;120:4316–31.
39. Jia YL, Xu M, Dou CW, Liu ZK, Xue YM, Yao BW, et al. P300/CBP-associated factor (PCAF) inhibits the growth of hepatocellular carcinoma by promoting cell autophagy. Cell Death Dis. 2016;7:e2400.
40. Feng D, Liu T, Sun Z, Bugge A, Mullican SE, Alenghat T, et al. A circadian rhythm orchestrated by histone deacetylase 3 controls hepatic lipid metabolism. Science. 2011;331:1315–9.
41. Bae HJ, Jung KH, Eun JW, Shen Q, Kim HS, Park SJ, et al. MicroRNA-221 governs tumor suppressor HDAC6 to potentiate malignant progression of liver cancer. J Hepatol. 2015;63:408–19.
42. Blander G, Guarente L. The Sir2 family of protein deacetylases. Annu Rev Biochem. 2004;73:417–35.
43. Herranz D, Serrano M. SIRT1: recent lessons from mouse models. Nat Rev Cancer. 2010;10:819–23.
44. Herranz D, Munoz-Martin M, Canamero M, Mulero F, Martinez-Pastor B, Fernandez-Capetillo O, et al. Sirt1 improves healthy ageing and protects from metabolic syndrome-associated cancer. Nat Commun. 2010;1:3.
45. Liu L, Liu C, Zhang Q, Shen J, Zhang H, Shan J, et al. SIRT1-mediated transcriptional regulation of SOX2 is important for self-renewal of liver cancer stem cells. Hepatology. 2016;64:814–27.
46. Li Y, Xu S, Li J, Zheng L, Feng M, Wang X, et al. SIRT1 facilitates hepatocellular carcinoma metastasis by promoting PGC-1alpha-mediated mitochondrial biogenesis. Oncotarget. 2016;7:29255–74.
47. Chen J, Chan AW, To KF, Chen W, Zhang Z, Ren J, et al. SIRT2 overexpression in hepatocellular carcinoma mediates epithelial to mesenchymal transition by protein kinase B/glycogen synthase kinase-3beta/beta-catenin signaling. Hepatology. 2013;57:2287–98.
48. Kim HS, Patel K, Muldoon-Jacobs K, Bisht KS, Aykin-Burns N, Pennington JD, et al. SIRT3 is a mitochondria-localized tumor suppressor required for maintenance of mitochondrial integrity and metabolism during stress. Cancer Cell. 2010;17:41–52.
49. Hirschey MD, Shimazu T, Jing E, Grueter CA, Collins AM, Aouizerat B, et al. SIRT3 deficiency and mitochondrial protein hyperacetylation accelerate the development of the metabolic syndrome. Mol Cell. 2011;44:177–90.
50. Rice JC, Briggs SD, Ueberheide B, Barber CM, Shabanowitz J, Hunt DF, et al. Histone methyltransferases direct different degrees of methylation to define distinct chromatin domains. Mol Cell. 2003;12:1591–8.
51. Fei Q, Shang K, Zhang J, Chuai S, Kong D, Zhou T, et al. Histone methyltransferase SETDB1 regulates liver cancer cell growth through methylation of p53. Nat Commun. 2015;6:8651.
52. Ueda K, Hayaishi O. ADP-ribosylation. Annu Rev Biochem. 1985;54:73–100.
53. Belenky P, Bogan KL, Brenner C. NAD+ metabolism in health and disease. Trends Biochem Sci. 2007;32:12–9.
54. Corda D, Di Girolamo M. Functional aspects of protein mono-ADP-ribosylation. EMBO J. 2003;22:1953–8.
55. Nomura F, Yaguchi M, Togawa A, Miyazaki M, Isobe K, Miyake M, et al. Enhancement of poly-adenosine diphosphate-ribosylation in human hepatocellular carcinoma. J Gastroenterol Hepatol. 2000;15:529–35.
56. Lampiasi N, Umezawa K, Montalto G, Poly CM. (ADP-ribose) polymerase inhibition synergizes with the NF-kappaB inhibitor DHMEQ to kill hepatocellular carcinoma cells. Biochim Biophys Acta. 2014;1843:2662–73.

57. Verger A, Perdomo J, Crossley M. Modification with SUMO. A role in transcriptional regulation. EMBO Rep. 2003;4:137–42.
58. Hay RT. SUMO: a history of modification. Mol Cell. 2005;18:1–12.
59. Muller S, Hoege C, Pyrowolakis G, Jentsch S. SUMO, ubiquitin's mysterious cousin. Nat Rev Mol Cell Biol. 2001;2:202–10.
60. Yeh ET. SUMOylation and De-SUMOylation: wrestling with life's processes. J Biol Chem. 2009;284:8223–7.
61. Shiio Y, Eisenman RN. Histone sumoylation is associated with transcriptional repression. Proc Natl Acad Sci U S A. 2003;100:13225–30.
62. Jin ZL, Pei H, Xu YH, Yu J, Deng T. The SUMO-specific protease SENP5 controls DNA damage response and promotes tumorigenesis in hepatocellular carcinoma. Eur Rev Med Pharmacol Sci. 2016;20:3566–73.
63. Liu J, Tao X, Zhang J, Wang P, Sha M, Ma Y, et al. Small ubiquitin-related modifier 1 is involved in hepatocellular carcinoma progression via mediating p65 nuclear translocation. Oncotarget. 2016;7:22206–18.
64. Rinn JL, Chang HY. Genome regulation by long noncoding RNAs. Annu Rev Biochem. 2012;81:145–66.
65. Chaudhuri K, Chatterjee R. MicroRNA detection and target prediction: integration of computational and experimental approaches. DNA Cell Biol. 2007;26:321–37.
66. Alvarez-Garcia I, Miska EA. MicroRNA functions in animal development and human disease. Development. 2005;132:4653–62.
67. Borchert GM, Lanier W, Davidson BL. RNA polymerase III transcribes human microRNAs. Nat Struct Mol Biol. 2006;13:1097–101.
68. Inui M, Martello G, Piccolo S. MicroRNA control of signal transduction. Nat Rev Mol Cell Biol. 2010;11:252–63.
69. Brennecke J, Stark A, Russell RB, Cohen SM. Principles of microRNA-target recognition. PLoS Biol. 2005;3:e85.
70. Mraz M, Pospisilova S. MicroRNAs in chronic lymphocytic leukemia: from causality to associations and back. Expert Rev Hematol. 2012;5:579–81.
71. Wang F, Zheng Z, Guo J, Ding X. Correlation and quantitation of microRNA aberrant expression in tissues and sera from patients with breast tumor. Gynecol Oncol. 2010;119:586–93.
72. Sotiropoulou G, Pampalakis G, Lianidou E, Mourelatos Z. Emerging roles of microRNAs as molecular switches in the integrated circuit of the cancer cell. RNA. 2009;15:1443–61.
73. Yang L, Belaguli N, Berger DH. MicroRNA and colorectal cancer. World J Surg. 2009;33:638–46.
74. Walter BA, Valera VA, Pinto PA, Merino MJ. Comprehensive microRNA profiling of prostate cancer. J Cancer. 2013;4:350–7.
75. Iorio MV, Visone R, Di Leva G, Donati V, Petrocca F, Casalini P, et al. MicroRNA signatures in human ovarian cancer. Cancer Res. 2007;67:8699–707.
76. Rottiers V, Naar AM. MicroRNAs in metabolism and metabolic disorders. Nat Rev Mol Cell Biol. 2012;13:239–50.
77. Celikbilek M, Baskol M, Taheri S, Deniz K, Dogan S, Zararsiz G, et al. Circulating microRNAs in patients with non-alcoholic fatty liver disease. World J Hepatol. 2014;6:613–20.
78. Lewis AP, Jopling CL. Regulation and biological function of the liver-specific miR-122. Biochem Soc Trans. 2010;38:1553–7.
79. Krutzfeldt J, Rajewsky N, Braich R, Rajeev KG, Tuschl T, Manoharan M, et al. Silencing of microRNAs in vivo with 'antagomirs'. Nature. 2005;438:685–9.
80. Esau C, Davis S, Murray SF, Yu XX, Pandey SK, Pear M, et al. miR-122 regulation of lipid metabolism revealed by in vivo antisense targeting. Cell Metab. 2006;3:87–98.
81. Tsai WC, Hsu SD, Hsu CS, Lai TC, Chen SJ, Shen R, et al. MicroRNA-122 plays a critical role in liver homeostasis and hepatocarcinogenesis. J Clin Invest. 2012;122:2884–97.
82. Csak T, Bala S, Lippai D, Satishchandran A, Catalano D, Kodys K, et al. microRNA-122 regulates hypoxia-inducible factor-1 and vimentin in hepatocytes and correlates with fibrosis in diet-induced steatohepatitis. Liver Int. 2015;35:532–41.
83. Coulouarn C, Factor VM, Andersen JB, Durkin ME, Thorgeirsson SS. Loss of miR-122 expression in liver cancer correlates with suppression of the hepatic phenotype and gain of metastatic properties. Oncogene. 2009;28:3526–36.
84. Kishikawa T, Otsuka M, Tan PS, Ohno M, Sun X, Yoshikawa T, et al. Decreased miR122 in hepatocellular carcinoma leads to chemoresistance with increased arginine. Oncotarget. 2015;6:8339–52.
85. Boix L, Lopez-Oliva JM, Rhodes AC, Bruix J. Restoring mir122 in human stem-like hepatocarcinoma cells, prompts tumor dormancy through smad-independent TGF-beta pathway. Oncotarget. 2016;7:71309.
86. Cheung O, Puri P, Eicken C, Contos MJ, Mirshahi F, Maher JW, et al. Nonalcoholic steatohepatitis is associated with altered hepatic MicroRNA expression. Hepatology. 2008;48:1810–20.
87. Gori M, Arciello M, Balsano C. MicroRNAs in nonalcoholic fatty liver disease: novel biomarkers and prognostic tools during the transition from steatosis to hepatocarcinoma. Biomed Res Int. 2014;2014:741465.
88. Loyer X, Paradis V, Henique C, Vion AC, Colnot N, Guerin CL, et al. Liver microRNA-21 is overexpressed in non-alcoholic steatohepatitis and contributes to the disease in experimental models by inhibiting PPARalpha expression. Gut. 2016;65:1882–94.

89. Vinciguerra M, Sgroi A, Veyrat-Durebex C, Rubbia-Brandt L, Buhler LH, Foti M. Unsaturated fatty acids inhibit the expression of tumor suppressor phosphatase and tensin homolog (PTEN) via microRNA-21 up-regulation in hepatocytes. Hepatology. 2009;49:1176–84.
90. Zhang N, Duan WD, Leng JJ, Zhou L, Wang X, Xu YZ, et al. STAT3 regulates the migration and invasion of a stemlike subpopulation through microRNA21 and multiple targets in hepatocellular carcinoma. Oncol Rep. 2015;33:1493–8.
91. Castro RE, Ferreira DM, Afonso MB, Borralho PM, Machado MV, Cortez-Pinto H, et al. miR-34a/SIRT1/p53 is suppressed by ursodeoxycholic acid in the rat liver and activated by disease severity in human non-alcoholic fatty liver disease. J Hepatol. 2013;58:119–25.
92. Derdak Z, Villegas KA, Harb R, Wu AM, Sousa A, Wands JR. Inhibition of p53 attenuates steatosis and liver injury in a mouse model of non-alcoholic fatty liver disease. J Hepatol. 2013;58:785–91.
93. Xiao Z, Li CH, Chan SL, Xu F, Feng L, Wang Y, et al. A small-molecule modulator of the tumor-suppressor miR34a inhibits the growth of hepatocellular carcinoma. Cancer Res. 2014;74:6236–47.
94. Hur W, Lee JH, Kim SW, Kim JH, Bae SH, Kim M, et al. Downregulation of microRNA-451 in non-alcoholic steatohepatitis inhibits fatty acid-induced proinflammatory cytokine production through the AMPK/AKT pathway. Int J Biochem Cell Biol. 2015;64:265–76.
95. Liu X, Zhang A, Xiang J, Lv Y, Zhang X. miR-451 acts as a suppressor of angiogenesis in hepatocellular carcinoma by targeting the IL-6R-STAT3 pathway. Oncol Rep. 2016;36:1385–92.
96. Ogawa T, Enomoto M, Fujii H, Sekiya Y, Yoshizato K, Ikeda K, et al. MicroRNA-221/222 upregulation indicates the activation of stellate cells and the progression of liver fibrosis. Gut. 2012;61:1600–9.
97. Callegari E, Elamin BK, Giannone F, Milazzo M, Altavilla G, Fornari F, et al. Liver tumorigenicity promoted by microRNA-221 in a mouse transgenic model. Hepatology. 2012;56:1025–33.
98. Hardy T, Mann DA. Epigenetics in liver disease: from biology to therapeutics. Gut. 2016;65:1895.
99. Zhao J, Sun BK, Erwin JA, Song JJ, Lee JT. Polycomb proteins targeted by a short repeat RNA to the mouse X chromosome. Science. 2008;322:750–6.
100. Chen G, Yu D, Nian X, Liu J, Koenig RJ, Xu B, et al. LncRNA SRA promotes hepatic steatosis through repressing the expression of adipose triglyceride lipase (ATGL). Sci Rep. 2016;6:35531.
101. Panzitt K, Tschernatsch MM, Guelly C, Moustafa T, Stradner M, Strohmaier HM, et al. Characterization of HULC, a novel gene with striking up-regulation in hepatocellular carcinoma, as noncoding RNA. Gastroenterology. 2007;132:330–42.
102. Yang Z, Zhou L, Wu LM, Lai MC, Xie HY, Zhang F, et al. Overexpression of long non-coding RNA HOTAIR predicts tumor recurrence in hepatocellular carcinoma patients following liver transplantation. Ann Surg Oncol. 2011;18:1243–50.
103. Fu WM, Zhu X, Wang WM, Lu YF, Hu BG, Wang H, et al. Hotair mediates hepatocarcinogenesis through suppressing miRNA-218 expression and activating P14 and P16 signaling. J Hepatol. 2015;63:886–95.
104. Malakar P, Shilo A, Mogilavsky A, Stein I, Pikarsky E, Nevo Y, et al. Long noncoding RNA MALAT1 promotes hepatocellular carcinoma development by SRSF1 up-regulation and mTOR activation. Cancer Res. 2017;77(5):1155–67.
105. Wu L, Candille SI, Choi Y, Xie D, Jiang L, Li-Pook-Than J, et al. Variation and genetic control of protein abundance in humans. Nature. 2013;499:79–82.
106. Machnicka MA, Milanowska K, Osman Oglou O, Purta E, Kurkowska M, Olchowik A, et al. MODOMICS: a database of RNA modification pathways--2013 update. Nucleic Acids Res. 2013;41:D262–7.
107. Wei CM, Moss B. Methylated nucleotides block 5′-terminus of vaccinia virus messenger RNA. Proc Natl Acad Sci U S A. 1975;72:318–22.
108. Rottman FM, Desrosiers RC, Friderici K. Nucleotide methylation patterns in eukaryotic mRNA. Prog Nucleic Acid Res Mol Biol. 1976;19:21–38.
109. Cao G, Li HB, Yin Z, Flavell RA. Recent advances in dynamic m6A RNA modification. Open Biol. 2016;6:160003.
110. Jia G, Fu Y, Zhao X, Dai Q, Zheng G, Yang Y, et al. N6-methyladenosine in nuclear RNA is a major substrate of the obesity-associated FTO. Nat Chem Biol. 2011;7:885–7.
111. Meyer KD, Saletore Y, Zumbo P, Elemento O, Mason CE, Jaffrey SR. Comprehensive analysis of mRNA methylation reveals enrichment in 3′ UTRs and near stop codons. Cell. 2012;149:1635–46.
112. Dominissini D, Moshitch-Moshkovitz S, Schwartz S, Salmon-Divon M, Ungar L, Osenberg S, et al. Topology of the human and mouse m6A RNA methylomes revealed by m6A-seq. Nature. 2012;485:201–6.
113. Batista PJ, Molinie B, Wang J, Qu K, Zhang J, Li L, et al. m(6)A RNA modification controls cell fate transition in mammalian embryonic stem cells. Cell Stem Cell. 2014;15:707–19.
114. Bokar JA, Rath-Shambaugh ME, Ludwiczak R, Narayan P, Rottman F. Characterization and artial purification of mRNA N6-adenosine methyltransferase from HeLa cell nuclei. Internal mRNA methylation requires a multisubunit complex. J Biol Chem. 1994;269:17697–704.
115. Bokar JA, Shambaugh ME, Polayes D, Matera AG, Purification RFM. cDNA cloning of the AdoMet-binding subunit of the human mRNA (N6-adenosine)-methyltransferase. RNA. 1997;3:1233–47.
116. Chen T, Hao YJ, Zhang Y, Li MM, Wang M, Han W, et al. m(6)A RNA methylation is regulated by microRNAs and promotes reprogramming to pluripotency. Cell Stem Cell. 2015;16:289–301.

117. Liu J, Yue Y, Han D, Wang X, Fu Y, Zhang L, et al. A METTL3-METTL14 complex mediates mammalian nuclear RNA N6-adenosine methylation. Nat Chem Biol. 2014;10:93–5.
118. Zheng G, Dahl JA, Niu Y, Fedorcsak P, Huang CM, Li CJ, et al. ALKBH5 is a mammalian RNA demethylase that impacts RNA metabolism and mouse fertility. Mol Cell. 2013;49:18–29.
119. Boissel S, Reish O, Proulx K, Kawagoe-Takaki H, Sedgwick B, Yeo GS, et al. Loss-of-function mutation in the dioxygenase-encoding FTO gene causes severe growth retardation and multiple malformations. Am J Hum Genet. 2009;85:106–11.
120. Klungland A, Dahl JA. Dynamic RNA modifications in disease. Curr Opin Genet Dev. 2014;26:47–52.
121. Blanco S, Frye M. Role of RNA methyltransferases in tissue renewal and pathology. Curr Opin Cell Biol. 2014;31:1–7.
122. Lim A, Zhou J, Sinha RA, Singh BK, Ghosh S, Lim KH, et al. Hepatic FTO expression is increased in NASH and its silencing attenuates palmitic acid-induced lipotoxicity. Biochem Biophys Res Commun. 2016;479:476–81.
123. Zhang C, Samanta D, Lu H, Bullen JW, Zhang H, Chen I, et al. Hypoxia induces the breast cancer stem cell phenotype by HIF-dependent and ALKBH5-mediated m(6)A-demethylation of NANOG mRNA. Proc Natl Acad Sci U S A. 2016;113:E2047–56.
124. Lin S, Choe J, Du P, Triboulet R, Gregory RI. The m(6)A methyltransferase METTL3 promotes translation in human cancer cells. Mol Cell. 2016;62:335–45.
125. Ma JZ, Yang F, Zhou CC, Liu F, Yuan JH, Wang F, et al. METTL14 suppresses the metastatic potential of hepatocellular carcinoma by modulating N6-methyladenosine-dependent primary MicroRNA processing. Hepatology. 2017;65:529–43.

The Influence of Gut Microbial Metabolism on the Development and Progression of Non-alcoholic Fatty Liver Disease

8

Wei Jia and Cynthia Rajani

Abstract

Non-alcoholic fatty liver disease (NAFLD) is defined as the presence of excess fat in the liver parenchyma in the absence of excess alcohol consumption and overt inflammation. It has also been described as the hepatic manifestation of metabolic syndrome (Than NN, Newsome PN, Atherosclerosis. 239:192–202, 2015). The incidence of NAFLD has been reported to be 43–60% in diabetics, ~90% in patients with hyperlipidemia and 91% in morbidly obese patients (Than NN, Newsome PN, Atherosclerosis. 239:192–202, 2015, Machado M, Marques-Vidal P, Cortez-Pinto H, J Hepatol, 45:600–606, 2006, Vernon G, Baranova A, Younossi ZM, Aliment Pharmacol Ther, 34:274–285, 2011). The risk factors that have been associated with the development of NAFLD include male gender, increasing age, obesity, insulin resistance, diabetes and hyperlipidemia (Attar BM, Van Thiel DH, Sci World J, 2013:481893, 2013, Gaggini M, Morelli M, Buzzigoli E, DeFronzo RA, Bugianesi E, Gastaldelli A, Forum Nutr, 5:1544–1460, 2013). All of these risk factors have been linked to alterations of the gut microbiota, ie., gut dysbiosis (He X, Ji G, Jia W, Li H, Int J Mol Sci, 17:300, 2016). However, it must be pointed out that the prevalence of NAFLD in normal weight individuals without metabolic risk factors is ~16% (Than NN, Newsome PN, Atherosclerosis. 239:192–202, 2015). This fact has led some investigators to hypothesize that the gut microbiota can impact lipid metabolism in the liver independently of obesity-related metabolic factors (Marchesi JR, Adams DH, Fava F, Hermes GD, Hirschfield GM, Hold g, et al., Gut, 65:330 339, 2016) (Le Roy T, Llopis M, Lepage P, Bruneau A, Rabot S, Bevilacqua C, et al., Gut, 62:1787–1794, 2013). In this chapter, we will explore the effect of the gut microbiota on hepatic lipid metabolism and how this affects the development of NAFLD.

Keywords

Non-alcoholic fatty liver disease · Gut microbiota · Diabetes · Steatosis · Metabolic syndrome · Bile acids

W. Jia (✉)
University of Hawaii Cancer Center, Honolulu, HI, USA

Shanghai Jiao Tong University School of Medicine, Shanghai, China
e-mail: wjia@cc.hawaii.edu

C. Rajani
University of Hawaii Cancer Center, Honolulu, HI, USA
e-mail: crajani@cc.hawaii.edu

J. Yu (ed.), *Obesity, Fatty Liver and Liver Cancer*, Advances in Experimental Medicine and Biology 1061, https://doi.org/10.1007/978-981-10-8684-7_8

8.1 Introduction

Non-alcoholic fatty liver disease (NAFLD) is defined as the presence of excess fat in the liver parenchyma in the absence of excess alcohol consumption and overt inflammation. It has also been described as the hepatic manifestation of metabolic syndrome. A much broader definition of NAFLD that has come into common use is that it can be considered as the entire spectrum of liver disease which progresses from simple steatosis → steatohepatitis → fibrosis → cirrhosis and finally leading to either liver transplantation or hepatocarcinoma (HCC) [1]. The incidence of NAFLD has been reported to be 43–60% in diabetics, ~90% in patients with hyperlipidemia and 91% in morbidly obese patients [1–3]. The risk factors that have been associated with the development of NAFLD include male gender, increasing age, obesity, insulin resistance, diabetes and hyperlipidemia [4, 5]. All of these risk factors have been linked to alterations of the gut microbiota, ie., gut dysbiosis [6]. The gut microbiota are considered to be an additional organ in the body which, as a collection of many different cells, works together with the host to promote health but can also malfunction and initiate disease [7]. Although gut microbiota have been implicated as part of the etiology of the risk factors leading to NAFLD, it must be pointed out that the prevalence of NAFLD in normal weight individuals without metabolic risk factors is ~16% [1]. The fact that not all persons with NAFLD are obese or have other associated metabolic risk factors has led some investigators to hypothesize that the gut microbiota can impact lipid metabolism in the liver independently of obesity-related metabolic factors [8]. In this chapter, we will explore the effect of the gut microbiota on hepatic lipid metabolism and how this affects the development of NAFLD.

8.2 The Gut Microbiota and Development of NAFLD

NAFLD is prevalent among obese persons, however, not all obese people develop NAFLD. In this section, we will discuss the evidence from pre-clinical and clinical studies that provide evidence for gut microbiota involvement in the etiology of NAFLD. High fat diet (HFD) is a standard method for inducing obesity, steatosis and insulin resistance in mice [9]. Early studies showed that germ-free (GF) mice treated with HFD gained less weight and exhibited less glycaemia, insulinemia, and better glucose tolerance and insulin sensitivity relative to conventional mice [10]. These differences in metabolism may be partially explained by the increased fatty acid (FA) oxidation and decreased lipogenesis observed in germ-free (GF) mice [11]. It has also been shown that diabetes-susceptible and resistant mice of the same genetic background are associated with different gut microbiota [12]. A recent study, which will be discussed below, was undertaken to examine NAFLD with the hypothesis that NAFLD could be dissociated from the degree of obesity and diabetes via the gut microbiota in mice [8].

In order to understand the role of the gut microbiota in NAFLD development, a conventional strain of C57BL/6J mice were fed a common high fat diet (HFD) for 16 weeks [8]. Within the same mouse strain, HFD treatment produced mice that responded to the diet by developing high levels of glycaemia, systemic inflammation and steatosis (responders) and also several mice that did not develop metabolic disorders (non-responders). From these two groups of mice, one responder and one non-responder was chosen that had similar body weight, fat pad mass and food intake to become a fecal donor mouse. Two groups of germ-free (GF) C57BL/6J mice were then submitted to fecal transplantation from either the responder mouse or the non-responder to generate RR mice and NRR mice, respectively. The RR and NRR groups were fed the same HFD for 16 weeks. Both NRR and RR groups exhibited similar food intake, weight gain and size of epididymal fat pads, but the RR group had enhanced levels of fasting glycaemia and insulinemia. The HOMO-IR index was 2.4-fold greater in the RR group indicating development of much more insulin resistance. Total caecal concentrations of short-chain fatty acids (SCFAs) were similar between NRR and RR but isobutyrate and isovalerate, bacterial fermentation products of valine and leucine were significantly higher in the caecum of RR mice. The NRR group developed slight to mild steatosis while the RR group developed marked steatosis with a 30% higher triglyceride (TG) level. The transcription factors, sterol regulatory binding protein (SREBP) 1c and carbohydrate response element binding protein (ChREBP) were found to be increased ~2-fold in RR *vs.* NRR mice. Both of these factors affect hepatic *de novo* lipogenesis (DNL) [13].

The microbiota of the mice on HFD showed a clustering pattern with two bacterial species, *Lachnospiraceae bacterium 609* and *Barnesiella intestinihominis*, higher in RR mice at both week 3 and 16, and *Bacteroides vulgates* was higher in NRR mice [8]. *Barnesiella intestinihominis* belongs to the family Porphyromonadaceae which was shown previously to be increased in inflammasome deficient mice that developed marked steatosis and inflammation and also in a clinical study of obese NAFLD patients relative to healthy lean [14]. On the other hand, *Bacteroides vulgates* was previously found to be decreased in patients with type-2 diabetes (T2D) suggesting this bacterium may exert protective effects against T2D [15]. More generally, *Barnesiella* and *Roseburia* genera were found to be more represented in RR mice while *Allobaculum* was increased in the NRR group. RR mice had significantly increased Firmicutes species than NRR mice even though the degree of adiposity was the same for both groups.

Other findings that were remarkable in this study were that there was no significant difference in systemic and hepatic inflammation or in body and liver weights between RR and NRR indicating that the gut microbiota can impact hepatic lipid metabolism independently of a systemic pro-inflammatory state and that insulin resistance does not depend on a greater degree of obesity [8]. Based on this study, the impact of microbiota on steatosis and NAFLD may be explained by their function in regulating glucose homeostasis via the transcription factors ChREBP and SREBP, which control transcription of lipogenic genes. Both ChREBP and SREBP transcription factor activities are under the control of another important hepatic transcription factor, the bile acid (BA) sensitive farnesoid X receptor (FXR). In the next section, we shall briefly review hepatic lipid metabolism and its connectivity with glucose metabolism and how BA activation of FXR influences lipid and glucose metabolism in the liver.

8.3 Hepatic Lipid Metabolism and Its Interface with Glucose Metabolism in NAFLD

Lipid metabolism begins in the intestine where lipids are emulsified by bile acids (BAs). Lipid emulsification allows them to become hydrolyzed and subsequently absorbed by the enterocytes where they become converted to lipoprotein particles called nascent chylomicrons. Nascent chylomicrons then travel through the lymphatic system into the circulation where they are processed further via replacement of apoproteins A-I and IV (apoI,IV) with apoE and apoC-II which allows them to be broken down into free fatty acids (FFAs), glycerol and chylomicron fragments. FFAs are then partially removed from the blood by adipose tissue while the cholesteryl-ester enriched and TG depleted chylomicron fragments are endocytosed by the liver and broken down in the lysosomes into recyclable hepatic glycerol, FA, cholesterol, amino acid and phosphate residues [16]. Therefore, hepatic FAs come from four sources, (1) lipolysis of adipose tissue, (2) dietary ingestion, (3) endogenous production via *de novo* lipogenesis (DNL) and, (4) released from hepatic lysosomes by autophagy. In a clinical study of NAFLD patients, it was determined that ~50–60% of TGs in the liver were derived from nonesterified FFAs (from lipolysis of adipose tissue and chylomicron fragments), ~19–33% from DNL and 8–22% from dietary sources [16, 17]. The increase in DNL in NAFLD was thought to be due to dysregulation of SREBP1c and FoxO-modulation of insulin signaling, thereby providing a link between hepatic lipid and glucose metabolism [18]. Hepatic FA synthesis, on the other hand, is initi-

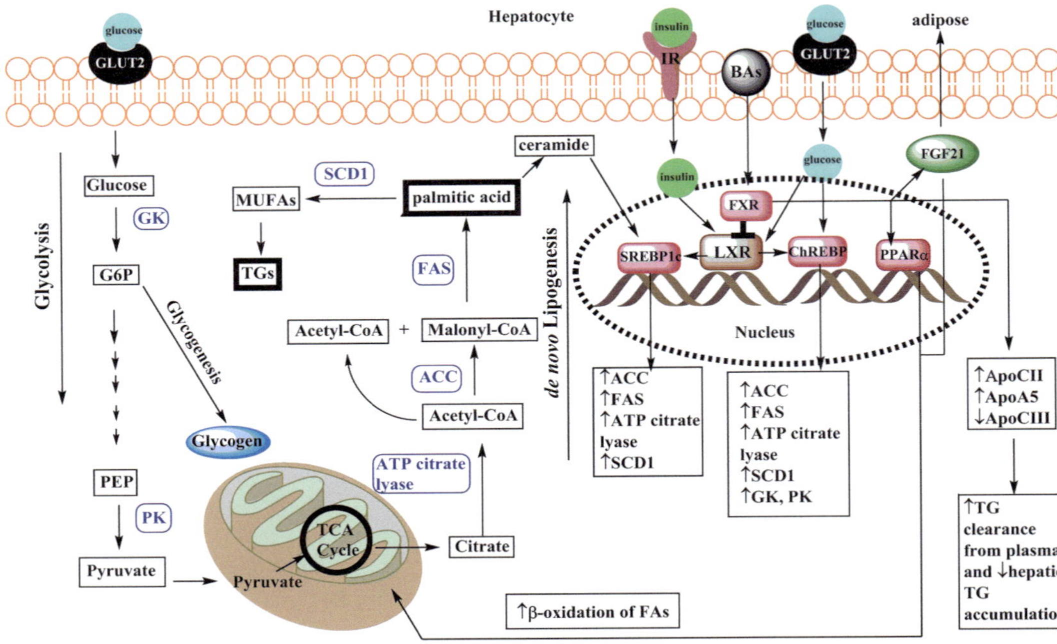

Fig. 8.1 The interface between hepatic lipid and glucose metabolis. Both glucose and insulin activate LXR and this causes increased expression and activation of SREBP1c and ChREBP which, in turn, increases *de novo* lipogenesis. In addition to LXR, glucose can also directly activate ChREBP and ceramide, a product of lipogenesis can directly activate SRBEP1c. ChREBP transcribes key enzymes for the glycolysis/glycogenesis cycles (GK, PK) and both ChREBP and SREBP1c synergistically transcribe important enzymes for *de novo* lipogenesis (ATP citrate lyase, ACC, FAS, SCD1). BAs activate the nuclear receptor FXR which modulates both glycolysis/glycogenesis and *de novo* lipogenesis cycles via it inhibitory effect on LXR. FXR activation also leads to increased expression of PPARα which in turn, transcribes genes for the increase of mitochondrial β-oxidation of FAs. Therefore, hepatic FXR activation leads to a decrease in the glycolysis → *de novo* lipogenesis → TG axis and reduces hepatic lipid accumulation and also increases the use of FAs for energy expenditure in the liver via upregulation of PPARα. Both of these FXR mediated effects reduce hepatic lipid accumulation to forestall NAFLD [16, 19, 20, 22, 23, 25] *Abbreviations: GLUT2* glucose receptor-2, *GK* glucokinase, *G6P* glucose-6-phospate, *PEP* phosphenolpyruvate, *PK* pyruvate kinase, *ACC* acetyl-CoA carboxylase, *FAS* fatty acid synthase, *FAs* fatty acid, *SCD1* steroyl-CoA-desaturase-1, *IR* insulin receptor. *BAs* bile acids, *FXR* farnesoid X receptor, *LXR* liver X receptor, *PPARα* peroxisome proliferator-activated receptor-α, *ChREBP1c* carbohydrate response element binding protein-1c, *SREBP* sterol response element binding protein, *FGF21* fibroblast growth factor-21

ated via two enzymes, acetyl-CoA carboxylase (ACC) and fatty acid synthase (FAS). The lipid sensitive SREBP1c and the glucose sensitive ChREBP transcription factors together induce expression of FAS and ACC in a synergistic way thus giving increased support to the idea of an interface between glucose and lipid metabolism in the liver [19, 20].

Figure 8.1 is a diagram depicting a brief overview of the interface between hepatic glucose and lipid metabolism in a normal liver. Glucose uptake via GLUT2 transporters can be shunted into either glycolysis or glycogenolysis. Activation of ChREBP results in the increased transcription of genes for glucokinase (GK) which phosphorylates glucose to become glucose-6-phophate which, in turn, can be used as a substrate for either glycolysis or glycogenesis. ChREBP also acts to upregulate pyruvate kinase (PK) which is a key enzyme in glycolysis that converts phosphoenolpyruvate into pyruvate. Pyruvate is then taken into the mitochondria where it enters TCA cycle. The result of this is the production of citrate which is converted into acetyl-CoA via the enzyme ATP citrate lyase, an enzyme that is controlled by both ChREBP and SREBP-1c. ChREBP and SRBEP-1c are regulated by glucose and insulin, respectively. Together, ChREBP and SRBEP-1c transcribe genes for enzymes involved in *de novo* lipogenesis (Fig. 8.1). Acetyl-CoA formed previously from citrate is then catalyzed by acetyl-CoA carboxylase (ACC) to form malonyl Co-A. Malonyl CoA and acetyl-CoA together can then be reacted with fatty acid synthase (FAS) to form palmitic acid, an important FA that is the substrate for production of monounsaturated FAs (MUFAs) via steroyl-CoA-desaturase-1 (SCD1). MUFAs are then eventually packaged into TGs or else undergo β-oxidation in the mitochondria [16, 19, 21].

Both SREBP1c and ChREBP expression are regulated by the BA sensitive nuclear receptor, farnesoid X receptor (FXR) via inhibition of liver X receptor (LXR) [22]. The primary evidence for FXR involvement in hepatic lipid metabolism came from studies of FXR KO mice which clearly showed that FXR deletion resulted in hepatic lipid accumulation and elevated plasma TGs. On the contrary, activation of FXR by either BAs or an agonist such as GW4064 or INT-747 reduced both glycolysis and de novo lipogenesis, leading to a reduction in hepatic TGs in mice [23, 24]. FXR activation also leads to the increased expression of peroxisome proliferator-activated receptor-α (PPARα) resulting in increased β-oxidation of FAs for energy expenditure and decreased hepatic TGs in mice [21]. This was shown in PPARα$^{-/-}$ mice which are incapable of upregulating FA oxidation in the liver and develop severe steatosis [25, 26]. When placed on a methionine/choline deficient diet, PPARα$^{-/-}$ mice develop NASH [26]. Furthermore, administration of PPARα agonists prevented the development of methionine- and choline-deficient diet-induced NASH in mice [27]. Clinical data is inconclusive in humans in the use of PPARα agonists for prevention of steatosis in NAFLD which has been attributed to small sample size and the use of combined treatments [28]. Lastly, hepatic FXR activation leads to the increased expression of fibroblast growth factor -21 (FGF21) which is secreted from the liver and acts mainly in adipose tissue via binding to fibroblast growth receptor-4 (FGFR4) (Fig. 8.2) to increase expression of adiponectin, a beneficial adipokine that has been shown to reduce the level of ceramide [29]. FGF21 has also been shown to activate an extracellular signal-related kinase ½ (ERK1/2) signaling pathway in adipose tissue (Fig. 8.2) that leads to increased expression of GLUT1 glucose transporters resulting in increased glucose uptake by adipose tissue and a lowering of blood glucose levels thus protecting against hyperglycemia, hyperinsulinemia and insulin resistance [30].

FXR activation also plays a critical role in VLDL clearance from the plasma. VLDL TGs are cleared from the plasma via their hydrolysis by lipoprotein lipase (LPL), an enzyme which lines the endothelial cells of extrahepatic tissues. FXR induces apoCII and apoA5 which are activators of LPL and suppresses apoCIII which is an LPL inhibitor [22, 31, 32]. FGF21 produced by FXR activation also acts in an endocrine way in the liver mitochondria to increase β-oxidation of FAs into acetyl-CoA for use in the ketogenesis pathway [22, 33] (Figs. 8.1 and 8.2).

FXR activation in the intestine has consequences for hepatic lipid metabolism and progression to NAFLD as shown in Fig. 8.2. In the intestine, FXR is known to target the expression of genes that lead to the synthesis of ceramide. This was shown in mice using an intestine specific FXR inhibitor, glyco-muricholic acid (G-MCA), which cannot be hydrolyzed by the gut microbiota. The G-MCA treatment protected the mice that were exposed to HFD from adiposity, hyperglycemia, insulin resistance and hepatic steatosis by decreasing the expression of ceramide and the ceramide synthetic enzymes, sphingomyelin phosphodiesterase 3 (Smpd3) and serine palmitoyltransferase long-chain base subunit 2 (Sptlc2) [34]. Increased ceramide activates three different signaling pathways in the liver, inhibitor of nuclear factor κB kinase subunit β (IKK2), c-Jun N-terminal kinase (JNK) and protein kinase C-ζ (PKCζ) that all result in insulin resistance (Fig. 8.2) [35]. However, FXR activation in the ileum exerts a hepatoprotective effect by increasing the production of FGF19/(15 in mice), a hormone that when secreted into the circulation binds to the hepatic FGFR4 receptor. Hepatic FGF19/15-FGFR4 binding decreases

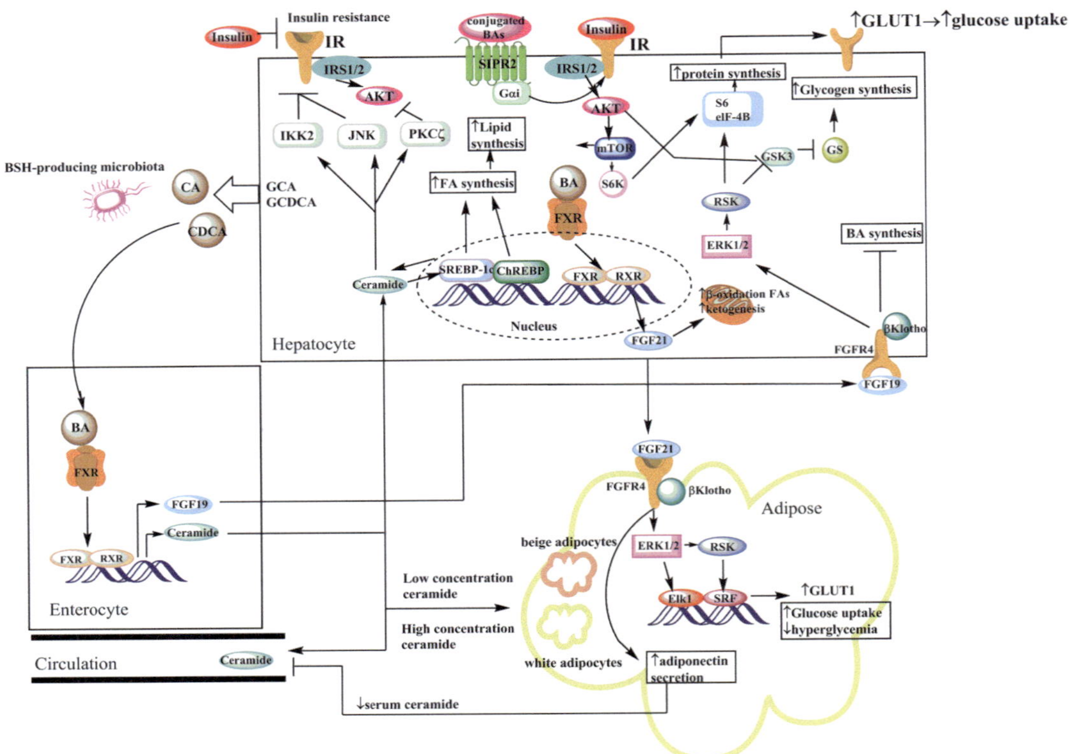

Fig. 8.2 The gut microbiota-BA-FXR- FGF21/FGF19-adiponectin-ceramide pathway role in metabolic diseases, including NAFLD. BSH producing microbiota deconjugate BAs secreted from the liver. Unconjugated, primary BAs (CA, CDCA) then activate intestinal FXR which leads to the production of FGF19. FXR activation also targets two genes for enzymes important for the synthesis of ceramide, *Smpd3* and *Sptlc2* and thus causes an increase in ceramide. FGF19 subsequently binds to FGFR4/β-Klotho which causes, (1) inhibition of BA synthesis, (2) activation of ERK1/2 → ↑protein (ie., GLUT1 glucose transporters) and glycogen synthesis. Ceramide, on the other hand, (1) activates SREBP-1c to ↑FA synthesis, (2) activates IKK2, JNK and PKCζ which effectively block the effects of insulin on its receptor, ie., insulin resistance. Insulin, also shown in this diagram, can be activated by the BA sensitive G-protein-coupled receptor SIPR2 and shows some parallel activity to the effects of FGF19 in that it augments the effect of insulin via the pathway leading to increased S6/elF-4B which causes increased protein (GLUT1) and glycogen synthesis. In addition, insulin targets mTOR to cause ↑lipid synthesis. FXR activation in the liver causes production of FGF21 which, after secretion, targets FGFR4/β-Klotho in WAT where it, (1) activates the ERK 1/2 → RSK → Elk1/SRF pathway that leads to increased expression of GLUT1 transporters which in turn cause enhanced uptake of glucose into WAT and a decrease in hyperglycemia, (2) causes an increase in adiponectin secretion that in turn, lowers serum ceramide. Lower serum ceramide means more beige adipocytes and increased energy utilization to fight obesity while high serum ceramide means more WAT and less energy expenditure [29, 30, 35–37]

Abbreviations: BA bile acid, *CA* cholic acid, *CDCA* chenodeoxycholic acid , *FXR* farnesoid X receptor, *RXR* retinoid X receptor, *FGF19/21* fibroblast growth factor-19/21, *IR* insulin receptor, *IRS1/2* insulin receptor substrate ½, *IKK2* inhibitor of nuclear factor κB kinase subunit beta, *JNK* c-Jun N-terminal kinase, *PKC* protein kinase C, *FA* fatty acid, *AKT* protein kinase B, *SREBP-1c* sterol response element binding protein-1c, *ChREBP* carbohydrate responsive element binding protein, *mTOR* mammalian target of rapamycin, *S6K* S6 ribosomal protein kinase-beta-1, *S6* S6 ribosomal protein, *elF-4B* eukaryotic translation initiator factor -4B, *GSK3* glycogen synthase kinase 3, *GS* glycogen synthase, *RSK* ribosomal S6 kinase, *ERK1/2* extracellular signal-related kinase ½, *FGFR4* fibroblast growth factor receptor-4, *Elk1* ETS domain containing protein-1, *SRF* serum response factor, *BSH* bile salt hydrolase, *WAT* white adipose tissue, *SIPR2* sphingosine-1-phosphate receptor-2

BA synthesis but activates ERK1/2 signaling pathways, increasing protein (GLUT1) and glycogen synthesis. These activities increase glucose uptake and storage of excess glucose as glycogen, conferring protection against hyperglycemia and hepatic insulin resistance [36]. Conjugated BAs also bind to another hepatic BA sensitive G-protein coupled receptor, sphingosine-1-phosphate receptor-2 (SIPR2), which has been shown to transactivate the insulin receptor (IR) to augment insulin signaling, the result is protein kinase B activation (AKT) which stimulates mammalian target of rapamycin (mTOR) to increase glycogenesis and protein synthesis (ie. GLUT1) [37].

In summary of this section, we have reviewed hepatic lipid metabolism and the signaling pathways that mediate it. Further we have discussed how BAs impact these signaling pathways and hepatic lipid metabolism via the nuclear receptor, FXR and the G-protein coupled receptor SIPR2 which not only directly impact transcription factors the govern lipogenesis, glycolysis and glycogenesis, but also cause transcription of important FGF hormones that positively affect metabolism. The gut microbiota is responsible for the composition of the BA pool which are the endogenous agonists for FXR and SIPR2. In the next section, we will discuss the gut microbiota-BA axis and its effect on NAFLD development.

8.4 The Gut Microbiota-BA Axis and Development of NAFLD

The gut microbiota shapes the composition of the BA pool producing the endogenous ligands for the BA sensitive receptors discussed so far in this chapter, FXR and SIPR2. Early evidence for the existence of a gut microbiota-BA axis came from examination of the BA pool in GF mice/rats. GF rodents have only primary conjugated BAs, an expanded intestinal BA pool, increased BA synthesis and decreased BA reabsorption [25]. Gut microbiota are essential for modifying the structure of the primary BAs produced in the liver and these modifications include deconjugation of the primary BAs, GCDCA (or TCDCA) and GCA (or TCA) into CDCA and CA, which must precede subsequent, multiple 7α-dehydroxylation steps to produce the secondary BAs, deoxycholic acid (DCA) and lithocholic acid (LCA). These gut microbiota transformed BA have been shown to be high affinity ligands for FXR and their affinities have been ranked as CDCA> LCA = DCA > CA [24, 38, 39]. Reconjugation in the liver of the secondary BAs LCA and DCA to TLCA (or GLCA)and TDCA (or GDCA) gives rise to the most potent ligands for the intestinal BA sensitive G-protein coupled receptor, Takeda G-protein coupled receptor 5 (TGR5) (TLCA > GLCA>LCA >TDCA> GDCA> DCA > TCDCA> GCDCA >CDCS > TCA > GCA > CA) [24, 37, 40, 41]. The hepatic BA sensitive G-protein coupled receptor, SIPR2, is only activated by conjugated Bas [37]. Notably, the genes for the two conjugating enzymes for BAs, BA-CoA synthase (BACS) and BA-CoA:amino acid N-acyltransferase (BAT) are FXR targets [22, 42]. Thus, the gut microbiota, by modifying the BA pool control FXR and SIPR2 signaling and the accumulation of TGs in the liver that lead to NAFLD.

A recent study nicely demonstrated the alteration of the BA pool that occurs with metabolic changes in mice [43]. A group of obesity-prone (129S6/SvEvTac=129T) and obesity resistant mice (129S6/SvlmJ=129J) from the same strain were treated with HFD along with another group of obesity-prone mice from a different strain (C571BL/6J=B6J). Both B6J and 129T mice gained a significant and similar amount of weight while the 129J mice remained lean. However, both 129T and 129J groups maintained normal blood glucose and insulin levels and remained insulin sensitive despite their significantly different BMIs. The B6J mice developed hyperinsulinemia, hyperglycemia and insulin resistance. Insulin resistance is strongly associated with the development of NAFLD [44]. The investigators then used a metabolomic technique to analyze the BAs in all of the mice with the following results. The BA profiles indicated a unique baseline (no HFD) gut microbiota for each group based on the differences in the BA abundances found which was altered by HFD in a unique way for each

Table 8.1 BA profiles reflect changes in microbiota

Mouse strain	Treatment	BA profile + dominant bacterial phlya
B6J	Chow + placebo	HDCA/UDCA > MCA = CDCA > DCA > CA > LCA
	HFD + placebo	CA > > MCA > DCA > HDCA/UDCA > CDCA >LCA
		Firmicutes >> Bacteroidetes >>>>> Actinobacteria
	HFD + V	CA > MCA > HDCA/UDCA > CDCA (no LCA, DCA)
		Proteobacteria >> Firmicutes >>> Tenericules
	HFD + M	MCA >> CA > HDCA/UDCA > CDCA > DCA (no LCA)
		Firmicutes > Proteobacteria >>>> unclassified
129T	Chow + placebo	CA > MCA >> HDCA/UDCA = CDCA >> CA > LCA
	HFD + placebo	CA > MCA > DCA > HDCA/UDCA > CDCA > LCA
		Firmicutes >> Bacteroidetes~ Verrucomicrobia >> Deferribacteres
	HFD + V	CA > MCA >> HDCA/UDCA > CDCA > DCA (no LCA)
		Firmicutes > Proteobacteria >> Deferribacteres>>> Tenericutes
	HFD + M	MCA > CA >>> HDCA/UDCA > CDCA (no DCA, LCA)
		Firmicuttes > > Proteobacteria >>>>> Actinobacteria
129J	Chow + placebo	MCA >> HDCA/UDCA > DCA = CDCA >> CA > LCA
	HFD + placebo	MCA > CA >> HDCA/UDCA > CDCA (no DCA, LCA)
		Verrucomicrobia >>> Firmicutes >> Bacteroidetes>>>> Proteobacteria
	HFD + V	CA > MCA >> HDCA/UDCA > CDCA (no DCA, LCA)
		Proteobacteria (2/3) >> Firmicutes (1/3)
	HFD + M	MCA >>> HDCA/UDCA > CDCA > CA (no DCA, LCA)
		Firmicutes >> Proteobacteria = Verrucomicrobia

group (Table 8.1). Both mouse [45] and human [46] obesity phenotypes have been associated with an decrease in the ratio of the two dominant phyla in the microbiota, Bacteroidetes/ Firmicutes relative to lean controls and thus the next strategy was to administer two antibiotics to two groups of HFD mice from each strain, metronidazole (M), a broad spectrum antibiotic that is absorbable by anaerobes and vancomycin (V) that is absorbable only by gram positive bacteria which would include *Firmicutes* and the third most common phylum in the gut, Actinobacteria [47]. Using the 129J strain (lean control) as a point of reference, the HFD treatment transformed the BA profile of 129T mice to be similar to the B6J in terms of rank ordering of BA abundance. The BA composition for both 129T and B6J mice on antibiotic treatment changed to become more similar to the 129J lean control. The gut microbiota differences among the different treatment groups showed an increase in Firmicutes with HFD only for the obesity-prone strains.

The V and M treated B6J mice showed improved glucose, glucose tolerance and insulin sensitivity with no changes in insulin levels. Finally, transplantation of fecal matter to HFD treated GF-B6J from V and M-treated B6J resulted in improved glucose, glucose tolerance and insulin sensitivity relative to the original HFD treated B6J mice, indicating that these differences were due to the transplanted microbiota. The major conclusions from this study are; (1) that development of metabolic syndrome does not depend on obesity but is strongly affected by the gut microbiota, (2) although 129T and 129J have the same genetic background, they can have different microbiota and therefore, different obesity tendencies, (3) changes in the gut microbiota may be visualized by changes in the BA pool composition. (Table 8.1).

8.5 Angiopoietin-Like Protein-4 and Development of NAFLD

BAs are not the only regulators of hepatic lipid accumulation under the control of the gut microbiota. In this section, we will examine the effect of the gut microbiota metabolites on the pathogenesis of NAFLD via their ability to impact LPL activity and alter the availability of choline. These pathways are summarized in Fig. 8.3.

The following pivotal study clearly revealed the involvement of the gut microbiota as a regulator of both hepatic and adipose lipid storage [48]. This experiment involved the comparison of GF C57BL/6J (B6J) mice with conventionalized mice (CONV-D) from a WT donor, as well as, conventionally raised WT mice (CONV-R). CONV-R mice contained 42% more total body fat than the GF mice. When the GF mice were conventionalized using a fecal transplant from the CONV-R mice (CONV-D), they increased their total body fat by 57% with a 61% increase in epididymal fat. The predominant caecal bacteria genera in both CONV-R and CONV-D were found to be Bacteroides and Clostridium. Relative to GF mice, CONV-D showed a 2.3-fold increase in hepatic TGs with no appreciable changes in liver FFAs or cholesterol. An increase in the mRNA for ChREBP and to a lesser extent, SREBP-1c, was observed along with mRNA increases for the enzymes ACC and FAS suggesting that these mice were displaying an increase in *de novo* lipogenesis. A doubling of capillary density in the small intestine was observed for CONV mice compared to GF and a single gavage of a mixture of glucose and 2-deoxyglucose and measurement 15 min. Later revealed 2-fold higher levels of 2-deoxy 6-phosphate in CONV-D mice relative to GF. Lipoprotein lipase (LPL) activity was increased and this was found to be due to less transcription of the gene for angiopoietin-like protein-4 (ANGPTL4), in the small intestine but not in the adipose tissue or liver confirmed by qRT-PCR of ANGTPL4 mRNA levels. The conclusions from these findings were proposed to be: (1) an increase in the processing of dietary polysaccharides by gut microbiota and increased delivery of monosaccharides to the liver resulted in increased TG synthesis and (2) a decrease in intestinal ANGTPL4 upon CONV resulted in increased LPL activity and thus increased FFA transport and subsequent storage as TGs in adipose. Both of these conclusions thus explained the observed increase in hepatic TGs and total body fat in CONV *vs.* GF mice [48].

The ability of the gut microbiota, independently of PPARs, to affect ANGTPL4 gene transcription in the intestine was confirmed in an experiment using specific pathogen-free (SPF) C57B/6J (B6J) treated with HFD and a probiotic bacterial strain thought to have anti-obesity effects, *Lactobacillus paracasei ssp paracasei F19* (F19) [49]. Relative to controls, F19 treated mice had elevated levels of ANGTPL4 and a significantly lower body fat. HCT116, LoVo, HT29 and SW480 colonocytes were then treated with F19 and all cell lines were stimulated by F19 to produce elevated levels of ANGTPL4. Heat-killed F19 could not produce a ANGTPL4 response while conditioned media from F19/cells, even if heat-killed, could produce a response. Supernatants of F19 cultured alone could also mount a ANGTPL4 response when added to colonocytes. When PPARα and PPARγ specific ligands were applied to colonocytes, an increase in ANGTPL4 was observed indicating that there is also regulation of ANGTPL4 by PPAR nuclear factors. The PPAR that is highly expressed in the intestine is PPARγ [22, 49].

Pursuing the idea of a gut microbiota secretion factor as a control of ANGTPL4 expression, another group used imaging to determine that ANGTPL4 was most highly expressed in enteroendocrine cells (EEC) and thus did experiments on the intestinal EEC cell line HuTu-80, a line known to express high levels of ANGTPL4 [50]. They then treated the cells with various nutrients and found that the short chain fatty acids (SCFAs) butyrate and propionate but not acetate, significantly induced AGTPL4 secretion into the medium and that this was accompanied by an increase in AGPTL4 mRNA. Some BAs were also tested and CDCA and DCA were found to inhibit AGTPL4 secretion. Therefore, from the three experiments discussed above, it would

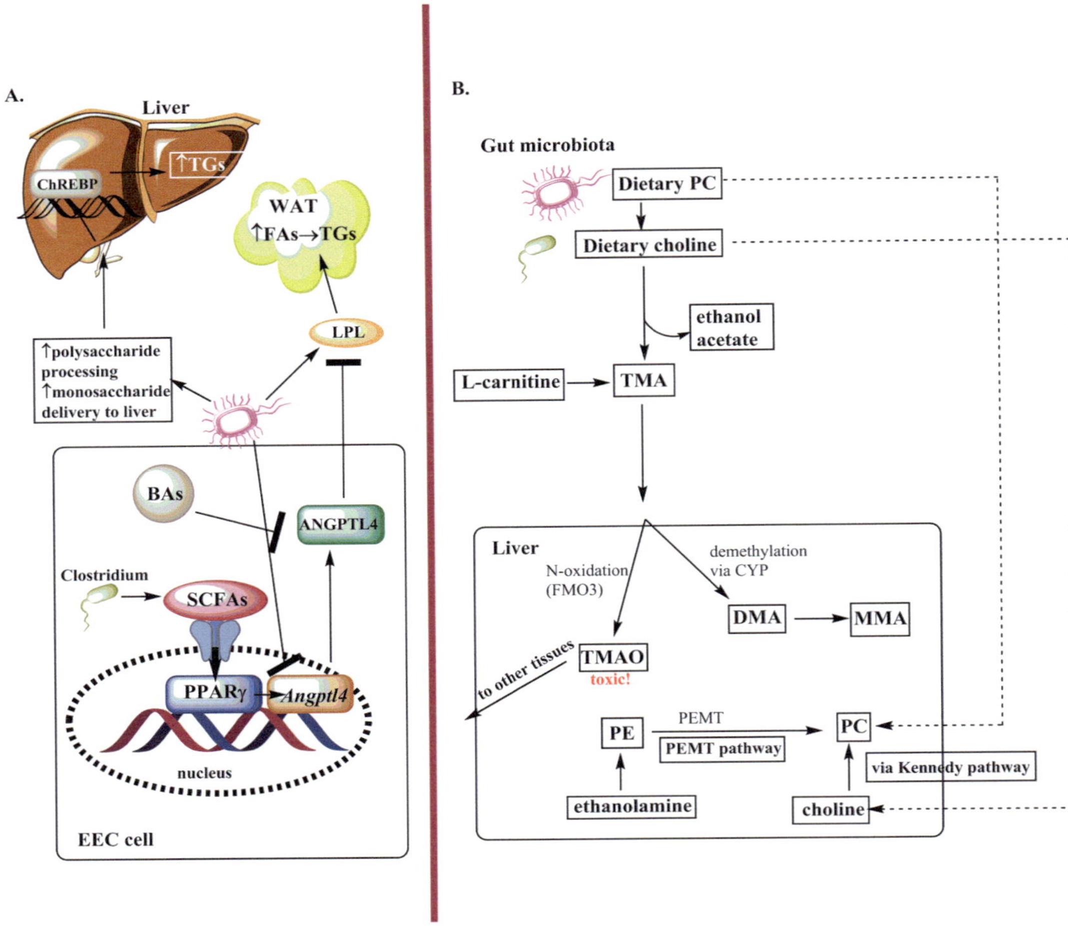

Fig. 8.3 (a) **The effect of gut microbiota on fat storage in NAFLD.** Gut microbiota in the colon that are capable of fermenting polysaccharides to provide an increased energy harvest are abundant in obesity and NAFLD. NAFLD is associated with increased capillary density which allows rapid transit of monosaccharides to be transported to the liver where they activate ChREBP which in turn, initiates *de novo* lipogenesis to produce more TGs to accumulate in the liver. The gut microbiota have also been shown to block transcription of the *Angptyl4* gene and thus increase activity of LPL to cause more FFAs to enter adipose for storage as TGs. Other types of gut microbiota such as *Clostridium sp.* produce SCFAs as a metabolite and these were found to increase secretion of ANGPTL4 presumably via a PPAR nuclear factor. Increased ANGPTL4 would cause a decrease in LPL activity and a decrease in fat storage. BAs, on the other hand were found to inhibit ANGPTL4 secretion from the EECs. This mechanism was proposed to explain the observed transmission of an NAFLD phenotype via gut microbiota [6, 27, 48–51]. (**b**) **The metabolism of dietary choline and PC by gut microbiota prevents PC synthesis in the liver resulting in NAFLD.** Dietary PC can be metabolized to choline in the gut. All choline in the gut can then be metabolized to TMA by certain species of gut microbiota. Diversion of choline into this metabolic pathway results in diminished synthesis of PC in the liver via the mammalian Kennedy pathway and PEMT pathways. In the liver, TMA can be demethylated by CYP enzymes to DMA and MMA or it can be N-oxidized by FMO3 enzymes to produce TMAO, a toxic substance that can be secreted to other tissues such as macrophages and arterial epithelium where it causes inflammation and atherosclerosis, respectively. If the microbiota cause choline deficiency in the liver via excess TMAO synthesis, then not enough PC can be produced to export VLDL and TGs accumulate in the liver and NAFLD results. A polymorphism in the PEMT gene causes the PEMT pathway to shut down and mammalian synthesis of PC decrease by ~30%. The combination of a PEMT polymorphism and high abundance of gut microbiota that produce TMAO is a risk factor for the development of NAFLD [55, 56, 60] *Abbreviations: TGs* triglycerides, *ChREBP* carbohydrate responsive element binding protein, *WAT* white adipose tissue, *BAs* bile acids, *FAs* fatty acids, *ANGPTL4* angiopoietin-like protein-4, *PPARγ* peroxisome proliferator-activated receptor-γ, *SCFAs* short chain fatty acids, *PC* phophatidylcholine, *TMA* trimethylamine, *DMA* dimethylamine, *MMA* monomethylamine, *TMAO* trimethylamine-N-oxide, *PE* phosphoethanolamine, *FMO3* flavin mono-oxygenase enzyme-3, *PEMT* phosphatidylethanolamine-N-methyltransferase

seem that the gut microbiota mediates LPL activity via AGTPL4 induction or suppression with their metabolites SCFAs or BAs, respectively and this, in turn, impacts hepatic lipid and adipose TG accumulation. SCFAs are known to activate PPARγ in the intestine which may account for the effect of SCFAs on increased AGPTL4 secretion [51]. Gut microbiota that are known to be producers of SCFAs include the Clostridial clusters IV and XIVa of *Firmicutes*, including species of the genera *Eubacterium, Roseburia, Faecalibacterium* and *Coprococcus* [52]. Figure 8.3a summarizes the above discussion.

8.6 Gut Microbiota Choline Metabolism and Development of NAFLD

Choline deficiency has been associated with NALFD in both animal models and humans [53]. It is an essential nutrient as it is a major methyl donor for the biosynthesis of the important cell membrane lipids, phosphatidylcholine, lysophosphatidylcholine and sphingomyelin [54, 55]. (Fig. 8.3b) It is also necessary for the synthesis of the neurotransmitter, acetylcholine [55]. Phosphatidycholine (PC) deficiency increases *de novo* lipogenesis which causes an increase in TGs. Lack of PC in hepatic lipid droplets reduces their surfactant properties and larger lipid droplets that are less likely to undergo lipolysis are formed. PC is required for both VLDL synthesis and secretion from the liver [55, 56]. PC has also been identified as a cell wall component of ~10–15% of all bacteria [57].

Several experiments have been done to examine the role of the microbiota on the bioavailability of choline for the host. Metabolomic profiling of urine samples from the inbred mouse strain 129S6, a strain that is susceptible to HFD-induced NAFLD, revealed increased amounts of microbiota-derived methylamines including trimethylamine (TMA) and trimethylamine-N-oxide (TMAO) which are breakdown products of choline that are not derived from mammalian metabolism. Serum PC levels were also low in spite of the fact that the diet was supplemented with choline. This metabolic profile was not observed in another NAFLD-resistant strain, BALB/c and may be a distinct metabotype for NAFLD [54]. Figure 8.3 diagrams the three pathways for choline catabolism, two are pure mammalian and one is a bacterial pathway [54]. In a subsequent metabolomic study, human gut isolates were used to identify eight bacterial species from two different phyla, *Firmicutes* and *Proteobacteria*, and six genera that exhibited significant choline consumption and TMA accumulation: *Anaerococcus hydrogenalis, Clostridium, asparagiforme, Clostridium hathewayi, Clostridium sporogenes, Escherichia gergusonii, Proteus penneri, Providencia rettgeri,* and *Edwarsiella tarda*. These strains could be cultured *in vitro* in media containing deuterated choline where they consumed 60% of the provided choline. They also encoded component genes for the metabolism of choline. When these bacteria were gavaged into GF mice containing a core community of non-TMA producers, there was a significant decrease in the abundance of fecal choline and decreased levels of serum choline. Therefore, bioavailabilty of choline for the host was shown to be affected by the presence of TMA producing gut microbiota [58]. A rigorously controlled longitudinal study of the effect of choline deficiency on human gut microbiota was performed on 15 healthy women who were cooked in-house meals to assure dietary compliance and to control choline supplementation for 2 months [59]. Each subject was tested with three diets, (1) a standard research diet containing a recommended amount of choline (for 10 d), (2) a choline deficient diet (for 42 d) and (3) a choline recovery diet (for 10 d) that contained significant amounts of choline added to the standard research diet. Their liver fats were measured by MRI at the beginning and end of the baseline diet, at 21 and 42 d during the choline deficient diet and at the end of the diet recovery period. Patient urine and blood samples were taken for baseline values at day 1, at the end of every dietary phase and every 3–4 days in between to monitor the health status of the subjects. Stool samples were collected at the beginning and end of each dietary phase and at the middle of the choline deficient phase and recovery phase for pyrosequencing of 16S rRNA. Even though the gut microbiota remained distinct for each subject throughout the study, variations in the amounts of two classes of bacteria, *Gammaproteobacteria* and *Erysipelotrichi* showed significant increase in abundance in subjects with low level of choline and were negatively correlated with liver fat. The elevated abundances were reversed when choline was restored to the diet indicating that these two bacteria classes respond to choline levels and may potentially be used as a potential biomarker for the detection of choline deficiency which may lead to the development of NAFLD [59].

8.7 Therapeutic Intervention for NAFLD

Gut dysbiosis has been implicated in NAFLD pathogenesis and previous studies have highlighted several benefits of using probiotic strains and or prebiotic compounds to adjust the gut microbiota, which include reduction in liver TGs, as well as improvement in glucose/insulin homeostasis and inflammation. Table 8.2 is a summary of some of the pre-clinical studies in mice and clinical studies in humans that have provided evidence that probiotics and synbiotics may help to alleviate NAFLD.

8.8 The Metabolomic Approach to NAFLD

The research discussed in this chapter all made use of a technique called metabolomics. Metabolomics is quite literally, "the measurement of metabolites" and it is considered one of the system biological approaches capable of capturing the changes of an entire spectrum of metabolites (untargeted approach) or a set of specific metabolites (targeted approach). The most

Table 8.2 Summary of pre-clinical and clinical intervention studies of probiotics and synbiotics in NAFLD

Subjects	Strain/prebiotic	Time weeks	Outcome	References
20 obese children	*Lactobaculus rhamnous GG*	8 week	↓ALT	[61]
28 adults	*Lactobacillus bulgaris*	12 week	↓ALT and γ-GTP	[62]
	Streptococcus thermophilus			
72 adults	*Lactobacillus acidophilus*	8 week	↓ALT, ASP, TC, LDL-C	[63]
	Bifidobacterium breve			
44 obese children	*Bifidobacteria, lacrobacilli*	16 week	↓fatty liver index, BMI, ↑GLP1	[64]
	Streptococcus thermophila			
40 rats HFD induced NAFLD	*Bifidobacterium longum*	10 week	↓liver TGs	[65]
	Lactobacillus acidophilus		*B.longum* > *L.acidophilus*	
40 mice HFD induced NAFLD (C57BL/6 J)	*Lactobacillus rhamnous*	12 week	↓BMI, liver TGs, adipose macrophage infiltration	[66]
	Bifidobacterium animalis ssp. lactis		Improved glucose/insulin homeostasis	
	Lactobacillus paracasei			
22 adults	*VSL#3*	3 month	↑MDA, 4-HNE,S-NO	[67]
66 adults	*Bifidobacterium longum*	24 week	↓liver TGs, AST	[68]
	FOS			
52 adults	*L.casei, L. rhamnous, S. thermophilus, B. breve, L. acidophilus, B. longum, L. bulgaricus* and FOS	30 week	↓NF-κB, TNFα	[69]
50 adults	Synbiotic Protexin	28 week	↓FBS, TGs, ALT, AST, GGT,LDL, cholesterol	[70]

Abbreviations: *ALT* alanine aminotransferase, *LDL* low density lipoprotein, *AST* aspartate aminotransferase, *GGT* γ-glutamyltranspeptidase, *TNFα* tumor necrosis factor α, *NF-κB* nuclear factor –κB, *MDA* malondialdehyde, VSL#3 combination of *B. breve, B. infantis, L. casei, L. plantarum, L. acidophilus, L. delbrueckii ssp. bulgaricus, S. thermophiles*, *FBS* fasting blood sugar, *4-HNE* 4-hydroxynonenal, *S-NO* S-nitrothiols common platforms employed are gas chromatography (GC) or high-performance liquid chromatography (HPLC) interfaced to a mass spectrometer, commonly referred to as GC-MS or HPLC-MS [6]. By examining the end-products of metabolism between two treatment groups of mice, for example, one can distinguish between the two groups based on their metabotype rather than on phenotype. This was highlighted in this chapter when it was discovered that two obese strains of mice with comparable BMI were metabolically very different from one another in that one had insulin resistance and the other did not. The measurements of BAs, lipids, cytokines and bacterial metabolites such as TMA and butyrate all make use of the metabolomic techniques.

Metabolomis is also a way to condense a large amount of data into a more workable format. For example, there are many functional redundancies among the microbiota in that more than one species is capable of producing butyrate. Therefore, instead of putting the focus on which of more than one thousand bacteria are present in any given patient, it may be more cogent to think in terms of whether the patient has a healthy gut based on the amount of beneficial bacterial metabolite he or she has. Analysis of metabolic endpoints allows one to look at a patient's situation in terms of a functional metabolome rather than the actual physical microbiome when assessing the health of his/her gut microbiota.

The metabolomic approach also has the capability of being able to handle large numbers of samples and to generate data from multiple biochemical pathways occurring simultaneously either at one time point or a series of time points. The clinician can then visualize a more complete picture of the functional status of his patient's health. A practical application was highlighted in this chapter with respect to choline deficiency. If the amount of bacterial choline metabolites increases over time in a patient, this may signal additional choline supplementation as a treatment to forestall development of NAFLD. FDA recommendations for daily choline intake may not be effective for everyone. Metabolomic techniques thus open up the possibility of a more "personalized" medical approach to someone's health. Ultimately the goals of this approach are: (1) to realize a distinct metabotype for the progression of any human pathological condition, (2) to discover which metabolites signify a risk for development of any future health problems. In the case of NAFLD, early, effective intervention and subsequent monitoring of both host and microbiota metabolites may prevent progression to more serious chronic liver disease or metabolic syndrome such as diabetes.

References

1. Than NN, Newsome PN. A concise review of non-alcoholic fatty liver disease. Atherosclerosis. 2015;239:192–202.
2. Machado M, Marques-Vidal P, Cortez-Pinto H. Hepatic histology in obese patients undergoing bariatric surgery. J Hepatol. 2006;45:600–6.
3. Vernon G, Baranova A, Younossi ZM. Systematic review: the epidemiology and natural history of non-alcoholic fatty liver disease and non-alcoholic steatohepatitis in adults. Aliment Pharmacol Ther. 2011;34:274–85.
4. Attar BM, Van Thiel DH. Current concepts and management approaches in nonalcoholic fatty liver disease. Sci World J. 2013;2013:481893.
5. Gaggini M, Morelli M, Buzzigoli E, DeFronzo RA, Bugianesi E, Gastaldelli A. Non-alcoholic fatty liver disease (NAFLD) and its connection with insulin resistance, dyslipidemia, atherosclerosis and coronary heart disease. Forum Nutr. 2013;5:1544–60.
6. He X, Ji G, Jia W, Li H. Gut microbiota and nonalcoholic fatty liver disease: insights on mechanism and application of metabolomics. Int J Mol Sci. 2016;17:300.
7. Marchesi JR, Adams DH, Fava F, Hermes GD, Hirschfield GM, Hold G, et al. The gut microbiota and host health: a new clinical frontier. Gut. 2016;65:330–9.
8. Le Roy T, Llopis M, Lepage P, Bruneau A, Rabot S, Bevilacqua C, et al. Intestinal microbiota determines development of non-alcoholic fatty liver disease in mice. Gut. 2013;62:1787–94.
9. Fearnside JF, Dumas ME, Rothwell AR, Wilder SP, Cloarec O, Toye A, et al. Phylometabonomic patterns of adaptation to high fat diet feeding in inbred mice. PLoS One. 2008;3:e1668.
10. Rabot S, Membrez M, Bruneau A, Gerard P, Harach T, Moser M, et al. Germ-free C57BL/6J mice are resistant to high-fat-diet-induced insulin resistance and have altered cholesterol metabolism. FASEB J. 2010;24:4948–59.
11. Backhed F, Manchester JK, Semenkovich CF, Gordon JI. Mechanisms underlying the resistance to diet-

induced obesity in germ-free mice. Proc Natl Acad Sci U S A. 2007;104:979–84.
12. Serino M, Luche E, Gres S, Baylac A, Berge M, Cenac C, et al. Metabolic adaptation to a high-fat diet is associated with a change in the gut microbiota. Gut. 2012;61:543–53.
13. Musso G, Gambino R, Cassader M. Recent insights into hepatic lipid metabolism in non-alcoholic fatty liver disease (NAFLD). Prog Lipid Res. 2009;48:1–26.
14. Henao-Mejia J, Elinav E, Jin C, Hao L, Mehal WZ, Strowig T, et al. Inflammasome-mediated dysbiosis regulates progression of NAFLD and obesity. Nature. 2012;482:179–85.
15. Wu X, Ma C, Han L, Nawaz M, Gao F, Zhang X, et al. Molecular characterisation of the faecal microbiota in patients with type II diabetes. Curr Microbiol. 2010;61:69–78.
16. Bechmann LP, Hannivoort RA, Gerken G, Hotamisligil GS, Trauner M, Canbay A. The interaction of hepatic lipid and glucose metabolism in liver diseases. J Hepatol. 2012;56:952–64.
17. Donnelly KL, Smith CI, Schwarzenberg SJ, Jessurun J, Boldt MD, Parks EJ. Sources of fatty acids stored in liver and secreted via lipoproteins in patients with nonalcoholic fatty liver disease. J Clin Invest. 2005;115:1343–51.
18. Liu HY, Han J, Cao SY, Hong T, Zhuo D, Shi J, et al. Hepatic autophagy is suppressed in the presence of insulin resistance and hyperinsulinemia: inhibition of FoxO1-dependent expression of key autophagy genes by insulin. J Biol Chem. 2009;284:31484–92.
19. Dentin R, Girard J, Postic C. Carbohydrate responsive element binding protein (ChREBP) and sterol regulatory element binding protein-1c (SREBP-1c): two key regulators of glucose metabolism and lipid synthesis in liver. Biochimie. 2005;87:81–6.
20. Denechaud PD, Dentin R, Girard J, Postic C. Role of ChREBP in hepatic steatosis and insulin resistance. FEBS Lett. 2008;582:68–73.
21. Berlanga A, Guiu-Jurado E, Porras JA, Auguet T. Molecular pathways in non-alcoholic fatty liver disease. Clin Exp Gastroenterol. 2014;7:221–39.
22. Li T, Chiang JY. Bile acid signaling in metabolic disease and drug therapy. Pharmacol Rev. 2014;66:948–83.
23. Zhang Y, Lee FY, Barrera G, Lee H, Vales C, Gonzalez FJ, et al. Activation of the nuclear receptor FXR improves hyperglycemia and hyperlipidemia in diabetic mice. Proc Natl Acad Sci U S A. 2006;103:1006–11.
24. Li Y, Jadhav K, Zhang Y. Bile acid receptors in nonalcoholic fatty liver disease. Biochem Pharmacol. 2013;86:1517–24.
25. Ip E, Farrell GC, Robertson G, Hall P, Kirsch R, Leclercq I. Central role of PPARalpha-dependent hepatic lipid turnover in dietary steatohepatitis in mice. Hepatology. 2003;38:123–32.
26. Kashireddy PV, Rao MS. Lack of peroxisome proliferator-activated receptor alpha in mice enhances methionine and choline deficient diet-induced steatohepatitis. Hepatol Res. 2004;30:104–10.
27. Ip E, Farrell G, Hall P, Robertson G, Leclercq I. Administration of the potent PPARalpha agonist, Wy-14,643, reverses nutritional fibrosis and steatohepatitis in mice. Hepatology. 2004;39:1286–96.
28. Tailleux A, Wouters K, Staels B. Roles of PPARs in NAFLD: potential therapeutic targets. Biochim Biophys Acta. 2012;1821:809–18.
29. Holland WL, Adams AC, Brozinick JT, Bui HH, Miyauchi Y, Kusminski CM, et al. An FGF21-adiponectin-ceramide axis controls energy expenditure and insulin action in mice. Cell Metab. 2013;17:790–7.
30. Ge X, Chen C, Hui X, Wang Y, Lam KS, Xu A. Fibroblast growth factor 21 induces glucose transporter-1 expression through activation of the serum response factor/Ets-like protein-1 in adipocytes. J Biol Chem. 2011;286:34533–41.
31. Claudel T, Inoue Y, Barbier O, Duran-Sandoval D, Kosykh V, Fruchart J, et al. Farnesoid X receptor agonists suppress hepatic apolipoprotein CIII expression. Gastroenterology. 2003;125:544–55.
32. Claudel T, Sturm E, Duez H, Torra IP, Sirvent A, Kosykh V, et al. Bile acid-activated nuclear receptor FXR suppresses apolipoprotein A-I transcription via a negative FXR response element. J Clin Invest. 2002;109:961–71.
33. Inagaki T, Dutchak P, Zhao G, Ding X, Gautron L, Parameswara V, et al. Endocrine regulation of the fasting response by PPARalpha-mediated induction of fibroblast growth factor 21. Cell Metab. 2007;5:415–25.
34. Jiang C, Xie C, Lv Y, Li J, Krausz KW, Shi J, et al. Intestine-selective farnesoid X receptor inhibition improves obesity-related metabolic dysfunction. Nat Commun. 2015;6:10166.
35. Gonzalez FJ, Jiang C, Patterson AD. An intestinal microbiota-Farnesoid X receptor Axis modulates metabolic disease. Gastroenterology. 2016;151:845–59.
36. Kir S, Beddow SA, Samuel VT, Miller P, Previs SF, Suino-Powell K, et al. FGF19 as a postprandial, insulin-independent activator of hepatic protein and glycogen synthesis. Science. 2011;331:1621–4.
37. Copple BL, Li T. Pharmacology of bile acid receptors: evolution of bile acids from simple detergents to complex signaling molecules. Pharmacol Res. 2016;104:9–21.
38. Parks DJ, Blanchard SG, Bledsoe RK, Chandra G, Consler TG, Kliewer SA, et al. Bile acids: natural ligands for an orphan nuclear receptor. Science. 1999;284:1365–8.
39. Makishima M, Okamoto AY, Repa JJ, Tu H, Learned RM, Luk A, et al. Identification of a nuclear receptor for bile acids. Science. 1999;284:1362–5.
40. Kawamata Y, Fujii R, Hosoya M, Harada M, Yoshida H, Miwa M, et al. A G protein-coupled receptor responsive to bile acids. J Biol Chem. 2003;278:9435–40.

41. Maruyama T, Miyamoto Y, Nakamura T, Tamai Y, Okada H, Sugiyama E, et al. Identification of membrane-type receptor for bile acids (M-BAR). Biochem Biophys Res Commun. 2002;298:714–9.
42. Thomas C, Pellicciari R, Pruzanski M, Auwerx J, Schoonjans K. Targeting bile-acid signalling for metabolic diseases. Nat Rev Drug Discov. 2008;7:678–93.
43. Fujisaka S, Ussar S, Clish C, Devkota S, Dreyfuss JM, Sakaguchi M, et al. Antibiotic effects on gut microbiota and metabolism are host dependent. J Clin Invest. 2016;126:4430–43.
44. Moschen AR, Kaser S, Tilg H. Non-alcoholic steatohepatitis: a microbiota-driven disease. Trends Endocrinol Metab. 2013;24:537–45.
45. Ley RE, Backhed F, Turnbaugh P, Lozupone CA, Knight RD, Gordon JI. Obesity alters gut microbial ecology. Proc Natl Acad Sci U S A. 2005;102:11070–5.
46. Ley RE, Turnbaugh PJ, Klein S, Gordon JI. Microbial ecology: human gut microbes associated with obesity. Nature. 2006;444:1022–3.
47. Musso G, Gambino R, Cassader M. Obesity, diabetes, and gut microbiota: the hygiene hypothesis expanded? Diabetes Care. 2010;33:2277–84.
48. Backhed F, Ding H, Wang T, Hooper LV, Koh GY, Nagy A, et al. The gut microbiota as an environmental factor that regulates fat storage. Proc Natl Acad Sci U S A. 2004;101:15718–23.
49. Aronsson L, Huang Y, Parini P, Korach-Andre M, Hakansson J, Gustafsson JA, et al. Decreased fat storage by lactobacillus paracasei is associated with increased levels of angiopoietin-like 4 protein (ANGPTL4). PLoS One. 2010;5:e13087.
50. Alex S, Lichtenstein L, Dijk W, Mensink RP, Tan NS, Kersten S. ANGPTL4 is produced by entero-endocrine cells in the human intestinal tract. Histochem Cell Biol. 2014;141:383–91.
51. Alex S, Lange K, Amolo T, Grinstead JS, Haakonsson AK, Szalowska E, et al. Short-chain fatty acids stimulate angiopoietin-like 4 synthesis in human colon adenocarcinoma cells by activating peroxisome proliferator-activated receptor. gamma Mol Cell Biol. 2013;33:1303–16.
52. Nicholson JK, Holmes E, Kinross J, Burcelin R, Gibson G, Jia W, et al. Host-gut microbiota metabolic interactions. Science. 2012;336:1262–7.
53. Buchman AL, Dubin MD, Moukarzel AA, Jenden DJ, Roch M, Rice KM, et al. Choline deficiency: a cause of hepatic steatosis during parenteral nutrition that can be reversed with intravenous choline supplementation. Hepatology. 1995;22:1399–403.
54. Dumas ME, Barton RH, Toye A, Cloarec O, Blancher C, Rothwell A, et al. Metabolic profiling reveals a contribution of gut microbiota to fatty liver phenotype in insulin-resistant mice. Proc Natl Acad Sci U S A. 2006;103:12511–6.
55. Sherriff JL, O'Sullivan TA, Properzi C, Oddo JL, Adams LA. Choline, its potential role in nonalcoholic fatty liver disease, and the case for human and bacterial genes. Adv Nutr. 2016;7:5–13.
56. Krahmer N, Guo Y, Wilfling F, Hilger M, Lingrell S, Heger K, et al. Phosphatidylcholine synthesis for lipid droplet expansion is mediated by localized activation of CTP: phosphocholine cytidylyltransferase. Cell Metab. 2011;14:504–15.
57. Geiger O, Lopez-Lara IM, Sohlenkamp C. Phosphatidylcholine biosynthesis and function in bacteria. Biochim Biophys Acta. 2013;1831:503–13.
58. Romano KA, Vivas EI, Amador-Noguez D, Rey FE. Intestinal microbiota composition modulates choline bioavailability from diet and accumulation of the proatherogenic metabolite trimethylamine-N-oxide. MBio. 2015;6:e02481.
59. Spencer MD, Hamp TJ, Reid RW, Fischer LM, Zeisel SH, Fodor AA. Association between composition of the human gastrointestinal microbiome and development of fatty liver with choline deficiency. Gastroenterology. 2011;140:976–86.
60. Russell WR, Hoyles L, Flint HJ, Dumas ME. Colonic bacterial metabolites and human health. Curr Opin Microbiol. 2013;16:246–54.
61. Vajro P, Mandato C, Licenziati MR, Franzese A, Vitale DF, Lenta S, et al. Effects of lactobacillus rhamnosus strain GG in pediatric obesity-related liver disease. J Pediatr Gastroenterol Nutr. 2011;52:740–3.
62. Aller R, De Luis DA, Izaola O, Conde R, Gonzalez Sagrado M, Primo D, et al. Effect of a probiotic on liver aminotransferases in nonalcoholic fatty liver disease patients: a double blind randomized clinical trial. Eur Rev Med Pharmacol Sci. 2011;15:1090–5.
63. Nabavi S, Rafraf M, Somi MH, Homayouni-Rad A, Asghari-Jafarabadi M. Effects of probiotic yogurt consumption on metabolic factors in individuals with nonalcoholic fatty liver disease. J Dairy Sci. 2014;97:7386–93.
64. Alisi A, Bedogni G, Baviera G, Giorgio V, Porro E, Paris C, et al. Randomised clinical trial: the beneficial effects of VSL#3 in obese children with non-alcoholic steatohepatitis. Aliment Pharmacol Ther. 2014;39:1276–85.
65. Xu RY, Wan YP, Fang QY, Lu W, Cai W. Supplementation with probiotics modifies gut flora and attenuates liver fat accumulation in rat non-alcoholic fatty liver disease model. J Clin Biochem Nutr. 2012;50:72–7.
66. Wang J, Tang H, Zhang C, Zhao Y, Derrien M, Rocher E, et al. Modulation of gut microbiota during probiotic-mediated attenuation of metabolic syndrome in high fat diet-fed mice. ISME J. 2015;9:1–15.
67. Loguercio C, Federico A, Tuccillo C, Terracciano F, D'Auria MV, De Simone C, et al. Beneficial effects of a probiotic VSL#3 on parameters of liver dysfunction in chronic liver diseases. J Clin Gastroenterol. 2005;39:540–3.
68. Malaguarnera M, Vacante M, Antic T, Giordano M, Chisari G, Acquaviva R, et al. Bifidobacterium longum with fructo-oligosaccharides in patients with non alcoholic steatohepatitis. Dig Dis Sci. 2012;57:545–53.

69. Eslamparast T, Poustchi H, Zamani F, Sharafkhah M, Malekzadeh R, Hekmatdoost A. Synbiotic supplementation in nonalcoholic fatty liver disease: a randomized, double-blind, placebo-controlled pilot study. Am J Clin Nutr. 2014;99:535–42.
70. Mofidi F, Poustchi H, Yari Z, Nourinayyer B, Merat S, Sharafkhah M, et al. Synbiotic supplementation in lean patients with non-alcoholic fatty liver disease: a pilot, randomised, double-blind, placebo-controlled, clinical trial. Br J Nutr. 2017;117:662–8.

Microbiota, Obesity and NAFLD

9

Louis H. S. Lau and Sunny H. Wong

Abstract

Non-alcoholic fatty liver disease (NAFLD) is an increasingly important cause of chronic liver disease globally. Similar to metabolic syndrome and obesity, NAFLD is associated with alternations in the gut microbiota and its related biological pathways. While the exact pathophysiology of NAFLD remains largely unknown, changes in intestinal inflammation, gut permeability, energy harvest, anaerobic fermentation and insulin resistance have been described. In this chapter, we review the relationship between the gut microbiota, obesity and NAFLD, and highlight potential ways to modify the gut microbiota to help managing NAFLD patients.

Keywords

Fatty liver · Microbiota · Intestinal inflammation · Gut permeability · Energy harvest · Insulin resistance

L. H. S. Lau · S. H. Wong (✉)
Institute of Digestive Disease, State Key Laboratory of Digestive Diseases, Department of Medicine & Therapeutics and LKS Institute of Health Sciences, The Chinese University of Hong Kong, Hong Kong, Hong Kong
e-mail: wonghei@cuhk.edu.hk

9.1 Epidemiology and Risk Factors NAFLD

9.1.1 Epidemiology of NAFLD

Non-alcoholic fatty liver disease (NAFLD) has become one of the leading causes of chronic liver disease globally [1]. It covers a wide spectrum of disease severity, ranging from simple steatosis to non-alcoholic steatohepatitis (NASH), which often results in progression to cirrhosis and hepatocellular carcinoma (HCC).

NAFLD is characterized by excessive fat accumulation in liver, defined by the presence of steatosis in >5% of hepatocytes. It requires the exclusion of secondary causes including systemic diseases, drugs, and weekly alcohol consumption of over 140 g/week for men and 70 g/week for women in the last 12 months [2]. It is highly associated with metabolic syndrome, obesity, hypertension, dyslipidemia, diabetes mellitus and insulin resistance. Extra-hepatic manifestations including osteoporosis, thyroid dysfunction, chronic kidney disease, cardiovascular disease and colorectal cancer are also reported [3].

The prevalence of NAFLD has doubled during last 20 years. Epidemiological studies reported the world prevalence of NAFLD up to 25%, with highest burden of disease in the Middle East and South America [4]. Remarkably, the prevalence of NAFLD in children has reached to 10% [5]. It

J. Yu (ed.), *Obesity, Fatty Liver and Liver Cancer*, Advances in Experimental Medicine and Biology 1061, https://doi.org/10.1007/978-981-10-8684-7_9

affects up to 70% of patients with type 2 diabetes mellitus and 90% of patients with morbid obesity [6]. Among the patients with NAFLD, 23% of them would progress to NASH, a form of NAFD with active hepatocellular necrosis, liver inflammation and tissue injury, and is associated with more rapid fibrosis progression [7]. The incidence of HCC was doubled [8] and the overall mortality was increased among NAFLD patients [4].

In this era of pandemic of NAFLD, the concept of gut-liver axis has been proposed as one of the therapeutic targets [9]. In this article, the role of gut microbiota in NAFLD would be explored with the current knowledge and evidence.

9.1.2 Genetic and Dietary Factors of NAFLD

There is a spectrum of histological changes in NAFLD. In the beginning, lipids are accumulated in the hepatocytes resulting in simple steatosis. NASH comprises of additional histological changes, including hepatocellular injury, necroinflammation, hepatocyte ballooning and fibrosis. In some patients, NASH may further progress to cirrhosis of HCC.

The pathogenesis of NAFLD is incompletely understood. It is believed to be multi-factorial and contributed by several genetic, dietary, metabolic, immunological and microbiological factors. Data suggest that genetic factors play an important role in the pathogenesis and disease progression of NAFLD. Epidemiological studies have shown familial clustering of NAFLD [10, 11] and an adjusted heritability of liver fat fraction to be 39% [12]. The importance of genetic factors was further corroborated by recent large scale genome-wide association studies. In one study, an allele in the gene *PNPA3* was strongly associated with increased hepatic flat content and hepatic inflammation [13]. Subsequent studies further confirmed the role of *PNPA3* in the progression of NAFLD [14] and predisposition to HCC [15, 16] in different populations. Other genes that have been reported to be associated with NAFLD susceptibility or progression included *FDFT1* [17], *TM6SF2* [18], *GCKR* [19] and *MBAT7* [20].

Dietary factors also play an important role in NAFLD. Excessive calorie intake is a major risk factor for NAFLD, especially with over-consumption of high-fat diet [21] and fructose-containing beverages [22–24]. Importantly, dietary fructose promotes hepatic de novo lipogenesis [25], a central metabolic pathway that was abnormally raised in NAFLD [26–28] in an insulin-independent manner. Increased uptake of free fatty acids derived from adipose tissue lipolysis also contributes to NAFLD pathogenesis, as knockout of fatty acid transporters (FATP2 and FATP5) protects against NAFLD [29, 30] whereas overexpression of fatty acid translocase (CD36) accentuates the condition [31]. It was estimated that 60% of hepatic triglycerides came from adipose tissue [32]. Lastly, lower dietary balance of n-3 versus n-6 polyunsaturated fatty acids has been associated with NAFLD [33–35]. Taken these together, these dietary components and metabolic factors are important contributors to NAFLD.

9.2 Microbiota and NAFLD

9.2.1 Changes in Gut Microbiota in NAFLD Patients

The human gastrointestinal tract contains a complex community of trillions of microbes forming collectively known as the gut microbiome. These microbes carrying out important physiological functions such as nutrient metabolism, energy harvest, regulation of immunity, and maintenance of mucosal defense. Alterations in the gut microbiome have been associated with different diseases, including obesity, diabetes mellitus and NAFLD. With relevance to NAFLD, the liver receives majority of its blood supply via the portal vein and thus becomes the first filter of substances coming from the intestines.

Hepatologists have long appreciated the importance of gut microbiota to liver diseases. A report in the 1950s showed that non-absorbable antibiotics could prevent cirrhosis in an animal model of NASH [36]. Another early study also found small intestine bacterial overgrowth (SIBO) in patients with hepatic steatosis, which could regress upon receiving antibiotics [37]. These studies provided early evidence that the gut microbiota is important to NAFLD.

Multiple studies in animals have showed that the gut microbiota is important to the pathogenesis of NAFLD. Compared to conventionalized mice, germ-free mice receiving high-fat diets were resistant to hepatic steatosis and dyslipidemia, while displaying better glucose tolerance and insulin sensitivity profiles [38]. A direct evidence suggesting importance of gut microbiota was shown by the observation that NAFLD is transmissible upon fecal transplantation [39], which transferred the intestinal microbiota concomitant with the propensity for NAFLD in the recipient mice. Significant changes were observed with the *Lachnospiraceae* family and *Bacteroides vulgatus* species, with the former associated positively and the latter associated inversely with NAFLD development. These suggested possible divergent effects of these bacteria in the pathogenesis of NAFLD.

The advent of next-generation sequencing technologies has allowed detailed metagenomic analysis of the fecal composition. Limited numbers of sequencing studies in human has showed changes in gut microbiota in patients with NAFLD (Fig. 9.1). Similar to obese individuals, NAFLD patients especially those with steatohepatitis showed increased abundance of *Bacteroidetes* and decreased abundance of *Firmicutes* [40, 41], though some results varied between different studies [42, 43]. At genus level, a subsequent study involving showed higher abundance of *Bacteroides* and lower abundance of *Prevotella* [41]. These two genera have been shown to be competitors with an inverse correlation within an ecology [44]. Further sub-group analysis of the microbiota showed that *Ruminococcus* abundance was independently associated with more severe liver fibrosis [41]. Dietary components can affect the gut microbiota composition [45] and susceptibility to NASH [46], including fructose [22], bile acid like deoxycholic acid [47], and amino acid like citrulline [48]. The abundance of *Bacteroides* correlated with decreased levels of SCFAs and amino acids [49].

In the pediatric population, a study has showed changes similar to obesity in NAFLD patients with more abundant *Bacteroidetes* and less abundant *Firmicutes*, as well as higher proportions of the *Prevotella* and *Escherichia* genera [50]. One study looking at children with NAFLD showed higher abundance of Gammaproteobacteria and Epsilonproteobacteria than children without NAFLD. Other genera that were significantly difference in pediatric NASH patients included increased levels of *Ruminococcus*, *Dorea* and *Blautia* [51].

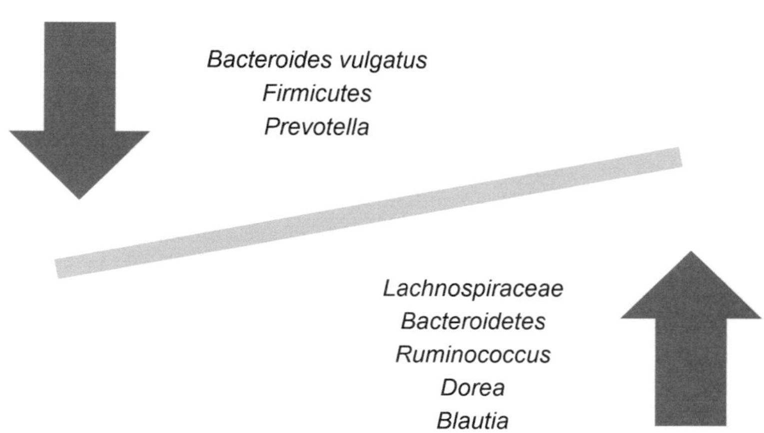

Fig. 9.1 Some putative bacterial genera or species that have been reported to change in NAFLD patients

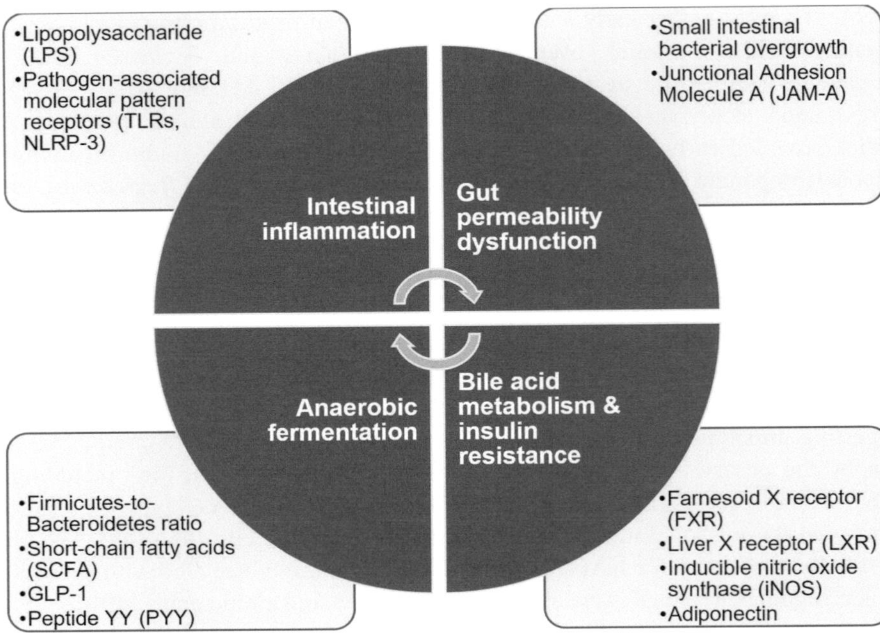

Fig. 9.2 Putative mechanisms and their molecular components relating gut microbiota and NAFLD

9.2.2 Importance of the Gut Microbiota Changes

Studies indicated that there are several mechanisms that gut microbiota can contribute to NAFLD [9, 52] (Fig. 9.2).

9.3 Intestinal Inflammation

Inflammation is a key component of steatohepatitis in which microbes play an important role. With this, our innate immunity likely plays a central role [53]. Bacterial products derived from the gut microbes, including lipopolysaccharide (endotoxin), peptidoglycan and bacterial DNA can travel up the portal vein to activate TLRs on Kupffer cells, leading to an inflammatory cascade that promotes NASH. Elevated levels of lipopolysaccharide were detected in NAFLD in mice [54] and in human [55], and has been associated with insulin resistance [56].

Pathogen-associated molecular pattern (PAMP) receptors, such as Toll-like receptors (TLRs), are involved in the pathogenesis of NASH by activating NF-kB, secreting macrophage chemokines, engaging Kupffer cells and recruiting them to the liver to cause inflammation [57]. Nod-like receptor protein (NLRP)-3 can stimulate the immunity through forming an inflammasome with ACS, an apoptosis-associated protein to activate pro-caspase 1 [58, 59]. Inflammasome dysfunction results in an aggravated liver inflammatory response, liver damage, fibrosis and cell death [60]. The role of NLRP3 has been suggested by mice on high-fat diet showing reduced liver steatosis by inhibition of NLRP3 inflammasome signaling [61].

Several TLRs have been shown to be of key importance. Mice deficient in TLR4 and myeloid-differentiation factor-2 (MD2) are protected from methionine- and choline-deficient diet induced liver inflammation and fat deposition [62]. Furthermore, plasma from patients with NASH contain high levels of mitochondrial DNA as a potent TLR9 activator. Mice deficient in TLR9 were protected from high-fat diet-induced hepatic steatosis and inflammation, reflecting the importance of TLR9 pathway in mediating the inflammatory component of NASH [60, 63]. Finally,

TLR5 may play a protective role in diet-induced steatohepatitis, as mice lacking TLR5 on hepatocytes showed exacerbated disease after given methionine- and choline-deficient diet [64]. These exemplify how PAMPs can give rise to liver inflammation, and suggest a possible communication with microbes in the pathogenesis of NASH.

9.4 Gut Permeability Dysfunction

Previous studies have demonstrated SIBO and increased intestinal permeability in patients with NASH [65, 66]. Culture with duodenal aspirates showed significant SIBO with colony count above 10^5 CFU/mL in 38% of patients with NAFLD, higher than that of healthy controls [67]. Disruptions in the gut wall integrity may influence the products to which the liver is exposed, and affect the progression of various liver diseases. The increased permeability is linked to dysregulation of epithelial tight junction function. Mice deficient in the tight Junctional Adhesion Molecule A (JAM-A) showed increased intestinal permeability and bacterial translocation to the liver, causing increased liver inflammation and steatohepatitis [68]. This increased permeability is linked with microbial dysbiosis, histological inflammation, changes in immune cell populations and cytokine levels [69, 70]. These observations suggest mechanistic relationships between gut microbiota, intestinal inflammation, mucosal permeability and steatohepatitis.

9.5 Energy Intake and Anaerobic Fermentation

Apart from direct effects in inducing liver inflammation, the gut microbiota can alter energy and metabolism of the host, leading to obesity and other diseases strongly associated with NAFLD. Experimental evidence came from gnotobiotic animal models, where germ-free mice gained less body weight compared to conventional mice despite given the same diet [71, 72]. Subsequent experiments showed that the obesity phenotype was transmissible with stool transplantation [73, 74], and similarly, microbial transfer can result in the development of exacerbated NASH in mice [60]. The increase in body weight was associated with a proportional increase in the Firmicutes-to-Bacteroidetes ratio [75]; conversely, this ratio could decrease upon weight loss with a calorie-restricted diet [75] or gastric bypass surgery [76].

Some bacteria provide the enzymes for breakdown of polysaccharides that are otherwise indigestible by the host, resulting in an increased energy extraction to the host [77]. Fermentation of polysaccharides by the gut microbiota into monosaccharides and short-chain fatty acids (SCFAs), including acetate, propionate and butyrate receptor which are linked with metabolic syndrome and NAFLD. Mice lacking GPR43, a receptor for these SCFAs, gained more weight and showed increased adiposity, insulin resistance and NAFLD upon given high fat diet, whereas GPR43 overexpression in mice exhibited no weight change or signs of liver steatosis [78]. These SCFAs can reduce weight gain, improve glucose tolerance and insulin sensitivity in animal models of obesity [79, 80]. These may be mediated through controlling satiety [81], promoting thermogenesis and energy expenditure [82], activating intestinal gluconeogenesis [80], modulating gut inflammation [83] and regulating intestinal hormones such as glucagon-like peptide (GLP)-1 and peptide YY (PYY) [84–86]. In particular, butyrate is a preferred energy substrate for colonocytes [87]. It can enhance glycogen synthesis, increase hepatic glycogen storage and decrease glucose oxidation, providing a link between dietary fiber consumption and improved glucose tolerance [87].

9.6 Energy Homeostasis and Bile Acid Metabolism

Apart from a role in enhancing dietary fat digestion, bile acids are recognized to be important for energy homeostasis and metabolism [88]. Gut microbiota can transform primary bile acids into conjugated bile acids. These bile acids can bind to the nuclear receptor Farnesoid X receptor (FXR), which can in turn controls bile acid synthesis, secretion and reabsorption through regulating genes involved in the relevant pathways [89, 90].

Bile acid metabolism has been linked to NAFLD in several ways. FXR-deficient animals displayed liver steatosis and inflammation [91], phenotypes which can be improved by natural [92] or synthetic [93, 94] FXR agonists in diet-induced liver steatosis models. Administration of antibiotics to mice, through affecting the gut microbiota, could alter bile acid composition, different FXR signaling and accumulation of triglycerides in the liver [95, 96]. The beneficial effects of bariatric surgery on metabolism were associated with changes in the gut microbiota and diminished in FXR-deficient mice [97]. In clinical studies looking at the effect of obeticholic acid in NAFLD and diabetes patients, obeticholic acid was effective in improving insulin sensitivity, reducing NAFLD activity score and ameliorating liver fibrosis [98, 99].

Taken together, these studies suggested a dominant role of the gut microbiota in regulating bile acids via FXR signaling, which in turn regulates obesity and its related metabolic manifestations including NAFLD.

9.7 Insulin Resistance

Insulin resistance is another important mechanism contributing to NAFLD and other components of metabolic syndrome. Insulin resistance promotes lipid accumulation in the liver, via mediating update of free fatty acids and free cholesterol via scavenge receptor CD36 [100]. Fat accumulation could also be mediated by the nuclear receptors liver X receptor (LXR) and intestinal farnesoid X receptor (FXR) [95, 101, 102]. These free cholesterol and fatty acids in the liver can activate JNK, and causes mitochondrial injury in a process called lipotoxicity. Molecules released from the damaged hepatocytes can activate innate immunity, promoting activation of proinflammatory pathways such as NF-kB to cause further injury.

The gut microbiota can affect insulin resistance in several ways. The stimulation of TLR4 by bacterial lipopolysaccharides can lead to activation of serine-kinases, which have important roles in induction of insulin resistance through serine phosphorylation of IRS-1 [103, 104]. This posttranslational modification of IRS-1 has been considered as an insulin resistance marker [105]. Furthermore, the increase in circulating lipopolysaccharides, via TLR4, leads to increased expression of inducible nitric oxide synthase (iNOS) [106]. The increase in iNOS expression induces S-nitrosation/S-nitrosylation of proteins in insulin-sensitive tissues, a central phenomenon in inducing ER stress and insulin resistance [107–109]. Genetic disruption of iNOS and its pharmacological inhibition attenuates insulin resistance in models of obesity or sepsis [110–112]. Conversely, adiponectin, a protein hormone secreted by adipose tissues, can mediate insulin sensitivity and its level is often decreased in patients with NAFLD [113].

9.7.1 Changes in Gut Microbiota in Cirrhosis Patients

In liver cirrhosis, the reduced secretion of bile acid and presence of portal hypertension could affect the composition of gut microbiota. Altered gut motility and small intestinal bacterial overgrowth has been observed in patients with liver cirrhosis [114].

Prior studies reported different fecal microbial communities in patients with cirrhosis in comparison with healthy individuals. *Bacteroidetes* was significantly reduced, whereas *Proteobacteria* and *Fusobacteria* were highly increased in the cirrhosis group. A positive correlation was observed between Child-Pugh score and *Streptococcaceae*, while a negative correlation was seen for *Lachnospiraceae* [115]. *Ruminococcus* abundance was associated with F2 or above liver fibrosis due to pro-inflammatory and ethanol-producing ability [41]. The concept of cirrhosis dysbiosis ratio (CDR) has also been reported to quantify the microbiome alterations in stool, which is associated with clinical decompensation and hepatic encephalopathy [116].

Another study analyzed the quantitative metagenomics of gut microbiomes in liver cirrhosis patients. It was found that *Streptococcus* and *Veillonella*, both of buccal origin, were enriched when compared to healthy individuals [117]. More evidence has shown that profound salivary dysbiosis is associated with liver cirrhosis [118]. Infection with *Porphyromonas gingivalis*, a major pathogen of periodontitis, was observed to be an additional risk factor of NAFLD [119].

These findings suggest a significant contribution of gut and oral microbiota to the development and prognosis of liver cirrhosis. It should be regarded as an important potential therapeutic target.

9.8 Modifying the Gut Microbiota for NAFLD Patients

9.8.1 Dietary Components

9.8.1.1 Fat, Cholesterol and Dietary Fiber

High-fat high-cholesterol diet has been identified to increase hepatic steatosis, inflammation and fibrosis with synergistic effect [120]. Chronic high fat diet feeding in mice was shown to increase *Firmicutes* but reduce *Bacterioidetes* species, known as the *Firmicutes*-to-*Bacterioidetes* ratio [121]. A bloom in a single class of the *Firmicutes* – the *Mollicutes* was observed in animal model for diet-induced obesity [122]. On the other hand, high-fibre diet was associated with protective effect against hepatic inflammation, with the reduced abundance of *Akkermansia* [123].

9.8.1.2 Fructose and Glycotoxins

Fructose does not stimulate insulin secretion with selective hepatic metabolism. It has been linked to dyslipidemia and insulin resistance. A study comparing fructose and glucose consumption reported increased visceral adipose volume, fasting plasma apoB, LDL and glucose levels, and most importantly hepatic de-novo lipogenesis, which was observed to be 3-fold higher in patients with NAFLD [26, 124, 125].

Glycotoxins, also known as advanced glycation end-products (AGE), are formed in food when sugars react with amino groups in protein. Its level is particularly high in baked and fried food under high-temperature cooking. Receptors of AGE (RAGE) were shown to be involved in Helicobacter pylori infection and Crohn's disease [126, 127]. An animal study reported high-AGE diet promoted liver steatosis and fibrosis [128].

9.8.1.3 Specific Food Substances

Caffeine consumption has been shown to inhibit the development of NAFLD and progression of liver fibrosis [129]. The possible mechanism of action includes reduction of fat accumulation, hepatic inflammation and oxidative stress [130]. It helps restore the *Firmicutes*-to-*Bacterioidetes* ratio [131]. It also helps by up-regulating Aquaporin-8 expression in proximal colon and enhancing the growth of *Bifidobacterium* species [132]. Recent evidence reported coffee consumption was associated with improvement in liver enzymes, reduced risk of liver cirrhosis, hepatocellular carcinoma and mortality, with a dose-dependent response [133–135].

Fermented green tea extract has been linked with alleviation of obesity and insulin resistance. It is hypothesized that the mechanisms of action are restoration of the *Firmicutes*-to-*Bacteroidetes* and *Bacteroides*-to-*Prevotella* ratios [136], together with the presence of epigallocatechin-3-gallate (EGCG) [137, 138]. In a recent trial, green tea extract recipients (notably containing 2.3% caffeine) had significant improvement in liver enzymes after 12 weeks in NAFLD patients [139]. Another study echoed the findings by demonstrating improvement of liver enzymes together with reduction in proportion of body fat in NAFLD patients [140].

Omega-3 polyunsaturated fatty acid (PUFA) is considered as another new promising option in NAFLD. It regulates the peroxisome proliferator-activated receptors (PPAR), and reduces pro-inflammatory cytokines and oxidative stress. In a recent meta-analysis, it was proposed that omega-3 PUFA could lead to improvement in liver enzymes and lipid profile [141]. Food rich in omega-3 PUFA are typically included in the Mediterranean diet, which is well known for its beneficial effects in preventing obesity, diabetes and cardiovascular events [142, 143].

9.8.2 Medical Interventions

9.8.2.1 Pharmacological Agents

Many pharmacological treatments have been proposed for management of NAFLD. Among them, thiazolidinediones, vitamin E, pentoxifylline and obeticholic acid are the most promising options [144]. However, none of them has been approved in clinical use currently.

9.8.2.2 Antibiotics

Antibiotics have been investigated as one of the therapeutic options. However, there is conflicting evidence about the efficacy of antimicrobial treatment. Use of norfloxacin and neomycin together with cisapride, a prokinetic, has been shown to improve liver function in cirrhotic patients by altering gut motility and bacterial overgrowth [145]. In the contrary, another study found no effect on liver function in NAFLD patients given norfloxacin [146]. Therefore, there is no established role for antibiotics in NAFLD. Its long-term use is also limited by potential side effects and drug resistance.

9.8.2.3 Probiotics, Prebiotics and Synbiotics

Probiotics represent a promising therapeutic option for NAFLD [147, 148]. It is defined as 'live microorganisms, when administered in adequate amounts, confer a health benefit on the host' by the World Health Organization. Prebiotics are defined as 'non-digestible food substances which can promote the growth of beneficial bacteria', while synbiotics refer to the combination of both probiotics and prebiotics.

Commercialized probiotics include lactic acid bacteria and spore-forming bacteria. Most of them included combinations of *Bifidiobacteria* and *Lactobacilli* [148]. The effectiveness of probiotic delivery to the intestine varies greatly depending on formulation. The micro-encapsulated formulation, in which probiotic bacteria enclosing in a coating material, appears to protect them until they reach the gut targets [149]. VSL#3 is one of the commercialized probiotic formulas. It is a probiotic combination of eight bacterial species. Various studies have shown the benefits of VSL#3 use in obese patients with NAFLD, in terms of sonographic outcome and parameters of liver function [150], through the upregulation of GLP-1 [151].

Apart from the traditional agents, a new group of newer probiotics is currently emerging. *Faecalibacterium prausnitzii*, one of the butyrate-producing *Clostridium* clusters, is called the 'probiotic of future' due to its strong anti-inflammatory characteristics [152]. An animal study has showed that this bacterium could decrease adipose tissue inflammation in mice and improve hepatic health [153]. Nevertheless, it is highly oxygen-sensitive and difficult to cultivate and preserve. Efforts has been made to preserve its viability by additional anti-oxidants cysteine, riboflavin and cryoprotectant inulin. Another potential probiotic is *Akkermansia muciniphila* [154, 155], a mucin-degrading bacterium. It has been shown to reduce fat mass, improve insulin sensitivity and dyslipidemia in mice [156, 157].

Meta-analyses also supported the use of probiotics in NAFLD, after demonstrating significant improvement in metabolic and inflammatory parameters [158, 159]. Its combined use with Metformin also produced better outcomes than monotherapy in terms of liver enzymes and sonographic features [160].

9.8.2.4 Fecal Microbiota Transplantation

Fecal microbiota transplantation (FMT) has been reported in clinical use for different gastrointestinal and extra-intestinal diseases, including *Clostridium difficile* infection, inflammatory bowel disease, metabolic syndrome, hepatic encephalopathy and other diseases [161–164].

The potential role of FMT in metabolic syndrome was studied. Transient improvement of insulin resistance in recipients was observed at week 6 after FMT infusion, but the effect weaned off after 12 weeks [165]. Recent animal study also demonstrated positive effect on hepatic lipid accumulation and histology after FMT [166]. The success rate of FMT is determined by the donor characteristics, especially fecal microbiome diversity, richness and compatibility [167]. The concept of 'super donor' with pre-screening is therefore proposed [168]. Further ongoing trials are essential to evaluate the long-term efficacy and safety.

9.8.3 Concluding Remarks

NAFLD is an important cause of chronic liver disease. Increasing evidence supports that the gut microbiota plays an important part in its pathophysiology. While the exact mechanisms of NAFLD remain unknown, studies have looked at intestinal inflammation, insulin resistance, and changes in gut permeability and energy homeostasis as parts of the pathogenic mechanisms. In this chapter, we have summarized the relationship between the gut microbiota and NAFLD, and have highlighted potential ways to modify the gut microbiota. Further mechanistic works will help us further design new therapies for NAFLD.

References

1. Loomba R, Sanyal AJ. The global NAFLD epidemic. Nat Rev Gastroenterol Hepatol. 2013;10:686–90.
2. Neuschwander-Tetri BA, Caldwell SH. Nonalcoholic steatohepatitis: summary of an AASLD Single Topic Conference. Hepatology. 2003;37:1202–19.
3. Armstrong MJ, Adams LA, Canbay A, Syn WK. Extrahepatic complications of nonalcoholic fatty liver disease. Hepatology. 2014;59:1174–97.
4. Younossi ZM, Koenig AB, Abdelatif D, Fazel Y, Henry L, Wymer M. Global epidemiology of nonalcoholic fatty liver disease-Meta-analytic assessment of prevalence, incidence, and outcomes. Hepatology. 2016;64:73–84.
5. Clemente MG, Mandato C, Poeta M, Vajro P. Pediatric non-alcoholic fatty liver disease: recent solutions, unresolved issues, and future research directions. World J Gastroenterol. 2016;22:8078–93.
6. Pappachan JM, Antonio FA, Edavalath M, Mukherjee A. Non-alcoholic fatty liver disease: a diabetologist's perspective. Endocrine. 2014;45:344–53.
7. Vernon G, Baranova A, Younossi ZM. Systematic review: the epidemiology and natural history of non-alcoholic fatty liver disease and non-alcoholic steatohepatitis in adults. Aliment Pharmacol Ther. 2011;34:274–85.
8. El-Serag HB, Tran T, Everhart JE. Diabetes increases the risk of chronic liver disease and hepatocellular carcinoma. Gastroenterology. 2004;126:460–8.
9. Kirpich IA, Marsano LS, McClain CJ. Gut-liver axis, nutrition, and non-alcoholic fatty liver disease. Clin Biochem. 2015;48:923–30.
10. Abdelmalek MF, Liu C, Shuster J, Nelson DR, Asal NR. Familial aggregation of insulin resistance in first-degree relatives of patients with nonalcoholic fatty liver disease. Clin Gastroenterol Hepatol. 2006;4:1162–9.
11. Loomba R, Hwang SJ, O'Donnell CJ, Ellison RC, Vasan RS, RB D'A Sr, et al. Parental obesity and offspring serum alanine and aspartate aminotransferase levels: the Framingham heart study. Gastroenterology. 2008;134:953–9.
12. Schwimmer JB, Celedon MA, Lavine JE, Salem R, Campbell N, Schork NJ, et al. Heritability of nonalcoholic fatty liver disease. Gastroenterology. 2009;136:1585–92.
13. Romeo S, Kozlitina J, Xing C, Pertsemlidis A, Cox D, Pennacchio LA, et al. Genetic variation in PNPLA3 confers susceptibility to nonalcoholic fatty liver disease. Nat Genet. 2008;40:1461–5.
14. Sookoian S, Pirola CJ. Meta-analysis of the influence of I148M variant of patatin-like phospholipase domain containing 3 gene (PNPLA3) on the susceptibility and histological severity of nonalcoholic fatty liver disease. Hepatology. 2011;53:1883–94.
15. Trepo E, Nahon P, Bontempi G, Valenti L, Falleti E, Nischalke HD, et al. Association between the PNPLA3 (rs738409 C>G) variant and hepatocellular carcinoma: evidence from a meta-analysis of individual participant data. Hepatology. 2014;59:2170–7.
16. Falleti E, Fabris C, Cmet S, Cussigh A, Bitetto D, Fontanini E, et al. PNPLA3 rs738409C/G polymorphism in cirrhosis: relationship with the aetiology of liver disease and hepatocellular carcinoma occurrence. Liver Int. 2011;31:1137–43.
17. Chalasani N, Guo X, Loomba R, Goodarzi MO, Haritunians T, Kwon S, et al. Genome-wide association study identifies variants associated with histologic features of nonalcoholic Fatty liver disease. Gastroenterology. 2010;139:1567–76, 1576 e1561–1566
18. Kozlitina J, Smagris E, Stender S, Nordestgaard BG, Zhou HH, Tybjaerg-Hansen A, et al. Exome-wide association study identifies a TM6SF2 variant that confers susceptibility to nonalcoholic fatty liver disease. Nat Genet. 2014;46:352–6.

19. Petta S, Miele L, Bugianesi E, Camma C, Rosso C, Boccia S, et al. Glucokinase regulatory protein gene polymorphism affects liver fibrosis in non-alcoholic fatty liver disease. PLoS One. 2014;9:e87523.
20. Mancina RM, Dongiovanni P, Petta S, Pingitore P, Meroni M, Rametta R, et al. The MBOAT7-TMC4 variant rs641738 increases risk of nonalcoholic fatty liver disease in individuals of European descent. Gastroenterology. 2016;150:1219–1230 e1216.
21. Vilar L, Oliveira CP, Faintuch J, Mello ES, Nogueira MA, Santos TE, et al. High-fat diet: a trigger of non-alcoholic steatohepatitis? Preliminary findings in obese subjects. Nutrition. 2008;24:1097–102.
22. Abdelmalek MF, Suzuki A, Guy C, Unalp-Arida A, Colvin R, Johnson RJ, et al. Increased fructose consumption is associated with fibrosis severity in patients with nonalcoholic fatty liver disease. Hepatology. 2010;51:1961–71.
23. Zelber-Sagi S, Nitzan-Kaluski D, Goldsmith R, Webb M, Blendis L, Halpern Z, et al. Long term nutritional intake and the risk for non-alcoholic fatty liver disease (NAFLD): a population based study. J Hepatol. 2007;47:711–7.
24. Ouyang X, Cirillo P, Sautin Y, McCall S, Bruchette JL, Diehl AM, et al. Fructose consumption as a risk factor for non-alcoholic fatty liver disease. J Hepatol. 2008;48:993–9.
25. Softic S, Cohen DE, Kahn CR. Role of dietary fructose and hepatic de novo lipogenesis in fatty liver disease. Dig Dis Sci. 2016;61:1282–93.
26. Lambert JE, Ramos-Roman MA, Browning JD, Parks EJ. Increased de novo lipogenesis is a distinct characteristic of individuals with nonalcoholic fatty liver disease. Gastroenterology. 2014;146:726–35.
27. Diraison F, Moulin P, Beylot M. Contribution of hepatic de novo lipogenesis and reesterification of plasma non esterified fatty acids to plasma triglyceride synthesis during non-alcoholic fatty liver disease. Diabetes Metab. 2003;29:478–85.
28. Chong MF, Fielding BA, Frayn KN. Mechanisms for the acute effect of fructose on postprandial lipemia. Am J Clin Nutr. 2007;85:1511–20.
29. Falcon A, Doege H, Fluitt A, Tsang B, Watson N, Kay MA, et al. FATP2 is a hepatic fatty acid transporter and peroxisomal very long-chain acyl-CoA synthetase. Am J Physiol Endocrinol Metab. 2010;299:E384–93.
30. Doege H, Grimm D, Falcon A, Tsang B, Storm TA, Xu H, et al. Silencing of hepatic fatty acid transporter protein 5 in vivo reverses diet-induced non-alcoholic fatty liver disease and improves hyperglycemia. J Biol Chem. 2008;283:22186–92.
31. Koonen DP, Jacobs RL, Febbraio M, Young ME, Soltys CL, Ong H, et al. Increased hepatic CD36 expression contributes to dyslipidemia associated with diet-induced obesity. Diabetes. 2007;56:2863–71.
32. Donnelly KL, Smith CI, Schwarzenberg SJ, Jessurun J, Boldt MD, Parks EJ. Sources of fatty acids stored in liver and secreted via lipoproteins in patients with nonalcoholic fatty liver disease. J Clin Invest. 2005;115:1343–51.
33. Araya J, Rodrigo R, Videla LA, Thielemann L, Orellana M, Pettinelli P, et al. Increase in long-chain polyunsaturated fatty acid n-6/n-3 ratio in relation to hepatic steatosis in patients with non-alcoholic fatty liver disease. Clin Sci (Lond). 2004;106:635–43.
34. Cortez-Pinto H, Jesus L, Barros H, Lopes C, Moura MC, Camilo ME. How different is the dietary pattern in non-alcoholic steatohepatitis patients? Clin Nutr. 2006;25:816–23.
35. Puri P, Baillie RA, Wiest MM, Mirshahi F, Choudhury J, Cheung O, et al. A lipidomic analysis of nonalcoholic fatty liver disease. Hepatology. 2007;46:1081–90.
36. Rutenburg AM, Sonnenblick E, Koven I, Aprahamian HA, Reiner L, Fine J. The role of intestinal bacteria in the development of dietary cirrhosis in rats. J Exp Med. 1957;106:1–14.
37. Drenick EJ, Fisler J, Johnson D. Hepatic steatosis after intestinal bypass—prevention and reversal by metronidazole, irrespective of protein-calorie malnutrition. Gastroenterology. 1982;82:535–48.
38. Rabot S, Membrez M, Bruneau A, Gerard P, Harach T, Moser M, et al. Germ-free C57BL/6J mice are resistant to high-fat-diet-induced insulin resistance and have altered cholesterol metabolism. FASEB J. 2010;24:4948–59.
39. Le Roy T, Llopis M, Lepage P, Bruneau A, Rabot S, Bevilacqua C, et al. Intestinal microbiota determines development of non-alcoholic fatty liver disease in mice. Gut. 2013;62:1787–94.
40. Wong VW, Tse CH, Lam TT, Wong GL, Chim AM, Chu WC, et al. Molecular characterization of the fecal microbiota in patients with nonalcoholic steatohepatitis—a longitudinal study. PLoS One. 2013;8:e62885.
41. Boursier J, Mueller O, Barret M, Machado M, Fizanne L, Araujo-Perez F, et al. The severity of nonalcoholic fatty liver disease is associated with gut dysbiosis and shift in the metabolic function of the gut microbiota. Hepatology. 2016;63:764–75.
42. Raman M, Ahmed I, Gillevet PM, Probert CS, Ratcliffe NM, Smith S, et al. Fecal microbiome and volatile organic compound metabolome in obese humans with nonalcoholic fatty liver disease. Clin Gastroenterol Hepatol. 2013;11:868–875 e861–863.
43. Mouzaki M, Comelli EM, Arendt BM, Bonengel J, Fung SK, Fischer SE, et al. Intestinal microbiota in patients with nonalcoholic fatty liver disease. Hepatology. 2013;58:120–7.
44. Yatsunenko T, Rey FE, Manary MJ, Trehan I, Dominguez-Bello MG, Contreras M, et al. Human gut microbiome viewed across age and geography. Nature. 2012;486:222–7.
45. David LA, Maurice CF, Carmody RN, Gootenberg DB, Button JE, Wolfe BE, et al. Diet rapidly and reproducibly alters the human gut microbiome. Nature. 2014;505:559–63.

46. Xie G, Wang X, Liu P, Wei R, Chen W, Rajani C, et al. Distinctly altered gut microbiota in the progression of liver disease. Oncotarget. 2016;7:19355–66.
47. Aranha MM, Cortez-Pinto H, Costa A, da Silva IB, Camilo ME, de Moura MC, et al. Bile acid levels are increased in the liver of patients with steatohepatitis. Eur J Gastroenterol Hepatol. 2008;20:519–25.
48. Jegatheesan P, Beutheu S, Freese K, Waligora-Dupriet AJ, Nubret E, Butel MJ, et al. Preventive effects of citrulline on Western diet-induced non-alcoholic fatty liver disease in rats. Br J Nutr. 2016;116:191–203.
49. Zhao Y, Wu J, Li JV, Zhou NY, Tang H, Wang Y. Gut microbiota composition modifies fecal metabolic profiles in mice. J Proteome Res. 2013;12:2987–99.
50. Zhu L, Baker SS, Gill C, Liu W, Alkhouri R, Baker RD, et al. Characterization of gut microbiomes in nonalcoholic steatohepatitis (NASH) patients: a connection between endogenous alcohol and NASH. Hepatology. 2013;57:601–9.
51. Del Chierico F, Nobili V, Vernocchi P, Russo A, Stefanis C, Gnani D, et al. Gut microbiota profiling of pediatric nonalcoholic fatty liver disease and obese patients unveiled by an integrated meta-omics-based approach. Hepatology. 2017;65:451–64.
52. Federico A, Dallio M, Godos J, Loguercio C, Salomone F. Targeting gut-liver axis for the treatment of nonalcoholic steatohepatitis: translational and clinical evidence. Transl Res. 2016;167:116–24.
53. Tilg H, Moschen AR, Szabo G. Interleukin-1 and inflammasomes in alcoholic liver disease/acute alcoholic hepatitis and nonalcoholic fatty liver disease/nonalcoholic steatohepatitis. Hepatology. 2016;64:955–65.
54. Rivera CA, Adegboyega P, van Rooijen N, Tagalicud A, Allman M, Wallace M. Toll-like receptor-4 signaling and Kupffer cells play pivotal roles in the pathogenesis of non-alcoholic steatohepatitis. J Hepatol. 2007;47:571–9.
55. Harte AL, da Silva NF, Creely SJ, McGee KC, Billyard T, Youssef-Elabd EM, et al. Elevated endotoxin levels in non-alcoholic fatty liver disease. J Inflamm (Lond). 2010;7:15.
56. Mehta NN, McGillicuddy FC, Anderson PD, Hinkle CC, Shah R, Pruscino L, et al. Experimental endotoxemia induces adipose inflammation and insulin resistance in humans. Diabetes. 2010;59:172–81.
57. Wu R, Nakatsu G, Zhang X, Yu J. Pathophysiological mechanisms and therapeutic potentials of macrophages in non-alcoholic steatohepatitis. Expert Opin Ther Targets. 2016;20:615–26.
58. Schroder K, Tschopp J. The inflammasomes. Cell. 2010;140:821–32.
59. Stienstra R, van Diepen JA, Tack CJ, Zaki MH, van de Veerdonk FL, Perera D, et al. Inflammasome is a central player in the induction of obesity and insulin resistance. Proc Natl Acad Sci U S A. 2011;108:15324–9.
60. Henao-Mejia J, Elinav E, Jin C, Hao L, Mehal WZ, Strowig T, et al. Inflammasome-mediated dysbiosis regulates progression of NAFLD and obesity. Nature. 2012;482:179–85.
61. Yang G, Lee HE, Lee JY. A pharmacological inhibitor of NLRP3 inflammasome prevents non-alcoholic fatty liver disease in a mouse model induced by high fat diet. Sci Rep. 2016;6:24399.
62. Csak T, Velayudham A, Hritz I, Petrasek J, Levin I, Lippai D, et al. Deficiency in myeloid differentiation factor-2 and toll-like receptor 4 expression attenuates nonalcoholic steatohepatitis and fibrosis in mice. Am J Physiol Gastrointest Liver Physiol. 2011;300:G433–41.
63. Garcia-Martinez I, Santoro N, Chen Y, Hoque R, Ouyang X, Caprio S, et al. Hepatocyte mitochondrial DNA drives nonalcoholic steatohepatitis by activation of TLR9. J Clin Invest. 2016;126:859–64.
64. Singh V, Chassaing B, Zhang L, San Yeoh B, Xiao X, Kumar M, et al. Microbiota-dependent hepatic lipogenesis mediated by stearoyl CoA desaturase 1 (SCD1) promotes metabolic syndrome in TLR5-deficient mice. Cell Metab. 2015;22:983–96.
65. Miele L, Valenza V, La Torre G, Montalto M, Cammarota G, Ricci R, et al. Increased intestinal permeability and tight junction alterations in nonalcoholic fatty liver disease. Hepatology. 2009;49:1877–87.
66. Giorgio V, Miele L, Principessa L, Ferretti F, Villa MP, Negro V, et al. Intestinal permeability is increased in children with non-alcoholic fatty liver disease, and correlates with liver disease severity. Dig Liver Dis. 2014;46:556–60.
67. Kapil S, Duseja A, Sharma BK, Singla B, Chakraborti A, Das A, et al. Small intestinal bacterial overgrowth and toll-like receptor signaling in patients with non-alcoholic fatty liver disease. J Gastroenterol Hepatol. 2016;31:213–21.
68. Rahman K, Desai C, Iyer SS, Thorn NE, Kumar P, Liu Y, et al. Loss of junctional adhesion molecule a promotes severe steatohepatitis in mice on a diet high in saturated fat, fructose, and cholesterol. Gastroenterology. 2016;151:733–746 e712.
69. Jiang W, Wu N, Wang X, Chi Y, Zhang Y, Qiu X, et al. Dysbiosis gut microbiota associated with inflammation and impaired mucosal immune function in intestine of humans with non-alcoholic fatty liver disease. Sci Rep. 2015;5:8096.
70. Chen P, Starkel P, Turner JR, Ho SB, Schnabl B. Dysbiosis-induced intestinal inflammation activates tumor necrosis factor receptor I and mediates alcoholic liver disease in mice. Hepatology. 2015;61:883–94.
71. Backhed F, Manchester JK, Semenkovich CF, Gordon JI. Mechanisms underlying the resistance to diet-induced obesity in germ-free mice. Proc Natl Acad Sci U S A. 2007;104:979–84.
72. Backhed F, Ding H, Wang T, Hooper LV, Koh GY, Nagy A, et al. The gut microbiota as an environmental factor that regulates fat storage. Proc Natl Acad Sci U S A. 2004;101:15718–23.

73. Ridaura VK, Faith JJ, Rey FE, Cheng J, Duncan AE, Kau AL, et al. Gut microbiota from twins discordant for obesity modulate metabolism in mice. Science. 2013;341:1241214.
74. Turnbaugh PJ, Ley RE, Mahowald MA, Magrini V, Mardis ER, Gordon JI. An obesity-associated gut microbiome with increased capacity for energy harvest. Nature. 2006;444:1027–31.
75. Ley RE, Turnbaugh PJ, Klein S, Gordon JI. Microbial ecology: human gut microbes associated with obesity. Nature. 2006;444:1022–3.
76. Zhang H, DiBaise JK, Zuccolo A, Kudrna D, Braidotti M, Yu Y, et al. Human gut microbiota in obesity and after gastric bypass. Proc Natl Acad Sci U S A. 2009;106:2365–70.
77. Machado MV, Cortez-Pinto H. Diet, microbiota, obesity, and NAFLD: a dangerous quartet. Int J Mol Sci. 2016;17:481.
78. Kimura I, Ozawa K, Inoue D, Imamura T, Kimura K, Maeda T, et al. The gut microbiota suppresses insulin-mediated fat accumulation via the short-chain fatty acid receptor GPR43. Nat Commun. 2013;4:1829.
79. Chambers ES, Viardot A, Psichas A, Morrison DJ, Murphy KG, Zac-Varghese SE, et al. Effects of targeted delivery of propionate to the human colon on appetite regulation, body weight maintenance and adiposity in overweight adults. Gut. 2015;64:1744–54.
80. De Vadder F, Kovatcheva-Datchary P, Goncalves D, Vinera J, Zitoun C, Duchampt A, et al. Microbiota-generated metabolites promote metabolic benefits via gut-brain neural circuits. Cell. 2014;156:84–96.
81. Frost G, Sleeth ML, Sahuri-Arisoylu M, Lizarbe B, Cerdan S, Brody L, et al. The short-chain fatty acid acetate reduces appetite via a central homeostatic mechanism. Nat Commun. 2014;5:3611.
82. Gao Z, Yin J, Zhang J, Ward RE, Martin RJ, Lefevre M, et al. Butyrate improves insulin sensitivity and increases energy expenditure in mice. Diabetes. 2009;58:1509–17.
83. Maslowski KM, Vieira AT, Ng A, Kranich J, Sierro F, Yu D, et al. Regulation of inflammatory responses by gut microbiota and chemoattractant receptor GPR43. Nature. 2009;461:1282–6.
84. Freeland KR, Wilson C, Wolever TM. Adaptation of colonic fermentation and glucagon-like peptide-1 secretion with increased wheat fibre intake for 1 year in hyperinsulinaemic human subjects. Br J Nutr. 2010;103:82–90.
85. Venter CS, Vorster HH, Cummings JH. Effects of dietary propionate on carbohydrate and lipid metabolism in healthy volunteers. Am J Gastroenterol. 1990;85:549–53.
86. Flint HJ, Scott KP, Louis P, Duncan SH. The role of the gut microbiota in nutrition and health. Nat Rev Gastroenterol Hepatol. 2012;9:577–89.
87. Guilloteau P, Martin L, Eeckhaut V, Ducatelle R, Zabielski R, Van Immerseel F. From the gut to the peripheral tissues: the multiple effects of butyrate. Nutr Res Rev. 2010;23:366–84.
88. Thomas C, Gioiello A, Noriega L, Strehle A, Oury J, Rizzo G, et al. TGR5-mediated bile acid sensing controls glucose homeostasis. Cell Metab. 2009;10:167–77.
89. Lefebvre P, Cariou B, Lien F, Kuipers F, Staels B. Role of bile acids and bile acid receptors in metabolic regulation. Physiol Rev. 2009;89:147–91.
90. Thomas C, Pellicciari R, Pruzanski M, Auwerx J, Schoonjans K. Targeting bile-acid signalling for metabolic diseases. Nat Rev Drug Discov. 2008;7:678–93.
91. Bjursell M, Wedin M, Admyre T, Hermansson M, Bottcher G, Goransson M, et al. Ageing Fxr deficient mice develop increased energy expenditure, improved glucose control and liver damage resembling NASH. PLoS One. 2013;8:e64721.
92. Cipriani S, Mencarelli A, Palladino G, Fiorucci S. FXR activation reverses insulin resistance and lipid abnormalities and protects against liver steatosis in Zucker (fa/fa) obese rats. J Lipid Res. 2010;51:771–84.
93. Liu X, Xue R, Ji L, Zhang X, Wu J, Gu J, et al. Activation of farnesoid X receptor (FXR) protects against fructose-induced liver steatosis via inflammatory inhibition and ADRP reduction. Biochem Biophys Res Commun. 2014;450:117–23.
94. Xiong X, Wang X, Lu Y, Wang E, Zhang Z, Yang J, et al. Hepatic steatosis exacerbated by endoplasmic reticulum stress-mediated downregulation of FXR in aging mice. J Hepatol. 2014;60:847–54.
95. Jiang C, Xie C, Li F, Zhang L, Nichols RG, Krausz KW, et al. Intestinal farnesoid X receptor signaling promotes nonalcoholic fatty liver disease. J Clin Invest. 2015;125:386–402.
96. Park MY, Kim SJ, Ko EK, Ahn SH, Seo H, Sung MK. Gut microbiota-associated bile acid deconjugation accelerates hepatic steatosis in ob/ob mice. J Appl Microbiol. 2016;121:800–10.
97. Ryan KK, Tremaroli V, Clemmensen C, Kovatcheva-Datchary P, Myronovych A, Karns R, et al. FXR is a molecular target for the effects of vertical sleeve gastrectomy. Nature. 2014;509:183–8.
98. Mudaliar S, Henry RR, Sanyal AJ, Morrow L, Marschall HU, Kipnes M, et al. Efficacy and safety of the farnesoid X receptor agonist obeticholic acid in patients with type 2 diabetes and nonalcoholic fatty liver disease. Gastroenterology. 2013;145:574–582 e571.
99. Neuschwander-Tetri BA, Loomba R, Sanyal AJ, Lavine JE, Van Natta ML, Abdelmalek MF, et al. Farnesoid X nuclear receptor ligand obeticholic acid for non-cirrhotic, non-alcoholic steatohepatitis (FLINT): a multicentre, randomised, placebo-controlled trial. Lancet. 2015;385:956–65.
100. Kashyap SR, Ioachimescu AG, Gornik HL, Gopan T, Davidson MB, Makdissi A, et al. Lipid-induced insulin resistance is associated with increased monocyte expression of scavenger receptor CD36 and

internalization of oxidized LDL. Obesity (Silver Spring). 2009;17:2142–8.
101. Zhang X, Han J, Man K, Li X, Du J, Chu ES, et al. CXC chemokine receptor 3 promotes steatohepatitis in mice through mediating inflammatory cytokines, macrophages and autophagy. J Hepatol. 2016;64:160–70.
102. Yu J, Shen J, Sun TT, Zhang X, Wong N. Obesity, insulin resistance, NASH and hepatocellular carcinoma. Semin Cancer Biol. 2013;23:483–91.
103. Folli F, Kahn CR, Hansen H, Bouchie JL, Feener EP. Angiotensin II inhibits insulin signaling in aortic smooth muscle cells at multiple levels. A potential role for serine phosphorylation in insulin/angiotensin II crosstalk. J Clin Invest. 1997;100:2158–69.
104. Velloso LA, Folli F, Sun XJ, White MF, Saad MJ, Kahn CR. Cross-talk between the insulin and angiotensin signaling systems. Proc Natl Acad Sci U S A. 1996;93:12490–5.
105. Tsukumo DM, Carvalho-Filho MA, Carvalheira JB, Prada PO, Hirabara SM, Schenka AA, et al. Loss-of-function mutation in Toll-like receptor 4 prevents diet-induced obesity and insulin resistance. Diabetes. 2007;56:1986–98.
106. Sugita H, Kaneki M, Tokunaga E, Sugita M, Koike C, Yasuhara S, et al. Inducible nitric oxide synthase plays a role in LPS-induced hyperglycemia and insulin resistance. Am J Physiol Endocrinol Metab. 2002;282:E386–94.
107. Stamler JS, Jaraki O, Osborne J, Simon DI, Keaney J, Vita J, et al. Nitric oxide circulates in mammalian plasma primarily as an S-nitroso adduct of serum albumin. Proc Natl Acad Sci U S A. 1992;89:7674–7.
108. Carvalho-Filho MA, Ueno M, Hirabara SM, Seabra AB, Carvalheira JB, de Oliveira MG, et al. S-nitrosation of the insulin receptor, insulin receptor substrate 1, and protein kinase B/Akt: a novel mechanism of insulin resistance. Diabetes. 2005;54:959–67.
109. Shinozaki S, Choi CS, Shimizu N, Yamada M, Kim M, Zhang T, et al. Liver-specific inducible nitric-oxide synthase expression is sufficient to cause hepatic insulin resistance and mild hyperglycemia in mice. J Biol Chem. 2011;286:34959–75.
110. Carvalho-Filho MA, Ueno M, Carvalheira JB, Velloso LA, Saad MJ. Targeted disruption of iNOS prevents LPS-induced S-nitrosation of IRbeta/IRS-1 and Akt and insulin resistance in muscle of mice. Am J Physiol Endocrinol Metab. 2006;291:E476–82.
111. Carvalho-Filho MA, Ropelle ER, Pauli RJ, Cintra DE, Tsukumo DM, Silveira LR, et al. Aspirin attenuates insulin resistance in muscle of diet-induced obese rats by inhibiting inducible nitric oxide synthase production and S-nitrosylation of IRbeta/IRS-1 and Akt. Diabetologia. 2009;52:2425–34.
112. Ropelle ER, Pauli JR, Cintra DE, da Silva AS, De Souza CT, Guadagnini D, et al. Targeted disruption of inducible nitric oxide synthase protects against aging, S-nitrosation, and insulin resistance in muscle of male mice. Diabetes. 2013;62:466–70.
113. Polyzos SA, Mantzoros CS. Adiponectin as a target for the treatment of nonalcoholic steatohepatitis with thiazolidinediones: a systematic review. Metabolism. 2016;65:1297–306.
114. Gunnarsdottir SA, Sadik R, Shev S, Simren M, Sjovall H, Stotzer PO, et al. Small intestinal motility disturbances and bacterial overgrowth in patients with liver cirrhosis and portal hypertension. Am J Gastroenterol. 2003;98:1362–70.
115. Chen Y, Yang F, Lu H, Wang B, Chen Y, Lei D, et al. Characterization of fecal microbial communities in patients with liver cirrhosis. Hepatology. 2011;54:562–72.
116. Bajaj JS, Heuman DM, Hylemon PB, Sanyal AJ, White MB, Monteith P, et al. Altered profile of human gut microbiome is associated with cirrhosis and its complications. J Hepatol. 2014;60:940–7.
117. Qin N, Yang F, Li A, Prifti E, Chen Y, Shao L, et al. Alterations of the human gut microbiome in liver cirrhosis. Nature. 2014;513:59–64.
118. Bajaj JS, Betrapally NS, Hylemon PB, Heuman DM, Daita K, White MB, et al. Salivary microbiota reflects changes in gut microbiota in cirrhosis with hepatic encephalopathy. Hepatology. 2015;62:1260–71.
119. Yoneda M, Naka S, Nakano K, Wada K, Endo H, Mawatari H, et al. Involvement of a periodontal pathogen, Porphyromonas gingivalis on the pathogenesis of non-alcoholic fatty liver disease. BMC Gastroenterol. 2012;12:16.
120. Savard C, Tartaglione EV, Kuver R, Haigh WG, Farrell GC, Subramanian S, et al. Synergistic interaction of dietary cholesterol and dietary fat in inducing experimental steatohepatitis. Hepatology. 2013;57:81–92.
121. Murphy EF, Cotter PD, Healy S, Marques TM, O'Sullivan O, Fouhy F, et al. Composition and energy harvesting capacity of the gut microbiota: relationship to diet, obesity and time in mouse models. Gut. 2010;59:1635–42.
122. Turnbaugh PJ, Backhed F, Fulton L, Gordon JI. Diet-induced obesity is linked to marked but reversible alterations in the mouse distal gut microbiome. Cell Host Microbe. 2008;3:213–23.
123. Jakobsdottir G, Xu J, Molin G, Ahrne S, Nyman M. High-fat diet reduces the formation of butyrate, but increases succinate, inflammation, liver fat and cholesterol in rats, while dietary fibre counteracts these effects. PLoS One. 2013;8:e80476.
124. Stanhope KL, Schwarz JM, Keim NL, Griffen SC, Bremer AA, Graham JL, et al. Consuming fructose-sweetened, not glucose-sweetened, beverages increases visceral adiposity and lipids and decreases insulin sensitivity in overweight/obese humans. J Clin Invest. 2009;119:1322–34.
125. Basaranoglu M, Basaranoglu G, Sabuncu T, Senturk H. Fructose as a key player in the development of fatty liver disease. World J Gastroenterol. 2013;19:1166–72.
126. Rojas A, Gonzalez I, Rodriguez B, Romero J, Figueroa H, Llanos J, et al. Evidence of involvement

of the receptor for advanced glycation end-products (RAGE) in the adhesion of Helicobacter pylori to gastric epithelial cells. Microbes Infect. 2011;13:818–23.
127. Ciccocioppo R, Vanoli A, Klersy C, Imbesi V, Boccaccio V, Manca R, et al. Role of the advanced glycation end products receptor in Crohn's disease inflammation. World J Gastroenterol. 2013;19:8269–81.
128. Leung C, Herath CB, Jia Z, Andrikopoulos S, Brown BE, Davies MJ, et al. Dietary advanced glycation end-products aggravate non-alcoholic fatty liver disease. World J Gastroenterol. 2016;22:8026–40.
129. Molloy JW, Calcagno CJ, Williams CD, Jones FJ, Torres DM, Harrison SA. Association of coffee and caffeine consumption with fatty liver disease, nonalcoholic steatohepatitis, and degree of hepatic fibrosis. Hepatology. 2012;55:429–36.
130. Vitaglione P, Morisco F, Mazzone G, Amoruso DC, Ribecco MT, Romano A, et al. Coffee reduces liver damage in a rat model of steatohepatitis: the underlying mechanisms and the role of polyphenols and melanoidins. Hepatology. 2010;52:1652–61.
131. Cowan TE, Palmnas MS, Yang J, Bomhof MR, Ardell KL, Reimer RA, et al. Chronic coffee consumption in the diet-induced obese rat: impact on gut microbiota and serum metabolomics. J Nutr Biochem. 2014;25:489–95.
132. Nakayama T, Oishi K. Influence of coffee (Coffea arabica) and galacto-oligosaccharide consumption on intestinal microbiota and the host responses. FEMS Microbiol Lett. 2013;343:161–8.
133. Kennedy OJ, Roderick P, Buchanan R, Fallowfield JA, Hayes PC, Parkes J. Systematic review with meta-analysis: coffee consumption and the risk of cirrhosis. Aliment Pharmacol Ther. 2016;43:562–74.
134. Setiawan VW, Wilkens LR, Lu SC, Hernandez BY, Le Marchand L, Henderson BE. Association of coffee intake with reduced incidence of liver cancer and death from chronic liver disease in the US multiethnic cohort. Gastroenterology. 2015;148:118–25; quiz e115
135. Hodge A, Lim S, Goh E, Wong O, Marsh P, Knight V, Sievert W, de Courten B. Coffee intake is associated with a lower liver stiffness in patients with non-alcoholic fatty liver disease, Hepatitis C, and Hepatitis B. Nutrients. 2017;9(1):56. http://www.mdpi.com/2072-6643/9/1/56
136. Seo DB, Jeong HW, Cho D, Lee BJ, Lee JH, Choi JY, et al. Fermented green tea extract alleviates obesity and related complications and alters gut microbiota composition in diet-induced obese mice. J Med Food. 2015;18:549–56.
137. Zhou J, Farah BL, Sinha RA, Wu Y, Singh BK, Bay BH, et al. Epigallocatechin-3-gallate (EGCG), a green tea polyphenol, stimulates hepatic autophagy and lipid clearance. PLoS One. 2014;9:e87161.
138. Santamarina AB, Carvalho-Silva M, Gomes LM, Okuda MH, Santana AA, Streck EL, et al. Decaffeinated green tea extract rich in epigallocatechin-3-gallate prevents fatty liver disease by increased activities of mitochondrial respiratory chain complexes in diet-induced obesity mice. J Nutr Biochem. 2015;26:1348–56.
139. Pezeshki A, Safi S, Feizi A, Askari G, Karami F. The effect of green tea extract supplementation on liver enzymes in patients with nonalcoholic fatty liver disease. Int J Prev Med. 2016;7:28.
140. Sakata R, Nakamura T, Torimura T, Ueno T, Sata M. Green tea with high-density catechins improves liver function and fat infiltration in non-alcoholic fatty liver disease (NAFLD) patients: a double-blind placebo-controlled study. Int J Mol Med. 2013;32:989–94.
141. Lu W, Li S, Li J, Wang J, Zhang R, Zhou Y, et al. Effects of omega-3 fatty acid in nonalcoholic fatty liver disease: a meta-analysis. Gastroenterol Res Pract. 2016;2016:1459790.
142. Di Minno MN, Russolillo A, Lupoli R, Ambrosino P, Di Minno A, Tarantino G. Omega-3 fatty acids for the treatment of non-alcoholic fatty liver disease. World J Gastroenterol. 2012;18:5839–47.
143. Demarin V, Lisak M, Morovic S. Mediterranean diet in healthy lifestyle and prevention of stroke. Acta Clin Croat. 2011;50:67–77.
144. Doulberis M, Kotronis G, Gialamprinou D, Kountouras J, Katsinelos P. Non-alcoholic fatty liver disease: an update with special focus on the role of gut microbiota. Metabolism. 2017;71:182–97.
145. Madrid AM, Hurtado C, Venegas M, Cumsille F, Defilippi C. Long-Term treatment with cisapride and antibiotics in liver cirrhosis: effect on small intestinal motility, bacterial overgrowth, and liver function. Am J Gastroenterol. 2001;96:1251–5.
146. Soza A, Riquelme A, Gonzalez R, Alvarez M, Perez-Ayuso RM, Glasinovic JC, et al. Increased orocecal transit time in patients with nonalcoholic fatty liver disease. Dig Dis Sci. 2005;50:1136–40.
147. Bashiardes S, Shapiro H, Rozin S, Shibolet O, Elinav E. Non-alcoholic fatty liver and the gut microbiota. Mol Metab. 2016;5:782–94.
148. Paolella G, Mandato C, Pierri L, Poeta M, Di Stasi M, Vajro P. Gut-liver axis and probiotics: their role in non-alcoholic fatty liver disease. World J Gastroenterol. 2014;20:15518–31.
149. Govender M, Choonara YE, Kumar P, du Toit LC, van Vuuren S, Pillay V. A review of the advancements in probiotic delivery: conventional vs. non-conventional formulations for intestinal flora supplementation. AAPS PharmSciTech. 2014;15:29–43.
150. Alisi A, Bedogni G, Baviera G, Giorgio V, Porro E, Paris C, et al. Randomised clinical trial: the beneficial effects of VSL#3 in obese children with non-alcoholic steatohepatitis. Aliment Pharmacol Ther. 2014;39:1276–85.
151. Loguercio C, Federico A, Tuccillo C, Terracciano F, D'Auria MV, De Simone C, et al. Beneficial effects of a probiotic VSL#3 on parameters of liver dysfunc-

tion in chronic liver diseases. J Clin Gastroenterol. 2005;39:540–3.
152. Sokol H, Pigneur B, Watterlot L, Lakhdari O, Bermudez-Humaran LG, Gratadoux JJ, et al. Faecalibacterium prausnitzii is an anti-inflammatory commensal bacterium identified by gut microbiota analysis of Crohn disease patients. Proc Natl Acad Sci U S A. 2008;105:16731–6.
153. Munukka E, Rintala A, Toivonen R, Nylund M, Yang B, Takanen A, et al. Faecalibacterium prausnitzii treatment improves hepatic health and reduces adipose tissue inflammation in high-fat fed mice. ISME J. 2017;11:1667–79.
154. Gomez-Gallego C, Pohl S, Salminen S, De Vos WM, Kneifel W. Akkermansia muciniphila: a novel functional microbe with probiotic properties. Benef Microbes. 2016;7:571–84.
155. Stenman LK, Burcelin R, Lahtinen S. Establishing a causal link between gut microbes, body weight gain and glucose metabolism in humans – towards treatment with probiotics. Benef Microbes. 2016;7:11–22.
156. Plovier H, Everard A, Druart C, Depommier C, Van Hul M, Geurts L, et al. A purified membrane protein from Akkermansia muciniphila or the pasteurized bacterium improves metabolism in obese and diabetic mice. Nat Med. 2017;23:107–13.
157. Zhao S, Liu W, Wang J, Shi J, Sun Y, Wang W, et al. Akkermansia muciniphila improves metabolic profiles by reducing inflammation in chow diet-fed mice. J Mol Endocrinol. 2017;58:1–14.
158. Gao X, Zhu Y, Wen Y, Liu G, Wan C. Efficacy of probiotics in non-alcoholic fatty liver disease in adult and children: a meta-analysis of randomized controlled trials. Hepatol Res. 2016;46:1226–33.
159. Ma YY, Li L, Yu CH, Shen Z, Chen LH, Li YM. Effects of probiotics on nonalcoholic fatty liver disease: a meta-analysis. World J Gastroenterol. 2013;19:6911–8.
160. Shavakhi A, Minakari M, Firouzian H, Assali R, Hekmatdoost A, Ferns G. Effect of a probiotic and metformin on liver aminotransferases in non-alcoholic steatohepatitis: a double blind randomized clinical trial. Int J Prev Med. 2013;4:531–7.
161. van Nood E, Vrieze A, Nieuwdorp M, Fuentes S, Zoetendal EG, de Vos WM, et al. Duodenal infusion of donor feces for recurrent Clostridium difficile. N Engl J Med. 2013;368:407–15.
162. Bajaj JS, Kassam Z, Fagan A, Gavis EA, Liu E, Cox IJ, et al. Fecal microbiota transplant from a rational stool donor improves hepatic encephalopathy: a randomized clinical trial. Hepatology. 2017;66(6):1727–38.
163. Kelly CR, Kim AM, Laine L, Wu GD. The AGA's fecal microbiota transplantation national registry: an important step toward understanding risks and benefits of microbiota therapeutics. Gastroenterology. 2017;152:681–4.
164. Reijnders D, Goossens GH, Hermes GD, Neis EP, van der Beek CM, Most J, et al. Effects of gut microbiota manipulation by antibiotics on host metabolism in obese humans: a randomized double-blind placebo-controlled trial. Cell Metab. 2016;24:63–74.
165. Vrieze A, Van Nood E, Holleman F, Salojarvi J, Kootte RS, Bartelsman JF, et al. Transfer of intestinal microbiota from lean donors increases insulin sensitivity in individuals with metabolic syndrome. Gastroenterology. 2012;143:913–916 e917.
166. Zhou D, Pan Q, Shen F, Cao HX, Ding WJ, Chen YW, et al. Total fecal microbiota transplantation alleviates high-fat diet-induced steatohepatitis in mice via beneficial regulation of gut microbiota. Sci Rep. 2017;7:1529.
167. Li SS, Zhu A, Benes V, Costea PI, Hercog R, Hildebrand F, et al. Durable coexistence of donor and recipient strains after fecal microbiota transplantation. Science. 2016;352:586–9.
168. Vermeire S, Joossens M, Verbeke K, Wang J, Machiels K, Sabino J, et al. Donor species richness determines faecal microbiota transplantation success in inflammatory bowel disease. J Crohns Colitis. 2016;10:387–94.

Autophagy, NAFLD and NAFLD-Related HCC

10

William K. K. Wu, Lin Zhang, and Matthew T. V. Chan

Abstract

Non-alcoholic fatty liver disease (NAFLD) will become a dominant cause of hepatocellular carcinoma (HCC) in the coming decade. Whereas the exact molecular mechanisms underlying the progression from simple steatosis, through steatohepatitis, to HCC remains largely unclear, emerging evidence has supported a central role of defective autophagy in the pathogenesis of NAFLD and its complications. Autophagy not only regulates lipid metabolism and insulin resistance, but also protects hepatocytes from injury and cell death. Nevertheless, in inflammation and tumorigenesis, the role of autophagy is more paradoxical. In NAFLD, defective hepatic autophagy occurs at multiple levels through numerous mechanisms and is causally linked to NAFLD-related HCC. In this chapter, we summarize the regulation and function of autophagy in NAFLD and highlight recent identification of potential pharmacological agents for restoring autophagic flux in NAFLD.

W. K. K. Wu (✉) · L. Zhang
Department of Anaesthesia and Intensive Care, The Chinese University of Hong Kong, Hong Kong, Hong Kong

State Key Laboratory of Digestive Diseases, Department of Medicine & Therapeutics and LKS Institute of Health Sciences, The Chinese University of Hong Kong, Hong Kong, Hong Kong
e-mail: wukakei@cuhk.edu.hk

M. T. V. Chan
Department of Anaesthesia and Intensive Care, The Chinese University of Hong Kong, Hong Kong, Hong Kong
e-mail: mtvchan@cuhk.edu.hk

Keywords

Fatty liver · Macroautophagy · Tumor suppression · Signaling

10.1 Epidemiology and General Mechanism of NAFLD and NAFLD-Related HCC

10.1.1 Epidemiology of NAFLD and NAFLD-Related HCC

The community prevalence of non-alcoholic fatty liver disease (NAFLD) has increased from less than 10% in the 1980s to current rates of 15–30% or higher. NAFLD affects 15–40% of the general population in Asia [1]. The pathological spectrum of NAFLD comprises hepatic steatosis alone, hepatic steatosis with lobular inflammation, and non-alcoholic steatohepatitis (NASH). More than 30% of people with NAFLD may have NASH, which may progress to cirrhosis (in 10–29% of NASH patients) and ultimately hepatocellular carcinoma (HCC) (in 4–27% of NASH-induced cirrhosis patients) [1]. NAFLD is

J. Yu (ed.), *Obesity, Fatty Liver and Liver Cancer*, Advances in Experimental Medicine and Biology 1061, https://doi.org/10.1007/978-981-10-8684-7_10

strongly associated with metabolic syndrome (i.e. obesity, diabetes, insulin resistance and dyslipidemia). The relative risk for HCC in obese men with body mass index (BMI) >35 was 4.52 compared to those with BMI between 18.5 and 24.9. Type II diabetes is also found to double the risk of HCC. With the increasing prevalence of obesity in children and adolescents, it is expected that NASH will become a dominant cause of HCC in the future with increasing number of patients presenting at an earlier age [1].

10.1.2 Molecular Basis of NASH and NAFLD-Related HCC

The current paradigm of NASH pathogenesis is that "toxic lipid species", including free fatty acids or free cholesterol, trigger cell death and inflammatory response. Such changes are accompanied by metabolic alterations, such as insulin resistance, and overproduction of free radicals from the mitochondria, causing lipid peroxidation, cytokine production, and necrosis [1, 2]. Some advances have also been made in understanding the molecular characteristics of NAFLD-related HCC. Hyperinsulinemia associated with type II diabetes could activate IRS-1 and the downstream mitogen-activated protein kinases (MAPK) and phosphoinositide-3-kinase (PI3K)/Akt pathways to promote cell proliferation and survival. Pro-inflammatory cytokines, such as interleukin (IL)-6 and tumor necrosis factor (TNF) α, could also mediate activation of oncogenic transcription factors, including activator protein-1 (AP-1), nuclear factor-κB (NF-κB) and signal transducer and activator of transcription 3 (STAT3). Imbalance of adipokine signaling (i.e. hypoadiponectinemia and hyperlectinemia) associated with increased adiposity is also linked to malignant phenotypes, such as unchecked cell cycle progression, evasion of apoptosis, and enhanced invasiveness and metastasis [1, 2]. However, little is known about how the effect of aberrant fatty accumulation in the liver is directly converted to oncogenic signals. As a consequence, there is minimal intervention in the clinic to prevent HCC development in NASH patients at risk of such progression. Thus, there is a compelling need to elucidate the molecular mechanisms of NAFLD-related HCC and to identify potential therapeutic targets to control this disorder.

10.2 Mechanism and Functions of Autophagy

10.2.1 Cellular Mechanism of Autophagy

Macroautophagy (hereafter referred to as autophagy) is a major process in which the cell digests its own contents. This self-cannibalistic pathway is instigated by the sequestration of cytosolic cargos, such as proteins and damaged organelles, by the phagophore followed by the formation of double-membrane structures known as autophagosomes. In the late phase, autophagosomes merge with lysosomes to produce autolysosomes. The sequestered materials are then degraded by acidic hydrolases to release free amino acids [3]. In this way, autophagy serves as an important pathway for energy production in time of starvation. Autophagy has been shown to have crosstalk with diverse signaling pathways and possess the ability to regulate other cellular and tissue processes, such as cell proliferation, apoptosis, differentiation, and inflammation. In this regard, altered autophagosomal-lysosomal pathway has been connected to many pathological conditions, including such as cancer, infection, autoimmunity, inflammatory diseases, neurodegeneration and aging [4].

10.2.2 Molecular Checkpoints of Autophagy

Although autophagy could be regulated at multiple levels, its execution converges on multiple mediators collectively known as "autophagy-related proteins", which are involved in the abovementioned multi-step machinery [5]. The initiation of autophagosome formation is regulated by the nutrient-sensing mammalian target of rapamycin (mTOR) through the unc-51-like kinase 1/2 (ULK1/2)-mAtg13-focal adhesion kinase family interacting protein of 200 kDa (FIP200) complex. Under growth-permissive conditions, mTOR binds and represses the ULK1/2-mAtg13-FIP200 complex and thereby inhibiting FIP200 phosphorylation and recruitment of Atg proteins. However, under growth factor- or nutrient-deprived conditions, mTOR dissociates from the ULK1/2-mAtg13-FIP200 complex to unmask the kinase activities of ULK1/2, resulting in assembly of Atg proteins at the autophagosome formation site [6]. Beclin 1, the mammalian orthologue of the yeast Apg6/Vps30, could mediate multiple vesicle-trafficking pathways and plays a central role in autophagy. Beclin1 is a Bcl-2-interacting protein which exists in complexes of at least three different configurations: Beclin 1-hVps34-p150-Atg14, Beclin 1-hVps34-p150-UVRAG-Bif1 and Beclin 1-hVps34-p150-Rubicon-UVRAG [7]. The former functions at the early stage of autophagosome formation whereas the latter two complexes facilitate autophagosomal membrane curvature and the maturation phase, respectively [7]. LC3, an autophagosomal ortholog of yeast Atg8, is another major regulator of autophagy, in which conversion of a cytosolic truncated form of LC3 (LC3-I) to its lipidated, autophagosomal membrane-associated form (LC3-II) is required for autophagosome formation [8].

10.3 Roles of Autophagy in NAFLD-Associated Biological Processes

10.3.1 Lipid Metabolism

Autophagosomal sequestration of triglycerides and cholesterol derived from lipid droplets in liver has been described and termed lipophagy. In autolysosomes, triglycerides are broken down by acidic hydrolases to produce free fatty acid, which are utilized for mitochondrial β-oxidation. In this capacity, lipophagy functions to regulate intracellular lipid stores and energy homeostasis. Accordingly, blockade of autophagy by pharmacological inhibitor or silencing expression autophagy related genes caused the retention of triglycerides and lipid droplets [9], reduced free fatty acid oxidation, and lowered the secretion of very-low-density lipoprotein (VLDL) from hepatocytes. Induction of hepatic autophagy through liver specific overexpression of Atg7 thus has been shown to alleviate the metabolic stress and mitigate hepatic steatosis in ob/ob mice [10]. Two pro-autophagic transcription factors FOXO1 and transcription factor EB (TFEB) also alleviate steatosis [11, 12]. Short-term treatment with pharmacological activators of autophagy, namely carbamazepine and rapamycin could reduce liver steatosis and triglyceride levels in the liver and blood [13]. These findings support a lipolytic role of autophagy in the liver.

10.3.2 Insulin Resistance

Defective autophagy has been linked to the development of insulin resistance. FOXO1-mediated suppression of autophagy conferred insulin resistance in genetically obese mice or mice fed with high-fat diet. Deficient hepatic autophagy of obese mice also promoted ER stress to induce insulin resistance [10, 12]. Concordantly, restoration of autophagy by hepatocyte-specific overexpression of Atg7 in obese mice normalized the insulin sensitivity and improved glucose tolerance [10].

10.3.3 Hepatocellular Injury

Recurrent hepatocellular injury and necroinflammation could lead to progression of simple steatosis to NASH, cirrhosis or even HCC. Autophagy functions to clear damaged organelles and, in this capacity, protects against cell death by removing abnormal mitochondria, which produce oxidative stress or trigger apoptosis through the intrinsic pathway [14–16]. Consistently, silencing *Atg5* could blunt the cytoprotective function of autophagy and thereby enhancing hepatocyte death induced by menadione, which causes oxidative stress and mitochondrial cytochrome release [14]. Autophagy has also been shown to protect hepatocytes from extrinsic pathway of apoptosis, including death triggered by necrosis factor-related apoptosis-inducing ligand (TRAIL) [17]. Activating autophagy could also attenuate cell death in hepatocytes loaded with palmitic acid [18].

10.3.4 Inflammation

Autophagy could be a potent suppressor of inflammation. Findings from genetic and functional studies have pinpointed defective autophagy as a contributing factor to several autoimmune disorders, particularly in Crohn's disease of which inflammation plays a key role in its pathogenesis [19]. Mechanistically, autophagy clears damaged mitochondria that release reactive oxygen species and mitochondrial DNA, thereby suppressing the activation of inflammasomes and Toll-like receptor 9 [20, 21]. Autophagy is also required for the degradation of p62/SQSTM1, an activator of NF-κB that promotes the transcription of pro-inflammatory cytokines [22, 23]. Through these mechanisms, autophagy dampens the transcription and/or maturation of pro-inflammatory cytokines to suppress inflammation [24, 25].

However, it is noteworthy that autophagy could in some biological contexts paradoxically promote inflammation. For instance, autophagy mediates the production of pro-inflammatory cytokines induced by avian influenza H5N1 pseudotyped particle via NF-κB and p38 mitogen-activated protein kinase (MAPK) signaling pathways [26]. Autophagy also enhances lipopolysaccharides-induced lung inflammation and neutrophil recruitment [27]. Enforced expression of hepatitis B virus X (HBx) protein, an oncogenic and pro-inflammatory protein, also induces autophagy in normal hepatocytes, in which knockdown of ATG5 and ATG7 mitigated HBx-induced activation of NF-κB and production of pro-inflammatory cytokines IL-6, IL-8, and CXCL2 in cultured hepatocytes [28].

10.4 Autophagic Impairment in NAFLD

Emerging data suggests that obesity and long-term high-fat diet feeding might impair the autophagosomal-lysosomal system at multiple levels (Fig. 10.1), namely blockade of autophagosome formation, inhibition of autophagosome-lysosome fusion and mitigation of lysosome function [29].

10.4.1 Endoplasmic Reticulum Stress

The endoplasmic reticulum (ER) provides the oxidizing environment for synthesis, folding and posttranslational modification of cellular proteins and is the primary storage organelle for intracellular Ca^{2+}. Disruption of ER homeostasis could have severe cellular consequences. When the ER stress occurs as a result of accumulation of misfolded proteins, cells activate a protective called unfolded protein response (UPR), which is consisted three major molecular circuitries – [1] IRE-1 (inositol requiring enzyme 1)-mediated alternative splicing of XBP1 (X-box binding protein 1); [2] nuclear translocation and activation of ATF6 (activating transcription factor 6); activation of PERK (PKR-like ER kinase)-eIF2α (eukaryotic initiation factor 2 α)-ATF4 cascade. Activation of these pathways presumably helps to reduce the protein load and increase the folding capacity of the ER [30]. González-Rodríguez et al. recently demonstrated that the autophagic flux is impaired in cell-line and animal models of NAFLD as well as in clinical specimens of NAFLD patients. Interestingly, abrogation of endoplasmic reticulum (ER) could alleviate such impairment. In particular, knockdown of C/EBP homologous protein (CHOP), a pro-apoptotic mediator induced by both ATF4 and ATF6 upon ER stress, has been shown to partially alleviate autophagic impairment and hepatocyte apoptosis [18]. A subsequent mechanistic study by Wang and colleagues demonstrated that ER stress-induced asparagine synthetase overexpression contribute to increased generation of asparagine and thereby inhibiting lysosome acidification.

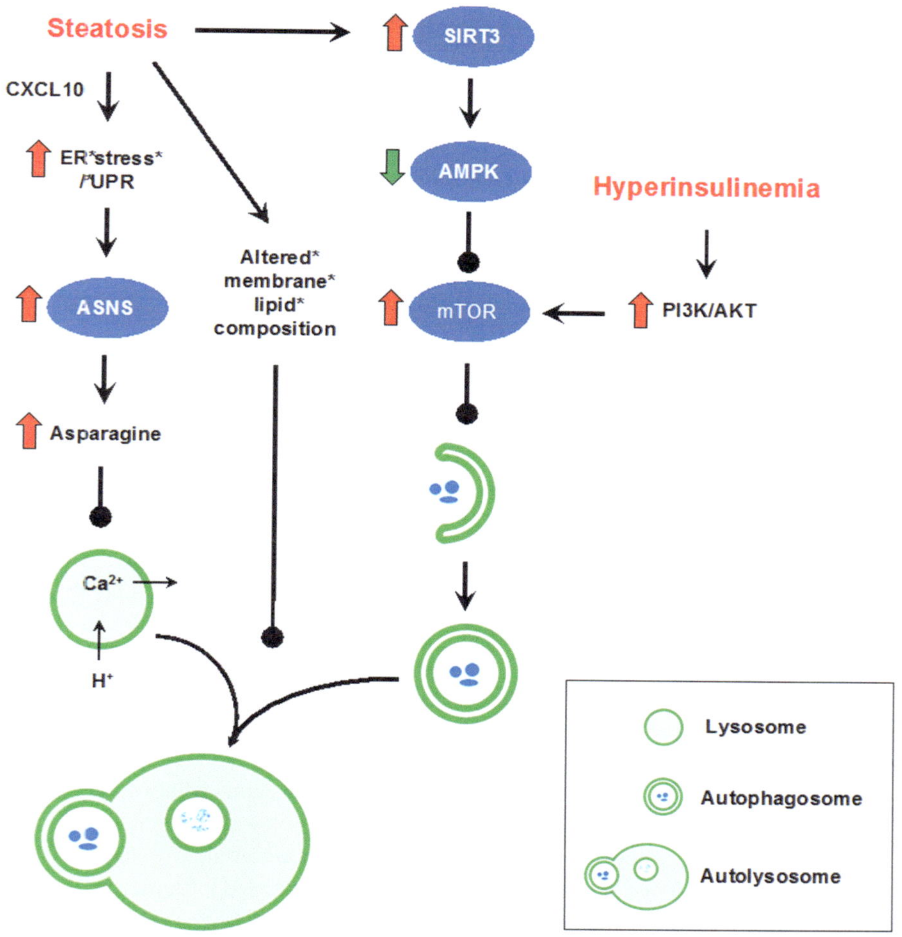

Fig. 10.1 Multi-level inhibition of autophagosome-lysosome system by steatosis in non-alcoholic fatty liver diseases

The induction of asparagine synthetase was mediated through the PERK (PKR-like ER kinase)-eIF2α-ATF4 cascade. Interestingly, both steatotic- and asparagine-treated hepatocytes showed reduced lysosomal acidity as evidenced by impaired cathepsin D cleavage and reduced number of acidic vesicular organelles. Such deficits were attributed to the retention of lysosomal Ca^{2+}, of which positive charge presumably prevents the transport of protons into lysosomes. Accordingly, knockdown of asparagine synthetase in steatotic hepatocytes restored autophagic flux [31]. These results also reverberated previous findings that cathepsin B, D, and L expression was significantly decreased in the liver from NAFLD patients [32].

10.4.2 Adipokines and Cytokines

Patients with NASH have been shown to exhibit dysregulated cytokine profiles in liver tissues, plasma and peripheral blood monocyte [33]. Reduced levels of adiponectin, an adipose-derived adipokine, are associated with obesity and NASH. Interestingly, adiponectin knockout attenuated high fat diet-induced autophagic defects, such as accumulation of p62/SQSTM1, and liver injury without reversing liver weights and hepatic steatosis, suggesting that reduced levels of adiponectin play an auto-protective role possibly through normalizing autophagy [34]. C-X-C motif chemokine 10 (CXCL10) is a crucial pro-inflammatory factor in chronic hepatitis.

In animal models of NASH, ablation of CXCL10 by neutralizing monoclonal antibody or gene knockout has been to protect against hepatocyte injury and steatohepatitis development. These protective effects were accompanied by rectification of autophagic flux impairment. Bafilomycin A1, an inhibitor of lysosomal vacuolar type H^+-ATPase and autolysosome formation, abolished the rectifying effect of CXCL10 ablation in cultured hepatocytes, indicating CXCL10 impaired late-stage autophagy in NAFLD [35].

10.4.3 Overactivation of mTOR Signaling

In both genetic and dietary models of obesity, a severe inhibition of autophagosome formation has been demonstrated. The mTOR signaling, which is a major suppressor of autophagosome formation, and FOXO1 downstream of AKT has been shown to be overactivated in steatotic liver, presumably owing to increased amino acid concentration and hyperinsulinemia [12, 36, 37]. High-fat diet rich in saturated fatty acids has been shown to elevate the expression and activity of Sirtuin 3 (Sirt3), which renders hepatocytes susceptible to palmitate-induced cell death. Mechanistically, Sirt3 upregulation results in manganese superoxide dismutase deacetylation and activation, which depleted intracellular superoxide contents, leading to AMP-activated protein kinase (AMPK) inhibition and mTOR complex 1 activation and thereby suppressing autophagy [38].

10.4.4 Altered Membrane Lipid Content

Koga and colleagues established an in vitro fusion assay using different lysosomal/autophagic compartments isolated from mouse liver. They found that altered membrane lipid composition induced by 25 mM methyl-beta-cyclodextrin *in vitro* or feeding animals with high-fat diet *in vivo* could reduce autophagosome-lysosome fusion up to 70% [39].

10.4.5 Foxo3a Downregulation

Autophagic impairment might occur in mesenchymal cells of steatotic livers. Palmitate and lipopolysaccharides have been shown to synergistically reduce Foxo3a expression in Kupffer cells, in which downregulation of Foxo3a increased blockage of autophagy flux. The protective effect of Foxo3a was found to be mediated through its transcriptional target Bim, whose overexpression also restored autophagy influx [40].

10.5 The Role of Autophagy in Tumorigenesis

10.5.1 Paradoxical Role of Autophagy in HCC

Autophagy plays a paradoxical role in hepatocarcinogenesis. Immunohistochemical staining has shown that the expression of Beclin-1, a key pro-autophagic protein, was significantly lower in HCC tissues than adjacent tissues and such downregulation was associated with more aggressive clinicopathological phenotypes and poorer overall survival [41]. Numerous tumor suppressors (e.g. XPD, Klotho, Tak1, PTPRO) have also been demonstrated to activate autophagy in HCC cells [42–45].

The tumor-suppressive function of autophagy was proposed to be mediated through degradation of oncogenic autophagic substrates (e.g. p62/STSTM1, microRNA-224) and maintenance of healthy mitochondria to reduce oxidative stress and DNA damage [46–48]. In this connection, gene targeting of p62/SQSTM1, a protein preferentially degraded through the autophagy pathway, has been shown to markedly abrogate the anchorage-independent growth of HCC cells, whereas overexpression of p62/SQSTM1 had opposite effects [48]. To this end, p62/SQSTM1 was reported to take part in the feedforward loop for inducing and sustaining NF-κB activity upon constitutive *KRAS* activation to promote the development of pancreatic ductal adenocarcinoma [22]. Moreover, knockdown of p62/

SQSTM1 inhibits cell migration and invasion in glioblastoma stem cells [49]. Autophagy mediates the degradation of the oncogenic microRNA-224, whose accumulation promotes HCC cell migration and tumor formation through silencing its target gene Smad4 [47]. Autophagy has also reported to mediate the growth-arresting and cytotoxic effects of interferon-γ in HCC cells [50].

Since autophagy is a major catabolic process, autophagy could paradoxically function as a pro-survival mechanism to generate nutrients, especially in time of nutrient deprivation and cellular stress. In this connection, autophagy has been shown to protects cancer cells from the accumulation of damaged organelles or protein aggregates, programmed cell death resulting from detachment from surrounding extracellular matrix (i.e. anoikis), and the toxicity of cancer therapies [3]. In HCC, autophagy inhibition by pharmacological inhibitors or siRNAs has been shown to sensitize cancer cells to the multikinase inhibitor linifanib [51]. MicroRNA-375-mediated inhibition of autophagy also impaired viability of HCC cells in response to hypoxia *in vitro* and *in vivo* [52]. Moreover, autophagy could suppress the expression of major tumor suppressors to promote the development of HCC [46].

It is generally believed that an optimal level of autophagy is key to tumor suppression in normal condition whereas this pathway could be subverted by cancer cells for tumor promotion in the later stages of hepatocarcinogenesis [3].

10.5.2 Crosstalk with Cancer-Related Signaling

Autophagy could be induced by Ras-Raf-MEK-ERK, IKK-nuclear factor (NF)-κB, transforming growth factor-β, platelet-derived growth factor, p16/p27/retinoblastoma protein (pRB), p53-DRAM, Ca^{2+}-CaMMKβ, reactive oxygen species (ROS)-ATM-AMPK signaling as well as endoplasmic reticulum stress mediators (e.g. PERK-eIF2α, GRP78/BiP, IRE1-JNK, HDAC6). In contrast, Autophagy is known to be negatively regulated by PI3K-Akt-mTOR signaling, anti-apoptotic members of Bcl-2 family, cytoplasmic p53, FLIP, BRCA1, Jumpy, Naf-1 and rubicon [3].

10.5.3 Emerging Evidence of Involvement of Autophagy in NAFLD-Related HCC

To date, only sporadic studies have directly examined the role of autophagy in NAFLD-related HCC with animal models. Inokuchi-Shimizu and colleagues reported that hepatocyte-specific deletion of the MAP kinase kinase kinase TGF β-activated kinase 1 (TAK1), a positive regulator of AMPK, increased mTOR activity and suppressed autophagy, accompanied by severe hepatosteatosis [44]. The expression of peroxisome proliferator-activated receptor α (PPARα) target genes and β-oxidation, which regulate hepatic lipid degradation, were also repressed. Interestingly, mice with hepatocyte-specific knockout of Tak1 developed spontaneous liver cancer, which expressed high levels of p62/SQSTM1. Inhibition of mTOR activity by rapamycin restored autophagy and prevented HCC development, indicating that induction of autophagy by Tak1 might inhibit fatty liver-associated HCC growth [44].

The tumor-suppressive function of autophagy could also be exemplified by another study reporting that genetic ablation of protein tyrosine phosphatase receptor type O (PTPRO), a known tumor suppressor, produced severe autophagy deficiency, liver injury, insulin resistance, hepatosteatosis and liver tumor formation upon feeding with high-fat diet after diethylnitrosamine (DEN) injection as compared with wild-type littermates [43]. Immunohistochemical staining demonstrated that hepatic PTPRO was reduced while p62/SQSTM1 was increased in NAFLD as compared with normal liver. These findings suggest that low expression of PTPRO in hepatocytes may contribute to the inhibition of autophagy and progression to NASH and NAFLD-related HCC [43].

10.6 Pharmacological Modulation of Autophagy for Treating NAFLD or Preventing NAFLD-Related HCC

Lysosome-dependent degradation of lipid through the autophagic pathway is growingly recognized as a crucial mechanism for lipid utilization whereas dysfunctional autophagy may contribute to NASH and NAFLD-related HCC development. Investigative efforts have thus been put forth to identify pharmacological agents that may restore autophagic functions in NAFLD and thus help to prevent NAFLD-related HCC.

10.6.1 Polyunsaturated Fatty Acids

Polyunsaturated fatty acids are fatty acids (PUFAs) that contain more than one double bond in their backbone. Shen and colleagues demonstrated that dietary PUFAs could increase LC3-II levels and attenuate IL-1β secretion and caspase-1 cleavage in response to lipopolysaccharides in cultured hepatocytes or liver tissues. Autophagy-dependent suppression of nucleotide-binding oligomerization domain leucine-rich repeat-containing receptor protein (NLRP3) inflammasome activation was proposed to mediate the beneficial effect of PUFAs [53].

10.6.2 4-Phenyl Butyric Acid

The chemical chaperone 4-phenyl butyric acid (4-PBA) has been shown to exhibit promising therapeutic effects in a variety of disease models, including metabolic syndrome, inflammatory diseases and cancer. Nissar and colleagues reported that 4-PBA could rectify the accumulation of p62/SQSTM1 and reduce lipid accumulation and apoptosis caused by palmitate in Huh7 hepatoma cells. Atg7 knockdown or pharmacological inhibition of autophagy with 3-methyladenine and chloroquine attenuated the lipid lowering effect of 4-PBA. These findings suggest that 4-PBA could reduce hepatocellular lipid accumulation and lipotoxicity through induction of autophagy [54].

10.6.3 Peretinoin

Peretinoin is an orally available, acyclic retinoid with potential antineoplastic and chemopreventive activities, presumably through activation of nuclear retinoic acid receptors (RAR). In two NASH-HCC mouse models, peretinoin has been shown to significantly improve liver histology and reduce the incidence of liver tumors. Peretinoin increased co-localized expression of LC3B-II and LAMP2, and increased autophagosome formation and autophagy flux in the liver through activating the promoter of *Atg16L1*, whose expression was reduced in the liver of patients with NASH. Atg16L1 overexpression was found to inhibit palmitate-induced NF-kB activation and IL-6-induced STAT3 activation by inducing the de-phosphorylation of Gp130, a receptor subunit of IL-6 family cytokines [55]. These findings suggest that peretinoin can prevent the development of NASH-HCC through activating autophagy by increasing Atg16L1 expression.

10.6.4 Carbon Monoxide

Carbon monoxide (CO), a reaction product of heme oxygenase activity, has been shown to protect against hepatic steatosis in mice. Subsequent mechanistic investigation demonstrated that carbon monoxide activated the PERK-eIF2α-ATF4 pathway to induce sestrin-2, which contributed to autophagy induction through activation of AMPK and inhibition of mTOR complex 1 [56].

10.6.5 Ginsenoside Rb2

Panax ginseng, a traditional Chinese medicine, has been widely used to treat a variety of metabolic diseases including hyperglycemia, hyperlipidemia, and hepatosteatosis. However, the active ingredient and molecular mechanisms underlying such effects remain largely unknown. Huang and colleagues found that ginsenoside Rb2, a major ginsenoside in Panax ginseng, can restore autophagy and prevent hepatic lipid accumulation *in vivo* and *in vitro* via induction of Sirt1 and activation of AMPK [57].

10.6.6 Thyroid Hormones

Iodothyronines are potential pharmacological compounds to treat NAFLD. Two iodothyronines, T_2 and T_3, both have shown efficacy in reducing the severity of NAFLD in cultured hepatocytes and animal models of NAFLD. Using a targeted metabolomics approach, Iannucci and colleagues found that both T_2 and T_3 could strongly induce hepatic autophagy and decrease hepatic fat content. However, only T_2 was able to rescue the impairment in AKT and MAPK/ERK pathways caused by short-term high-fat diet [58], indicating their differential effects.

10.6.7 Nicotinamide

Nicotinamide, the amide form of nicotinic acid (vitamin B3), could upregulate Sirt1 via the cAMP/PKA/CREB pathway to induce autophagy hepatocytes and thereby attenuating palmitate-induced ER stress and cytotoxicity [59]. These findings suggest that nicotinamide supplementation may represent a therapeutic choice for NAFLD.

10.6.8 Pectic Bee Pollen Polysaccharide

Bee pollen has been used as a nutraceutical against diabetes and obesity. Using high glucose and fatty acid-treated hepatocytes and high fat diet-fed mice, Li and colleagues found that pectic bee pollen polysaccharide from *Rosa rugosa* could alleviates hepatic steatosis and insulin resistance by promoting autophagy via an AMPK/mTOR-mediated signaling pathway [60], suggesting that this natural compound could be a novel therapeutic agent used for NAFLD.

10.6.9 Caffeine

Caffeine, a psychoactive component in coffee, tea and cola, is the world's most widely consumed drug. Through genetic, pharmacological, and metabolomic approaches, Sinha and colleagues demonstrated that caffeine could reduce intrahepatic lipid content and stimulate β-oxidation in hepatocytes via concomitantly increasing autophagy and lipid uptake in lysosomes. This beneficial effect was probably mediated through inhibition of mTOR signaling and paralleled with alterations in hepatic amino acids and sphingolipid levels [61].

10.6.10 Epigallocatechin Gallate

Epigallocatechin gallate (EGCG) is a major polyphenol in green tea with anti-inflammatory, anticancer, and anti-steatotic properties. EGCG has been shown to reduce hepatosteatosis and concomitantly increase autophagy in mice fed with high-fat diet. In this connection, EGCG increased phosphorylation of AMPK, whose knockdown abrogated autophagy induced by EGCG [62]. These findings suggest that AMPK-dependent induction of hepatic autophagy by EGCG might contribute to its beneficial effects in hepatosteatosis.

10.7 Concluding Remarks and Future Perspectives

NASH has become a dominant cause of HCC and its incidence is on the rise. Autophagy, a self-cannibalistic process, is a major pathway for lipid catabolism. Optimal and timely activation of autophagy also protects hepatocytes from injury and cell death as well as suppresses inflammation. In NAFLD, lipid accumulation, hyper-insulinemia, ER stress and deregulated cytokine expression have been shown to contribute to hepatic autophagy deficiency. Unfortunately, autophagic impairment further promotes these metabolic and molecular abnormalities, thereby creating a detrimental vicious circle. Defective autophagy is causally linked to NAFLD-related HCC, probably through accumulation of p62/SQSTM1, which induces and sustains the oncogenic NF-κB activity, and retention of damaged mitochondria, which produce reactive oxidative species to damage DNA. Nevertheless, it is noteworthy that autophagy could be subverted by HCC cells for opposing tumor suppression or as a pro-survival mechanism in response to therapies in the later stages of cancer development.

Pertinent to clinical practice, several pharmacological agents have been identified for their capacity to restore autophagic flux in NAFLD. These agents might also be promising prophylactics for preventing NALFD-related HCC if hepatocarcinogenesis has not yet been initiated. Nevertheless, the clinical utilization of these agents still awaits further validation in large-cohort human studies. Aside from therapy, recent discovery of circulating p62/SQSTM1 as serological marker [31] may open up a novel avenue for the use of autophagic markers for NAFLD diagnosis.

Acknowledgements The work was supported by Early Career Scheme (24115815) of the Research Grant Council Hong Kong; Shenzhen Science and Technology Programme (JCYJ20150630165236956, JCYC20140905151710921) of Shenzhen Science and Technology Innovation Commission; and Natural Science Foundation of Guangdong Province (2015A030313886) of Department of Science and Technology of Guangdong Province.

References

1. Yu J, Shen J, Sun TT, Zhang X, Wong N. Obesity, insulin resistance, NASH and hepatocellular carcinoma. Semin Cancer Biol. 2013;23(6 Pt B):483–91.
2. Tian Y, Wong VW, Chan HL, Cheng AS. Epigenetic regulation of hepatocellular carcinoma in non-alcoholic fatty liver disease. Semin Cancer Biol. 2013;23(6 Pt B):471–82.
3. Wu WK, Coffelt SB, Cho CH, Wang XJ, Lee CW, Chan FK, et al. The autophagic paradox in cancer therapy. Oncogene. 2012;31(8):939–53.
4. Levine B, Kroemer G. Autophagy in the pathogenesis of disease. Cell. 2008;132(1):27–42.
5. He C, Klionsky DJ. Regulation mechanisms and signaling pathways of autophagy. Annu Rev Genet. 2009;43:67–93.
6. Chan EY. mTORC1 phosphorylates the ULK1-mAtg13-FIP200 autophagy regulatory complex. Sci Signal. 2009;2(84):pe51.
7. Funderburk SF, Wang QJ, Yue Z. The Beclin 1-VPS34 complex—at the crossroads of autophagy and beyond. Trends Cell Biol. 2010;20(6):355–62.
8. Mizushima N, Yoshimori T. How to interpret LC3 immunoblotting. Autophagy. 2007;3(6):542–5.
9. Singh R, Kaushik S, Wang Y, Xiang Y, Novak I, Komatsu M, et al. Autophagy regulates lipid metabolism. Nature. 2009;458(7242):1131–5.
10. Yang L, Li P, Fu S, Calay ES, Hotamisligil GS. Defective hepatic autophagy in obesity promotes ER stress and causes insulin resistance. Cell Metab. 2010;11(6):467–78.
11. Settembre C, De Cegli R, Mansueto G, Saha PK, Vetrini F, Visvikis O, et al. TFEB controls cellular lipid metabolism through a starvation-induced autoregulatory loop. Nat Cell Biol. 2013;15(6):647–58.
12. Liu HY, Han J, Cao SY, Hong T, Zhuo D, Shi J, et al. Hepatic autophagy is suppressed in the presence of insulin resistance and hyperinsulinemia: inhibition of FoxO1-dependent expression of key autophagy genes by insulin. J Biol Chem. 2009;284(45):31484–92.
13. Lin CW, Zhang H, Li M, Xiong X, Chen X, Chen X, et al. Pharmacological promotion of autophagy alleviates steatosis and injury in alcoholic and non-alcoholic fatty liver conditions in mice. J Hepatol. 2013;58(5):993–9.
14. Wang Y, Singh R, Xiang Y, Czaja MJ. Macroautophagy and chaperone-mediated autophagy are required for hepatocyte resistance to oxidant stress. Hepatology. 2010;52(1):266–77.
15. Maiuri MC, Zalckvar E, Kimchi A, Kroemer G. Self-eating and self-killing: crosstalk between autophagy and apoptosis. Nat Rev Mol Cell Biol. 2007;8(9):741–52.
16. Lemasters JJ. Selective mitochondrial autophagy, or mitophagy, as a targeted defense against oxidative stress, mitochondrial dysfunction, and aging. Rejuvenation Res. 2005;8(1):3–5.
17. Lim SC, Jeon HJ, Kee KH, Lee MJ, Hong R, Han SI. Involvement of DR4/JNK pathway-mediated autophagy in acquired TRAIL resistance in HepG2 cells. Int J Oncol. 2016;49(5):1983–90.
18. Gonzalez-Rodriguez A, Mayoral R, Agra N, Valdecantos MP, Pardo V, Miquilena-Colina ME, et al. Impaired autophagic flux is associated with increased endoplasmic reticulum stress during the development of NAFLD. Cell Death Dis. 2014;5:e1179.
19. Jones SA, Mills KH, Harris J. Autophagy and inflammatory diseases. Immunol Cell Biol. 2013;91(3):250–8.
20. Oka T, Hikoso S, Yamaguchi O, Taneike M, Takeda T, Tamai T, et al. Mitochondrial DNA that escapes from autophagy causes inflammation and heart failure. Nature. 2012;485(7397):251–5.
21. Nakahira K, Haspel JA, Rathinam VA, Lee SJ, Dolinay T, Lam HC, et al. Autophagy proteins regulate innate

immune responses by inhibiting the release of mitochondrial DNA mediated by the NALP3 inflammasome. Nat Immunol. 2011;12(3):222–30.
22. Ling J, Kang Y, Zhao R, Xia Q, Lee DF, Chang Z, et al. KrasG12D-induced IKK2/beta/NF-kappaB activation by IL-1alpha and p62 feedforward loops is required for development of pancreatic ductal adenocarcinoma. Cancer Cell. 2012;21(1):105–20.
23. Sanz L, Sanchez P, Lallena MJ, Diaz-Meco MT, Moscat J. The interaction of p62 with RIP links the atypical PKCs to NF-kappaB activation. EMBO J. 1999;18(11):3044–53.
24. Lee HM, Shin DM, Yuk JM, Shi G, Choi DK, Lee SH, et al. Autophagy negatively regulates keratinocyte inflammatory responses via scaffolding protein p62/SQSTM1. J Immunol. 2011;186(2):1248–58.
25. Saitoh T, Fujita N, Jang MH, Uematsu S, Yang BG, Satoh T, et al. Loss of the autophagy protein Atg16L1 enhances endotoxin-induced IL-1beta production. Nature. 2008;456(7219):264–8.
26. Pan H, Zhang Y, Luo Z, Li P, Liu L, Wang C, et al. Autophagy mediates avian influenza H5N1 pseudotyped particle-induced lung inflammation through NF-kappaB and p38 MAPK signaling pathways. Am J Physiol Lung Cell Mol Physiol. 2014;306(2):L183–95.
27. Guo L, Stripay JL, Zhang X, Collage RD, Hulver M, Carchman EH, et al. CaMKIalpha regulates AMP kinase-dependent, TORC-1-independent autophagy during lipopolysaccharide-induced acute lung neutrophilic inflammation. J Immunol. 2013;190(7):3620–8.
28. Luo MX, Wong SH, Chan MT, Yu L, Yu SS, Wu F, et al. Autophagy mediates HBx-induced nuclear factor-kappaB activation and release of IL-6, IL-8, and CXCL2 in hepatocytes. J Cell Physiol. 2015;230(10):2382–9.
29. Lavallard VJ, Gual P. Autophagy and non-alcoholic fatty liver disease. Biomed Res Int. 2014;2014:120179.
30. Wu WK, Sakamoto KM, Milani M, Aldana-Masankgay G, Fan D, Wu K, et al. Macroautophagy modulates cellular response to proteasome inhibitors in cancer therapy. Drug Resist Updat. 2010;13(3):87–92.
31. Wang X, Zhang X, Chu ESH, Chen X, Kang W, Wu F, et al. Defective lysosomal clearance of autophagosomes and its clinical implications in nonalcoholic steatohepatitis. FASEB J. 2018;32(1):37–51.
32. Fukuo Y, Yamashina S, Sonoue H, Arakawa A, Nakadera E, Aoyama T, et al. Abnormality of autophagic function and cathepsin expression in the liver from patients with non-alcoholic fatty liver disease. Hepatol Res. 2014;44(9):1026–36.
33. Braunersreuther V, Viviani GL, Mach F, Montecucco F. Role of cytokines and chemokines in non-alcoholic fatty liver disease. World J Gastroenterol. 2012;18(8):727–35.
34. Guo R, Nair S, Zhang Y, Ren J. Adiponectin deficiency rescues high-fat diet-induced hepatic injury, apoptosis and autophagy loss despite persistent steatosis. Int J Obes. 2017;41(9):1403–12.
35. Zhang X, Wu WK, Xu W, Man K, Wang X, Han J, et al. C-X-C motif chemokine 10 impairs autophagy and autolysosome formation in non-alcoholic steatohepatitis. Theranostics. 2017;7(11):2822–36.
36. Tremblay F, Krebs M, Dombrowski L, Brehm A, Bernroider E, Roth E, et al. Overactivation of S6 kinase 1 as a cause of human insulin resistance during increased amino acid availability. Diabetes. 2005;54(9):2674–84.
37. Gual P, Le Marchand-Brustel Y, Tanti JF. Positive and negative regulation of insulin signaling through IRS-1 phosphorylation. Biochimie. 2005;87(1):99–109.
38. Li S, Dou X, Ning H, Song Q, Wei W, Zhang X, et al. Sirtuin 3 acts as a negative regulator of autophagy dictating hepatocyte susceptibility to lipotoxicity. Hepatology. 2017;66(3):936–52.
39. Koga H, Kaushik S, Cuervo AM. Altered lipid content inhibits autophagic vesicular fusion. FASEB J. 2010;24(8):3052–65.
40. Liu Y, Zhang W, Wu X, Gong J. Foxo3a-dependent Bim transcription protects mice from a high fat diet via inhibition of activation of the NLRP3 inflammasome by facilitating autophagy flux in Kupffer cells. Oncotarget. 2017;8(21):34258–67.
41. Qiu DM, Wang GL, Chen L, Xu YY, He S, Cao XL, et al. The expression of beclin-1, an autophagic gene, in hepatocellular carcinoma associated with clinical pathological and prognostic significance. BMC Cancer. 2014;14:327.
42. Zheng JF, Li LL, Lu J, Yan K, Guo WH, Zhang JX. XPD functions as a tumor suppressor and dysregulates autophagy in cultured HepG2 cells. Med Sci Monit. 2015;21:1562–8.
43. Zhang W, Hou J, Wang X, Jiang R, Yin Y, Ji J, et al. PTPRO-mediated autophagy prevents hepatosteatosis and tumorigenesis. Oncotarget. 2015;6(11):9420–33.
44. Inokuchi-Shimizu S, Park EJ, Roh YS, Yang L, Zhang B, Song J, et al. TAK1-mediated autophagy and fatty acid oxidation prevent hepatosteatosis and tumorigenesis. J Clin Invest. 2014;124(8):3566–78.
45. Shu G, Xie B, Ren F, Liu DC, Zhou J, Li Q, et al. Restoration of klotho expression induces apoptosis and autophagy in hepatocellular carcinoma cells. Cell Oncol (Dordr). 2013;36(2):121–9.
46. Tian Y, Kuo CF, Sir D, Wang L, Govindarajan S, Petrovic LM, et al. Autophagy inhibits oxidative stress and tumor suppressors to exert its dual effect on hepatocarcinogenesis. Cell Death Differ. 2015;22(6):1025–34.
47. Lan SH, Wu SY, Zuchini R, Lin XZ, Su IJ, Tsai TF, et al. Autophagy suppresses tumorigenesis of hepatitis B virus-associated hepatocellular carcinoma through degradation of microRNA-224. Hepatology. 2014;59(2):505–17.
48. Inami Y, Waguri S, Sakamoto A, Kouno T, Nakada K, Hino O, et al. Persistent activation of Nrf2 through p62 in hepatocellular carcinoma cells. J Cell Biol. 2011;193(2):275–84.
49. Galavotti S, Bartesaghi S, Faccenda D, Shaked-Rabi M, Sanzone S, McEvoy A, et al. The autophagy-

associated factors DRAM1 and p62 regulate cell migration and invasion in glioblastoma stem cells. Oncogene. 2013;32(6):699–712.
50. Li P, Du Q, Cao Z, Guo Z, Evankovich J, Yan W, et al. Interferon-gamma induces autophagy with growth inhibition and cell death in human hepatocellular carcinoma (HCC) cells through interferon-regulatory factor-1 (IRF-1). Cancer Lett. 2012;314(2):213–22.
51. Pan H, Wang Z, Jiang L, Sui X, You L, Shou J, et al. Autophagy inhibition sensitizes hepatocellular carcinoma to the multikinase inhibitor linifanib. Sci Rep. 2014;4:6683.
52. Chang Y, Yan W, He X, Zhang L, Li C, Huang H, et al. miR-375 inhibits autophagy and reduces viability of hepatocellular carcinoma cells under hypoxic conditions. Gastroenterology. 2012;143(1):177–87. e8
53. Shen L, Yang Y, Ou T, Key CC, Tong SH, Sequeira RC, et al. Dietary PUFAs attenuate NLRP3 inflammasome activation via enhancing macrophage autophagy. J Lipid Res. 2017;58(9):1808–21.
54. Nissar AU, Sharma L, Mudasir MA, Nazir LA, Umar SA, Sharma PR, et al. Chemical chaperone 4-phenyl butyric acid (4-PBA) reduces hepatocellular lipid accumulation and lipotoxicity through induction of autophagy. J Lipid Res. 2017;58(9):1855–68.
55. Okada H, Takabatake R, Honda M, Takegoshi K, Yamashita T, Nakamura M, et al. Peretinoin, an acyclic retinoid, suppresses steatohepatitis and tumorigenesis by activating autophagy in mice fed an atherogenic high-fat diet. Oncotarget. 2017;8(25):39978–93.
56. Kim HJ, Joe Y, Kim SK, Park SU, Park J, Chen Y, et al. Carbon monoxide protects against hepatic steatosis in mice by inducing sestrin-2 via the PERK-eIF2alpha-ATF4 pathway. Free Radic Biol Med. 2017;110:81–91.
57. Huang Q, Wang T, Yang L, Wang HY. Ginsenoside Rb2 alleviates hepatic lipid accumulation by restoring autophagy via induction of Sirt1 and activation of AMPK. Int J Mol Sci. 2017;18(5):1063.
58. Iannucci LF, Cioffi F, Senese R, Goglia F, Lanni A, Yen PM, et al. Metabolomic analysis shows differential hepatic effects of T2 and T3 in rats after short-term feeding with high fat diet. Sci Rep. 2017;7(1):2023.
59. Shen C, Dou X, Ma Y, Ma W, Li S, Song Z. Nicotinamide protects hepatocytes against palmitate-induced lipotoxicity via SIRT1-dependent autophagy induction. Nutr Res. 2017;40:40–7.
60. Li X, Gong H, Yang S, Yang L, Fan Y, Zhou Y. Pectic bee pollen polysaccharide from Rosa rugosa alleviates diet-induced hepatic steatosis and insulin resistance via induction of AMPK/mTOR-mediated autophagy. Molecules. 2017;22(5):699.
61. Sinha RA, Farah BL, Singh BK, Siddique MM, Li Y, Wu Y, et al. Caffeine stimulates hepatic lipid metabolism by the autophagy-lysosomal pathway in mice. Hepatology. 2014;59(4):1366–80.
62. Zhou J, Farah BL, Sinha RA, Wu Y, Singh BK, Bay BH, et al. Epigallocatechin-3-gallate (EGCG), a green tea polyphenol, stimulates hepatic autophagy and lipid clearance. PLoS One. 2014;9(1):e87161.

Animal Models of Non-alcoholic Fatty Liver Diseases and Its Associated Liver Cancer

11

Jennie Ka Ching Lau, Xiang Zhang, and Jun Yu

Abstract

Non-alcoholic fatty liver disease (NAFLD) is a spectrum of diseases, which include simple liver steatosis, non-alcoholic steatohepatitis (NASH), cirrhosis and hepatocellular carcinoma (HCC). It is a burgeoning health problem worldwide in line with the trend towards unhealthy diet and increased prevalence of obesity and type 2 diabetes mellitus (T2DM). Many animal models that illustrate both the histology and pathology of human NAFLD have been established. It is important to choose an animal model that best conforms to the aim of the study. This chapter presents a critical analysis of the histopathology and pathogenesis of NAFLD and the most commonly used and recently developed animal models of hepatic steatosis, NASH and NAFLD-induced hepatocellular carcinoma (NAFLD-HCC). The main mechanisms involved in the experimental pathogenesis of NAFLD in various animal models were also discussed. This chapter also includes a brief summary of recent therapeutic targets found using animal models. Although current animal models provide important guidance in understanding the pathogenesis and development of NAFLD, future study is essential to develop more precise models that better mimic the disease spectrum for both improved mechanistic understanding and identification of novel therapeutic options.

Keywords

Non-alcoholic fatty liver disease (NAFLD) · Liver cancer · Dietary animal model · Genetic animal model · Disease histopathology

J. K. C. Lau (✉)
Institute of Digestive Disease and Department of Medicine & Therapeutics, State Key Laboratory of Digestive Disease, LKS Institute of Health Sciences, The Chinese University of Hong Kong, Hong Kong, Hong Kong

SHHO College, The Chinese University of Hong Kong, Hong Kong, Hong Kong

X. Zhang · J. Yu
Institute of Digestive Disease and Department of Medicine & Therapeutics, State Key Laboratory of Digestive Disease, LKS Institute of Health Sciences, The Chinese University of Hong Kong, Hong Kong, Hong Kong
e-mail: jenniferzhang@link.cuhk.edu.hk; junyu@cuhk.edu.hk

11.1 Introduction

Non-alcoholic fatty liver disease (NAFLD) is recognized as the hepatic exhibition of the metabolic syndrome. With the growing epidemic of obesity and insulin resistance, the worldwide prevalence of NAFLD continues to increase and is becoming the most common cause of chronic liver disease

J. Yu (ed.), *Obesity, Fatty Liver and Liver Cancer*, Advances in Experimental Medicine and Biology 1061, https://doi.org/10.1007/978-981-10-8684-7_11

[1]. NAFLD can progresses from simple liver steatosis to non-alcoholic steatohepatitis (NASH), and even to liver fibrosis and cirrhosis. Fibrosing NASH leads to liver fibrosis and ultimately cirrhosis [2], increases risks for hepatocellular carcinoma (HCC) development [3]. Different stage of the NAFLD disease spectrum has distinctive histopathology features. Simple liver steatosis contains lipid accumulation in hepatocytes [4]. Hepatocellular injury, ballooning, and inflammation were present in NASH.

Excessive import or reduced export or oxidation of free fatty acids (FFAs) can induce hepatic steatosis. Lipid accumulation occurs when the rate of import or synthesis of FFAs by hepatocytes surpasses rate of export or catabolism [5]. Either of the following 4 can lead to triglyceride accumulation: [1] increased uptake of FFAs into hepatocytes due to excess lipolysis from adipose tissue stores or dietary intake, [2] increased de novo lipogenesis, [3] failure of FFA export through VLDL synthesis, and [4] failure of FFA elimination due to impaired β-oxidation. NAFLD occur where fat droplets accumulate in at least over 5% of hepatocytes [6]. The accumulation of fat droplets is usually macrovesicular, in which one large fat droplet or small well-defined droplets displace the nucleus from the cell center into the periphery. Microvesicular hepatic steatosis, though less common, may also occur concurrently in which very small fat droplets fill the hepatocytes without displacing the nucleus from the center of the cells. Pure microvesicular steatosis is a rare feature of NAFLD.

NASH is the resultant inflammatory response that is stimulated by various additional hits [2]. 1/3 of NAFLD patients could progress to NASH [7]. Liver steatosis, inflammatory cell infiltration and hepatocellular ballooning with or without fibrosis are the histopathology of NASH. The inflammation in NASH include lobular inflammation, which showed the infiltration of innate immune cells [8] and portal inflammation, which is usual and mild [9]. "Multiple-hit" hypothesis was reported recently for the pathogenesis of NASH, which include oxidative stress, inflammation, hyperinsulinemia, hyperleptinemia, and hypoadiponectinemia [10]. Of all these factors, oxidative stress and inflammation are two mechanisms pivotal to NASH genesis. The degree of oxidative stress is closely related with the severity of NASH [11, 12]. The imbalance of ROS generated by oxidative could induce lipid peroxidation and hepatocyte cellular damage. These damages affect plasmatic membranes, intracellular organelles, mitochondrial DNA, and respiratory chain-related proteins. Another consequence of increased ROS is that it may induce Fas ligand expression as it contains a binding site for nuclear factor-κB (NF-κB) and promote paracrine-induced apoptotic hepatocyte death. Excess FFA also leads to peroxisome proliferator-activated receptor alpha (PPAR-α)–mediated activation of the synthesis of enzymes responsible for extra-mitochondrial β-oxidation and ω-oxidation pathway. Chronic hepatic inflammation is closely related with NASH. The production of pro-inflammatory cytokines including TNF-α and interleukin-6 (IL-6) could affect adipokine levels, which induce perpetuation of the loop of chronic inflammation [13]. TNF-α increases FFA levels by inducing insulin resistance (IR), induces ROS formation by uncoupling mitochondrial respiration, and induces hepatocyte apoptosis and necrosis. Other reported pro-inflammatory cytokines that are elevated in NASH include IL-1α, IL-1β, and IL-18.

Nevertheless, the exact mechanism of NAFLD progression is still unclear. Further research for pathogenesis and therapeutic options are pivotal considering the increased incidence of NAFLD. Animal models that mirror the pathophysiology of each stage of human NAFLD progression provide important guidance in understanding the disease pathogenesis and progression. This chapter will summarize the current and most commonly used animal models. Moreover, it will briefly outline possible therapeutic options that have recently been identified using animal models.

11.2 Dietary Animal Models of NAFLD

11.2.1 High Fat Diet (HFD) Animal Model

The relationship between NAFLD and obesity induce the establishment of a high-fat diet that is similar with Western diets. In HFD animal models, 45–75% of the animals' total calorie intake is resulted from fat.

The traditional reported HFD comprised of 71% fat, 18% protein and 11% carbohydrates for 3 weeks, whereas a standard Lieber-DeCarli diet included 35% fat, 47% carbohydrates and 18% protein. Although no weight change in rats fed with control or HFD, insulin resistance was developed as indicated by increased plasma insulin levels [14].

Mice fed with HFD comprised of 45% fat, 35% carbohydrates and 20% protein showed hepatic steatosis as indicated by increased lipid accumulation, hepatocyte ballooning and Mallory bodies (Fig. 11.1a). HFD could result in a higher percentage of cells enriched in lipid. For example, Wistar male rats were fed diets with same quantity (15 g/rat/day) for 16 weeks but with different composition including high-fat, moderate-fat, high-sucrose, and high-fructose groups. The HF group had the highest body and liver weight and highest percentage of liver steatosis (40%) [15].

The advantage of HFD-fed animal model is that it mimic both the histopathology and pathogenesis of human NAFLD as they induce hallmark features observed in human NAFLD including metabolic syndrome. However, the degree of hepatic steatosis seems to depend upon various factors including rodent strain.

11.2.2 Methionine and Choline-deficient (MCD) Dietary Model

Feeding mice a lipogenic MCD diet is a frequently used and very reproducible nutritional model of NASH. The diet is deficient in methionine and choline with moderately fat. Choline is an essential nutrient that is stored and metabolized chiefly in the liver. Choline deficient impairs hepatic VLDL secretion and results in hepatosteatosis, oxidative stress, liver cell death, and the alteration of cytokines and adipocytokines [16], but only causes mild hepatic inflammation and fibrosis. In contrast, mice fed a diet lacking both choline and amino acid methionine develop severe hepatic inflammation at 2 weeks of MCD diet feeding [5, 17] (Fig. 11.1b). Alongside with ballooning degeneration of hepatocytes, serum alanine aminotransferase (ALT) levels also increase [18]. Recent studies suggest that the progression of steatosis to steatohepatitis in MCD mice models involve significant downregulation

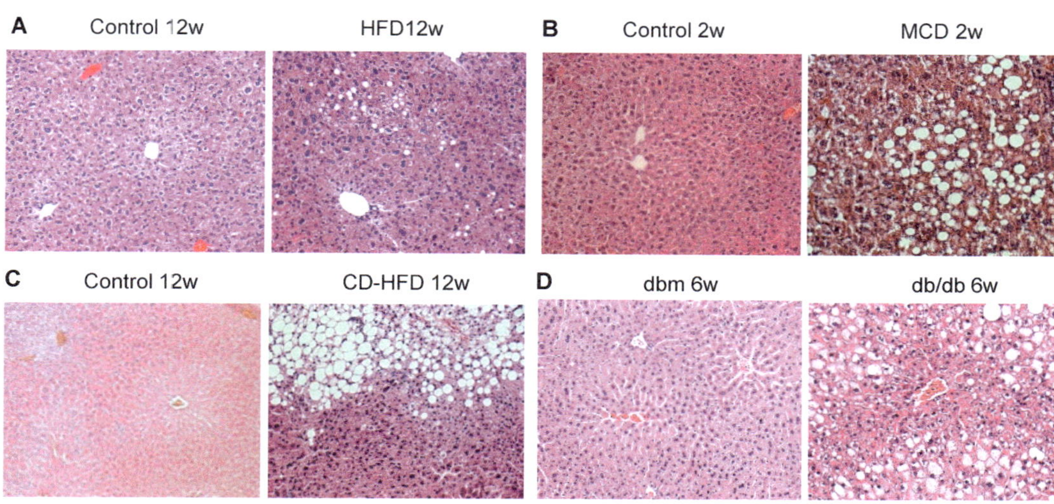

Fig. 11.1 Histopathological features of NAFLD in dietary and genetic animal models. Representative H&E staining from liver sections of (**a**) C57 BL/6 mice fed with control or high fat diet (HFD) for 12 weeks; (**b**) C57 BL/6 mice fed with control or methionine and choline-deficient (MCD) diet for 2 weeks; (**c**) C57 BL/6 mice fed with control or choline deficient high fat diet (CD-HFD) for 12 weeks; (**d**) *db/db* and dbm control mice fed with normal chow for 6 weeks

in expressions of proteins involved in Met metabolism and oxidative stress [19].

Compared with other dietary models, MCD mouse models better mimicked pathological findings of severe human NASH. The typical features of NAFLD include inflammation, fibrosis, and hepatocyte apoptosis were much more quickly and severely than mice fed HFD or Western diets. The diet also better models the mechanisms implicated in the pathogenesis of human NASH. Endoplasmic reticulum stress, oxidative stress, and autophagocytic stress are all substantially more active in MCD models than other dietary models [20]. Thus, this model is ideal for studying histologically advanced NASH and the mechanisms of inflammation and fibrosis in NASH. It must be noted that studies have shown that different mouse strains respond differently towards the MCD diet.

The disadvantage of MCD model is obvious. Instead of being obese, mice fed an MCD diet exhibit significant weight loss, cachexia, without metabolic profile of human NASH, and low serum insulin, fasting glucose, leptin and triglyceride levels [21]. Hence, MCD diets are often fed to *db/db* or *ob/ob* mice in order to better mimic human NASH. MCD diet fed *db/db* mice are obese and showed marked hepatic inflammation and fibrosis [22].

11.2.3 High Cholesterol Diet Model

Dietary cholesterol is an important factor in the progression of steatohepatitis and hepatic inflammation in both animal models [23–25] and humans [26]. Mice fed a high-cholesterol diet (HCD) (1%) alone show striking increases in serum insulin levels but only slight increases in liver weight, triglyceride, FFAs, and serum ALT [26]. However, when high-cholesterol is given in conjunction with high-fat or high-cholate, features of NASH are much more pronounced. Mice fed a high-fat (15%), high-cholesterol (1%) diet (HFHC) showed greater weight gain, greater hepatic lipid accumulation, elevated serum ALT level, decreased adiponectin, adipose tissue inflammation, and fibrosis, the features of which were much more severe in HFHC mice than HFD or HCD mice [26]. Similarly, mice fed a high-cholesterol (1.25%), high-cholate (0.5%) diet also showed greater steatosis, inflammation, hepatocellular ballooning and fibrosis [23, 27]. Mice fed with 23% fat, 424 g/Kg sucrose and1.9 g/kg cholesterol diet or choline-deficient high fat diet (CD-HFD) for 3 months developed pronounced steatohepatitis (Fig. 11.1c). Several studies suggest dietary cholesterol reduces VLDL synthesis and β-oxidation of fatty acids and increases apoptosis and hepatic oxidative stress [25, 26].

11.2.4 High Fructose Diet Model

Epidemiologic data suggests that humans consume a significant number of calories from fructose rich foods and this has been paralleled with the development of obesity and NASH in humans [28]. C57BL/6 mice a HFD or high-fat high-fructose (HFHF) diet showed similar fructose consumption [28]. In a study from our group, *CXCR3*-knockout and C57BL/6 wild-type mice were fed a similar HFHF diet comprising of a HFHC diet supplemented with 23 g/L of fructose in drinking water. Results showed that *CXCR3*-knockout mice had improved liver histology, significantly lower necroinflammation, and reduced lipid peroxidation. This suggests that CXCR3 plays a pivotal role in NASH development in HFHF mouse models [29].

11.3 Genetic Animal Models of NAFLD

11.3.1 *db/db* and *ob/ob* Genetic Animal Model

db/db mice are homozygous for the autosomal recessive diabetic gene (db). The db gene encodes for a point mutation of the leptin receptor (Ob-Rb), which leads to defective signaling of leptin hormone [30]. Thus, *db/db* mice have normal or elevated levels of leptin but are resistant to its effects. Leptin is responsible for regulating feeding behaviour by promoting satiety. These mice have persistent hyperphagia and are obese and diabetic [31]. They show severe hyperglycaemia, hyperinsulinemia, elevated serum leptin, and develop macrovesicular hepatic steatosis [5, 22, 32] (Fig. 11.1d). Prolonged calorie overconsumption (>1 month) may lead to slightly aggravated hepatic inflammation [30]. Nevertheless, *db/db* mice when fed a control diet rarely display features of NASH. Thus, *db/db* mice alone are good models of NAFLD but not of NASH.

Unlike *db/db* mice, *ob/ob* mice have functional leptin receptors but have truncated and non-functional leptin. Similarly, these mice are grossly overweight, hyperphagic, hyperinsulimenic, hyperglycemic, and resistant to insulin, and develop spontaneous marked liver steatosis [30] but not steatohepatitis. Secondary insults are also required to trigger steatohepatitis. This may be provided through exposure to MCD diet, HFD, small doses of lipopolysaccharide endotoxin [31], ethanol or hepatic ischaemia-reperfusion challenge [5]. *ob/ob* mice are essentially resistant to fibrosis because leptin is essential for hepatic fibrosis [32].

Unlike dietary models, *db/db* and *ob/ob* mouse models exhibit features of human metabolic syndrome. When fed a standard diet without an additional hit, these mice are useful models of NAFLD as they develop pronounced hepatic steatosis. With the addition of a second-hit like MCD diet, *db/db* mice can also be used to study the progression of steatosis to NASH. However, congenital leptin deficiency and leptin resistance caused by gene mutation in obese humans are extremely rare [33], so *db/db* and *ob/ob* mice models are limited in reflecting the aetiology of human obesity, insulin resistance and hepatic steatosis.

11.3.2 foz/foz Genetic Model

foz/foz mice have a mutated *Alms1* which have a possible role in intracellular transport and appetite regulation [34]. *foz/foz* mice are morbidly obese, hyperphagic, and develop IR, significantly reduced adiponectin levels, increased cholesterol levels, and steatosis. A HFD promotes the transition of steatosis to NASH with severe fibrosis in these mice by attenuating metabolic complications, resulting in further decreased adiponectin levels and elevated cholesterol levels. However, the severity of diet-induced NASH in *foz/foz* mice depends on the strain. When *foz/foz* BALB/c and C57BL6/J mice were fed a HFD, weight gain was equivalent, suggesting that the appetite defect in *foz/foz* mice is independent of strain, however NAFLD was much more severe in *foz/foz* C57BL6/J mice than in *foz/foz* BALB/c mice. IR, hyperinsulinaemia, obesity, and substantial NAFLD-related liver fibrosis were exhibited in *foz/foz* C57BL6/J mice but not in *foz/foz* BALB/c mice. These findings suggest that although obesity in *foz/foz* mice is equal, the responses to obesity including features of NASH are dependent on strain [35].

11.3.3 *db/db* Genetic Supplemented Dietary NASH Model

In addition to MCD diet, a recent study found that iron overload in *db/db* mice can also cause progression of NAFLD to NASH and fibrosis. Unlike *db/db* mice fed a normal chow diet, *db/db* mice fed a chow diet supplemented with high iron showed hepatocellular ballooning, fibrogenesis increased hepatic oxidative stress, inflammasome activation, hepatic inflammatory immune cell activation and impaired hepatic mitochondrial fatty acid β-oxidation [36].

11.4 Animal Models of NAFLD-Induced HCC

HCC is the third most common cause of cancer-related death worldwide. There is a weighty connection between NASH and HCC. Liver cirrhosis is the most important risk factor for HCC although HCC could occur in non-cirrhotic NASH [8]. Increased fat uptake, hepatic steatosis, and NASH are all incremental risk factors for HCC. 4–27% of patients with NASH-related cirrhosis ultimately progress to HCC [3]. Long-term follow up studies reveal that the prevalence of HCC in NASH patients is 0–2.8% [3, 37, 38].

Current mouse models of NAFLD and NASH do not replicate pathological process from fatty liver, NASH, and fibrosis to HCC. Various experimental mouse models for HCC are present but only a few of them represent NAFLD-induced HCC [39].

11.4.1 Diet NAFLD-Induced HCC Model

Models fed with only one type of diet have distinctive limitations. C57BL/6 mice fed MCD or CD diets is lean without insulin resistance. HFD-fed mice do not exhibit NASH-like pathology whereas mice fed a MCD or CD diet do. To solve this problem, Wolf *et al.* proposed a mixed diet model combining choline deficient diet and HFD for the investigation of NAFLD-induced HCC development. Liver steatosis, features of metabolic syndrome and liver damage reflected by elevated serum ALT and AST levels were present concurrently in this novel model. Features of liver damage were reminiscent of human NASH including oxidative stress, hepatocyte ballooning, immune cell infiltration, glycogeneated nuclei, and MDB. Liver analysis of HFD versus CD-HFD mice found that tumor incidence in HFD mice is only 2.5% while incidence in CD-HFD mice is 25% [40].

In another diet model, C57BL/6 mice are fed a choline-deficient L-amino-acid-defined-diet (CDAA). The mice develop liver injury that mimic NASH features that lead to HCC. Treatment of mice with CDAA induced insulin resistance, increase in hepatic steatosis, modifications of enzymes of carbohydrate and lipid metabolism, liver damage, and fibrosis. HCC developed after 9 months of feeding [41].

Asgharpour et al. recently reported a diet-induced animal model that recapitulates the key human NASH-HCC features. They generated an isogenic mouse strain B6/129 by repeating brother-sister mating of the C57BL/6 J and 129S1/SvlmK mice for over 4-years. B6/129 mice fed with high fat high carbohydrate diet will sequentially develop steatosis in 4–8 weeks, NASH in 16–24 weeks and HCC at week 52, which may be an ideal preclinical model of NASH-HCC investigation [42].

11.4.2 Combined Chemical & Dietary NAFLD- Induced HCC Model

CDAA diet C57BL/6 mice subjected to low dose intraperitoneal injections of Carbon Tetrachloride (CCl_4) have more marked features of NASH and HCC. Mice had greater steatosis, lobular inflammation, and fibrogenesis when compared with CDAA diet alone. In addition, CDAA C57BL/6 mice showed presence of HCC only in 35% of cases but CDAA + CCl_4 group showed presence of HCC in all mice and with a significantly higher average tumour diameter. Thus the CDAA+CCl_4 model better represents NASH and its progression to HCC than CDAA diet alone model [41].

In another combined chemical and dietary model, Mice fed a HFD and treated with Streptozotocin (STZ), a glucosamine-nitrosourea compound, is toxic towards pancreatic β cells and induces hypoinsulinemia, hyperglycaemia, and diabetes in mice. STZ-primed mice stimulated with HFD induced histological changes including steatosis, lobular inflammation, fibrosis and, at 20 weeks, tumor protrusion. Male STZ-HFD mice developed significant proliferation of hepatocytes at 16 weeks and eventually HCC. The model provides insight into the mechanism linking metabolic disorder, NASH and HCC [43].

11.4.3 Genetic NAFLD-Induced HCC Model

Phosphatase and tensin homolog (PTEN) is a tumor suppressor gene through its lipid phosphatase activity and is mutated in many human cancers [44]. PTEN is a putative tumor suppressor in liver and PTEN loss could promote cell proliferation, inhibit apoptosis and induce tumor formation. Mice with PTEN loss in hepatocytes develop features similar to human NASH and NASH-induced HCC [45]. Hepatocarcinogenesis is evident in PTEN-deficient mice as liver tumors were present in 66% of male and 30% of female

PTEN-deficient mice at 40–44 weeks and pathological examinations showed that HCC was present in 83% of male and 50% of females at 74–78 weeks [45]. Thus, this model is useful for not only the understanding of pathogenesis of NASH but also the progression to HCC.

11.4.4 Combined Genetic and Chemical NAFLD-Induced HCC Model

Shen *et al.* found that genetic obesity in *db/db* mice is a direct promoter of NASH-HCC development. Compared to wild-type lean mice, *db/db* mice treated with carcinogen diethylnitrosamine (DEN) had higher body weight, higher liver weight, hepatic steatosis, higher HCC incidence, and tumor nodules significantly higher in number and larger in size. Results also found that these mice had genetic alterations in inflammation-related pathways and mutations in *Cel,* which leads to endoplasmic reticulum (ER) stress and cell proliferation. Findings from this mouse model suggest that obesity and NASH increases susceptibility of HCC development [46].

11.5 Usage of Animal Models

Animal models are crucial in elucidating the mechanisms and pathways involved in the pathogenesis of the NAFLD progression. Often studies using the aforementioned animal models may provide encouraging results for future treatments for NAFLD and NASH.

Using HFD mice models, Jin et al. reported that Cyclin D3-cyclin-dependent kinase 4 (CDK4) activation is a crucial event in NAFLD progression [47]. C/EBPα and C/EBPβ are members of the C/EBP protein family, which control multiple functions in different tissues and are involved in the development of NAFLD. C/EBPα is a strong inhibitor of liver proliferation. Its functions and biological activities on the liver are controlled by post-translational modification at the Ser193 amino acid site. Cyclin D3-cyclin-dependent kinase 4 (cdk4) phosphorylates C/EBPα on Ser193 causing it to form a complex with chromatin remodeling protein p300. C/EBPα-p300 causes C/EBPα-dependent growth arrest. HFD activates cdk4 in wild-type mice, leading to an increase in C/EBPα-p300 complexes. Similarly, HFD-mediated steatosis, fibrosis, and liver injury are inhibited in Cdk-4 resistant C/EBPα-S193A mice. These findings suggest that elevation of cdk4 is a key event in the development of NAFLD and cdk4 inhibition can be considered as a possible treatment for NAFLD. Using *db/db* mice model, Li *et al.* demonstrated that Carboxylesterase 2 (CES2) is a novel triglyceride hydrolase in lipid regulation and NAFLD [48]. Glucagon-like peptide-1 (GLP-1) is a neuropeptide that induces pancreatic β-cells to release insulin in response to glucose, restores glucose sensitivity of β-cells, and promotes β-cells proliferation. Exendin-4 is a GLP-1 analogue that is resistant to such inactivation and is hence a target for the treatment of type 2 diabetes mellitus. Using MCD-fed *db/db* mice model, Yamamoto *et al.* showed that exendin-4 treatment prevented MCD-induced steatohepatitis with decreased lipid accumulation and FFA content. Results found that exendin-4 exerted such effects via three mechanisms. Firstly, exendin-4 could suppress SREBP-1c-related hepatic de novo lipogenesis. Secondly, it was observed that exendin-4 attenuated the MCD-diet induced decrease in levels of peroxisomal acyl-coenzyme A oxidase 1 (ACOX1) mRNA. This suggests that exendin-4 induces lipid oxidation, as ACOX1 is an enzyme involved in hepatic β-oxidation. Lastly, fatty acid transport protein 4 (FATP4) plays an important role in hepatic fatty acid uptake and exendin-4 administration attenuated the MCD-diet induced increase in liver FATP4 mRNA, thus suggesting a decrease in hepatic FFA influx. With regards to hepatic inflammation, exendin-4 reduced hepatic inflammation score, levels of a hepatic ROS marker namely MDA, and levels of pro-inflammatory cytokines and chemokines such as TNF-α and monocyte chemoattractant protein-1 (MCP-1). These data found using a MCD mice model shed light on the possible use of exendin-4 for the treatment of non-obese patients with NASH [49].

11.6 Conclusion

The animal models aforementioned in this chapter are useful tools in studying the pathogenesis of NAFLD and the identification of possible therapeutic options. However, they are not perfect to characterize all the features of NAFLD. Some replicate the histopathology of NAFLD remarkably but not the physiological properties, and others vice versa. Therefore, more accurate animal models that better mimic the disease spectrum are still essential and need further study.

Acknowledgment This chapter was modified from the paper published by our group in Journal of Pathology (Lau, Zhang and Yu 2017; 241:36–44). The related contents are re-used with the permission.

References

1. Alexander Wree LB, Canbay A, Hoffman HM, Feldstein AE. From NAFLD to NASH to cirrhosis—new insights into disease mechanisms. Nat Rev Gastroenterol Hepatol. 2013;10:627–36.
2. Dowman JK, Tomlinson JW, Newsome PN. Pathogenesis of non-alcoholic fatty liver disease. QJM. 2010;103:71–83.
3. Starley BQ, Calcagno CJ, Harrison SA. Nonalcoholic fatty liver disease and hepatocellular carcinoma: a weighty connection. Hepatology. 2010;51:1820–32.
4. Hubscher SG. Histological assessment of non-alcoholic fatty liver disease. Histopathology. 2006;49:450–65.
5. Anstee QM, Goldin RD. Mouse models in non-alcoholic fatty liver disease and steatohepatitis research. Int J Exp Pathol. 2006;87:1–16.
6. Tandra S, Yeh MM, Brunt EM, Vuppalanchi R, Cummings OW, Unalp-Arida A, et al. Presence and significance of microvesicular steatosis in nonalcoholic fatty liver disease. J Hepatol. 2011;55:654–9.
7. Farrell GC, Larter CZ. Nonalcoholic fatty liver disease: from steatosis to cirrhosis. Hepatology. 2006;43:S99–S112.
8. Brunt EM, Tiniakos DG. Histopathology of nonalcoholic fatty liver disease. World J Gastroenterol. 2010;16:5286–96.
9. Brunt EM, Kleiner DE, Wilson LA, Unalp A, Behling CE, Lavine JE, et al. Portal chronic inflammation in nonalcoholic fatty liver disease (NAFLD): a histologic marker of advanced NAFLD-Clinicopathologic correlations from the nonalcoholic steatohepatitis clinical research network. Hepatology. 2009;49:809–20.
10. Tilg H, Moschen AR. Evolution of inflammation in nonalcoholic fatty liver disease: the multiple parallel hits hypothesis. Hepatology. 2010;52:1836–46.
11. Sanyal AJ, Campbell-Sargent C, Mirshahi F, Rizzo WB, Contos MJ, Sterling RK, et al. Nonalcoholic steatohepatitis: association of insulin resistance and mitochondrial abnormalities. Gastroenterology. 2001;120:1183–92.
12. George J, Pera N, Phung N, Leclercq I, Yun Hou J, Farrell G. Lipid peroxidation, stellate cell activation and hepatic fibrogenesis in a rat model of chronic steatohepatitis. J Hepatol. 2003;39:756–64.
13. Tilg H. The role of cytokines in non-alcoholic fatty liver disease. Dig Dis. 2010;28:179–85.
14. Nieto-Vazquez I, Fernandez-Veledo S, Kramer DK, Vila-Bedmar R, Garcia-Guerra L, Lorenzo M. Insulin resistance associated to obesity: the link TNF-alpha. Arch Physiol Biochem. 2008;114:183–94.
15. Fakhoury-Sayegh N, Trak-Smayra V, Khazzaka A, Esseily F, Obeid O, Lahoud-Zouein M, et al. Characteristics of nonalcoholic fatty liver disease induced in wistar rats following four different diets. Nutr Res Pract. 2015;9:350–7.
16. Corbin KD, Zeisel SH. Choline metabolism provides novel insights into nonalcoholic fatty liver disease and its progression. Curr Opin Gastroenterol. 2012;28:159–65.
17. Yamada T, Obata A, Kashiwagi Y, Rokugawa T, Matsushima S, Hamada T, et al. Gd-EOB-DTPA-enhanced-MR imaging in the inflammation stage of nonalcoholic steatohepatitis (NASH) in mice. Magn Reson Imaging. 2016;34:724–9.
18. Larter CZ, Yeh MM, Williams J, Bell-Anderson KS, Farrell GC. MCD-induced steatohepatitis is associated with hepatic adiponectin resistance and adipogenic transformation of hepatocytes. J Hepatol. 2008;49:407–16.
19. Lee SJ, Kang JH, Iqbal W, Kwon OS. Proteomic analysis of mice fed methionine and choline deficient diet reveals marker proteins associated with steatohepatitis. PLoS One. 2015;10:e0120577.
20. Machado MV, Michelotti GA, Xie G, Almeida Pereira T, Boursier J, Bohnic B, et al. Mouse models of diet-induced nonalcoholic steatohepatitis reproduce the heterogeneity of the human disease. PLoS One. 2015;10:e0127991.
21. Rinella ME, Green RM. The methionine-choline deficient dietary model of steatohepatitis does not exhibit insulin resistance. J Hepatol. 2004;40:47–51.
22. Sahai A, Malladi P, Pan X, Paul R, Melin-Aldana H, Green RM, et al. Obese and diabetic db/db mice develop marked liver fibrosis in a model of nonalcoholic steatohepatitis: role of short-form leptin receptors and osteopontin. Am J Physiol Gastrointest Liver Physiol. 2004;287:G1035–43.
23. Matsuzawa N, Takamura T, Kurita S, Misu H, Ota T, Ando H, et al. Lipid-induced oxidative stress causes steatohepatitis in mice fed an atherogenic diet. Hepatology. 2007;46:1392–403.
24. Zheng S, Hoos L, Cook J, Tetzloff G, Davis H Jr, van Heek M, et al. Ezetimibe improves high fat and cholesterol diet-induced non-alcoholic fatty liver disease in mice. Eur J Pharmacol. 2008;584:118–24.

25. Subramanian S, Goodspeed L, Wang S, Kim J, Zeng L, Ioannou GN, et al. Dietary cholesterol exacerbates hepatic steatosis and inflammation in obese LDL receptor-deficient mice. J Lipid Res. 2011;52:1626–35.
26. Savard C, Tartaglione EV, Kuver R, Haigh WG, Farrell GC, Subramanian S, et al. Synergistic interaction of dietary cholesterol and dietary fat in inducing experimental steatohepatitis. Hepatology. 2013;57:81–92.
27. Takahashi Y, Soejima Y, Fukusato T. Animal models of nonalcoholic fatty liver disease/nonalcoholic steatohepatitis. World J Gastroenterol. 2012;18:2300–8.
28. Kohli R, Kirby M, Xanthakos SA, Softic S, Feldstein AE, Saxena V, et al. High-fructose, medium chain trans fat diet induces liver fibrosis and elevates plasma coenzyme Q9 in a novel murine model of obesity and nonalcoholic steatohepatitis. Hepatology. 2010;52:934–44.
29. Zhang X, Han J, Man K, Li X, Du J, Chu ES, et al. CXC chemokine receptor 3 promotes steatohepatitis in mice through mediating inflammatory cytokines, macrophages and autophagy. J Hepatol. 2016;64:160–70.
30. Trak-Smayra V, Paradis V, Massart J, Nasser S, Jebara V, Fromenty B. Pathology of the liver in obese and diabetic ob/ob and db/db mice fed a standard or high-calorie diet. Int J Exp Pathol. 2011;92:413–21.
31. Yang SQ, Lin HZ, Lane MD, Clemens M, Diehl AM. Obesity increases sensitivity to endotoxin liver injury: implications for the pathogenesis of steatohepatitis. Proc Natl Acad Sci U S A. 1997;94:2557–62.
32. Leclercq IA, Farrell GC, Schriemer R, Robertson GR. Leptin is essential for the hepatic fibrogenic response to chronic liver injury. J Hepatol. 2002;37:206–13.
33. Paz-Filho G, Mastronardi C, Delibasi T, Wong ML, Licinio J. Congenital leptin deficiency: diagnosis and effects of leptin replacement therapy. Arq Bras Endocrinol Metabol. 2010;54:690–7.
34. Bell-Anderson KS, Aouad L, Williams H, Sanz FR, Phuyal J, Larter CZ, et al. Coordinated improvement in glucose tolerance, liver steatosis and obesity-associated inflammation by cannabinoid 1 receptor antagonism in fat Aussie mice. Int J Obes (Lond). 2011;35:1539–48.
35. Farrell GC, Mridha AR, Yeh MM, Arsov T, Van Rooyen DM, Brooling J, et al. Strain dependence of diet-induced NASH and liver fibrosis in obese mice is linked to diabetes and inflammatory phenotype. Liver Int. 2014;34:1084–93.
36. Handa P, Morgan-Stevenson V, Maliken BD, Nelson JE, Washington S, Westerman M, et al. Iron overload results in hepatic oxidative stress, immune cell activation, and hepatocellular ballooning injury, leading to nonalcoholic steatohepatitis in genetically obese mice. Am J Physiol Gastrointest Liver Physiol. 2016;310:G117–27.
37. Rafiq N, Bai C, Fang Y, Srishord M, McCullough A, Gramlich T, et al. Long-term follow-up of patients with nonalcoholic fatty liver. Clin Gastroenterol Hepatol. 2009;7:234–8.
38. Ong JP, Pitts A, Younossi ZM. Increased overall mortality and liver-related mortality in non-alcoholic fatty liver disease. J Hepatol. 2008;49:608–12.
39. Heindryckx F, Colle I, Van Vlierberghe H. Experimental mouse models for hepatocellular carcinoma research. Int J Exp Pathol. 2009;90:367–86.
40. Wolf MJ, Adili A, Piotrowitz K, Abdullah Z, Boege Y, Stemmer K, et al. Metabolic activation of intrahepatic CD8+ T cells and NKT cells causes nonalcoholic steatohepatitis and liver cancer via cross-talk with hepatocytes. Cancer Cell. 2014;26:549–64.
41. De Minicis S, Agostinelli L, Rychlicki C, Sorice GP, Saccomanno S, Candelaresi C, Giaccari A, Trozzi L, Pierantonelli I, Mingarelli E, Marzioni M, Muscogiuri G, Gaggini M, Benedetti A, Gastaldelli A, Guido M, Svegliati-Baroni G. HCC development is associated to peripheral insulin resistance in a mouse model of NASH. PLoS One. 2014;9:e97136.
42. Asgharpour A, Cazanave SC, Pacana T, Seneshaw M, Vincent R, Banini BA, et al. A diet-induced animal model of non-alcoholic fatty liver disease and hepatocellular cancer. J Hepatol. 2016;65:579.
43. Fujii M, Shibazaki Y, Wakamatsu K, Honda Y, Kawauchi Y, Suzuki K, Arumugam S, Watanabe K, Ichida T, Asakura H, Yoneyama H. A murine model for non-alcoholic steatohepatitis showing evidence of association between diabetes and hepatocellular carcinoma. Med Mol Morphol. 2013;46:141–52.
44. Horie Y, Suzuki A, Kataoka E, Sasaki T, Hamada K, Sasaki J, et al. Hepatocyte-specific Pten deficiency results in steatohepatitis and hepatocellular carcinomas. J Clin Invest. 2004;113:1774–83.
45. Watanabe S, Horie Y, Kataoka E, Sato W, Dohmen T, Ohshima S, et al. Non-alcoholic steatohepatitis and hepatocellular carcinoma: lessons from hepatocyte-specific phosphatase and tensin homolog (PTEN)-deficient mice. J Gastroenterol Hepatol. 2007;22(Suppl 1):S96–S100.
46. Shen J, Tsoi H, Liang Q, Chu ES, Liu D, Yu AC, et al. Oncogenic mutations and dysregulated pathways in obesity-associated hepatocellular carcinoma. Oncogene. 2016;35:6271.
47. Jin J, Valanejad L, Nguyen TP, Lewis K, Wright M, Cast A, et al. Activation of CDK4 triggers development of non-alcoholic fatty liver disease. Cell Rep. 2016;16:744.
48. Li Y, Zalzala M, Jadhav K, Xu Y, Kasumov T, Yin L, et al. Carboxylesterase 2 prevents liver steatosis by modulating lipolysis, endoplasmic reticulum stress, and lipogenesis and is regulated by hepatocyte nuclear factor 4 alpha in mice. Hepatology. 2016;63:1860–74.
49. Yamamoto T, Nakade Y, Yamauchi T, Kobayashi Y, Ishii N, Ohashi T, et al. Glucagon-like peptide-1 analogue prevents nonalcoholic steatohepatitis in non-obese mice. World J Gastroenterol. 2016;22:2512–23.

Current Prevention and Treatment Options for NAFLD

12

Vincent Wai-Sun Wong

Abstract

Non-alcoholic fatty liver disease (NAFLD) is now the most common chronic liver disease worldwide and the second leading indication for liver transplantation and the third leading cause of hepatocellular carcinoma (HCC) in the United States. This chapter focuses on the prevention and management of NAFLD. Healthy lifestyle is the cornerstone for the prevention and management of NAFLD and should be recommended to every patient at risk or having established NAFLD. Despite the high prevalence of NAFLD, it should be recognized that the majority of patients will not develop liver-related complications; cardiovascular disease remains the leading cause of death in NAFLD patients. Until further data are available, pharmacological treatment should be restricted to selected patients with confirmed non-alcoholic steatohepatitis. As some agents with primarily anti-fibrotic effect are currently being tested in NAFLD patients, significant fibrosis and cirrhosis may become additional indications for treatment in the future. Because of the surgical morbidity, currently bariatric surgery should only be performed in patients with morbid obesity, although the long-term impact of bariatric surgery on the histology of NAFLD is favorable.

Keywords

non-alcoholic steatohepatitis; obeticholic acid; elafibranor; cenicriviroc; selonsertib

12.1 Introduction

Non-alcoholic fatty liver disease (NAFLD) is now the most common chronic liver disease worldwide [1, 2], and the second leading indication for liver transplantation and the third leading cause of hepatocellular carcinoma (HCC) in the United States [3, 4]. Its epidemiology and pathogenesis have been discussed in previous chapters. This chapter focuses on the prevention and management of NAFLD. Healthy lifestyle is the cornerstone for the prevention and management of NAFLD and should be recommended to every patient at risk or having established NAFLD. Despite the high prevalence of NAFLD, it should be recognized that the majority of patients will not develop liver-related complications; cardiovascular disease

V. W.-S. Wong (✉)
Department of Medicine and Therapeutics and State Key Laboratory of Digestive Disease, The Chinese University of Hong Kong, Hong Kong, Hong Kong
e-mail: wongv@cuhk.edu.hk

J. Yu (ed.), *Obesity, Fatty Liver and Liver Cancer*, Advances in Experimental Medicine and Biology 1061, https://doi.org/10.1007/978-981-10-8684-7_12

remains the leading cause of death in NAFLD patients [5]. Until further data are available, pharmacological treatment should be restricted to selected patients with confirmed non-alcoholic steatohepatitis (NASH). As some agents with primarily anti-fibrotic effect are currently being tested in NAFLD patients, significant fibrosis and cirrhosis may become additional indications for treatment in the future. Because of the surgical morbidity, currently bariatric surgery should only be performed in patients with morbid obesity, although the long-term impact of bariatric surgery on the histology of NAFLD is favorable.

While more than a dozen pharmacological agents are now being evaluated, this chapter focuses on existing agents and drugs in phase 2/3 development. It should be highlighted that the existing agents discussed in this chapter have not been specifically registered for the treatment of NASH [6]. Besides, because liver-related complications take years if not decades to develop, biochemical, radiological and histological endpoints have been used to evaluate NASH treatments. In other words, the impact of the treatments on clinical outcomes and survival is highly uncertain. This important question must be clarified in future long-term studies.

12.2 Lifestyle Changes

Lifestyle management is currently the only acceptable method to prevent NAFLD/NASH. Body weight and metabolic parameters are closely associated with NAFLD in epidemiological studies [7, 8]. Lifestyle management is also the cornerstone for the management of NAFLD/NASH. The degree of weight reduction is pivotal to the control of NAFLD/NASH. In a randomized controlled trial testing a 1-year lifestyle modification program versus usual care in 154 community NAFLD subjects, 97% of those who lost more than 10% of the baseline body weight had complete resolution of NAFLD as determined by proton-magnetic resonance spectroscopy and transient elastography, compared with 13% who lost <3% of the baseline body weight and 41–60% of those losing 3–10% (Fig. 12.1) [9]. In another prospective cohort study of 293 NAFLD patients from Cuba using paired liver biopsy, resolution of NASH was achieved in a substantial proportion of patients who lost more than 7% of the baseline body weight, whereas fibrosis regression was only apparent in those having ≥10% weight reduction [10]. While encouraging, it should be noted that significant weight reduction is not commonly achieved. In both studies, fewer than half of the patients lost ≥5% body weight (Fig. 12.1).

The optimal diet for the prevention and treatment of NAFLD/NASH has not been well defined. Low-carbohydrate, low-fat, low-glycemic-index and Mediterranean diets have all been shown to improve NAFLD in small studies of relatively short duration of follow-up. For example, although a low-carbohydrate diet reduces intrahepatic triglyceride content more promptly than a low-fat, high-carbohydrate diet at 48 h, the difference is no longer apparent in 2–3 months [11]. Caloric restriction and diet adherence according to personal preference are likely to be more important in the long run [12].

On the other hand, fructose consumption has been more consistently associated with NAFLD [13] and its histological severity [14]. Unlike glucose, fructose is not controlled by insulin and has a strong first-pass effect in the liver. It serves as the substrate for *de novo* lipogenesis and contributes to the development of insulin resistance [15]. The source of excessive fructose is usually from high fructose corn syrup, which is found in soft drinks and sweetened beverages.

An ongoing debate is whether modest alcohol consumption is protective. Data from the Third National Health and Nutrition Examination Survey suggest that modest wine drinking, but not other types of alcohol, reduces the risk of NAFLD inferred by elevated alanine aminotransferase level [16]. Among adult patients with biopsy-proven NAFLD in the NASH Clinical

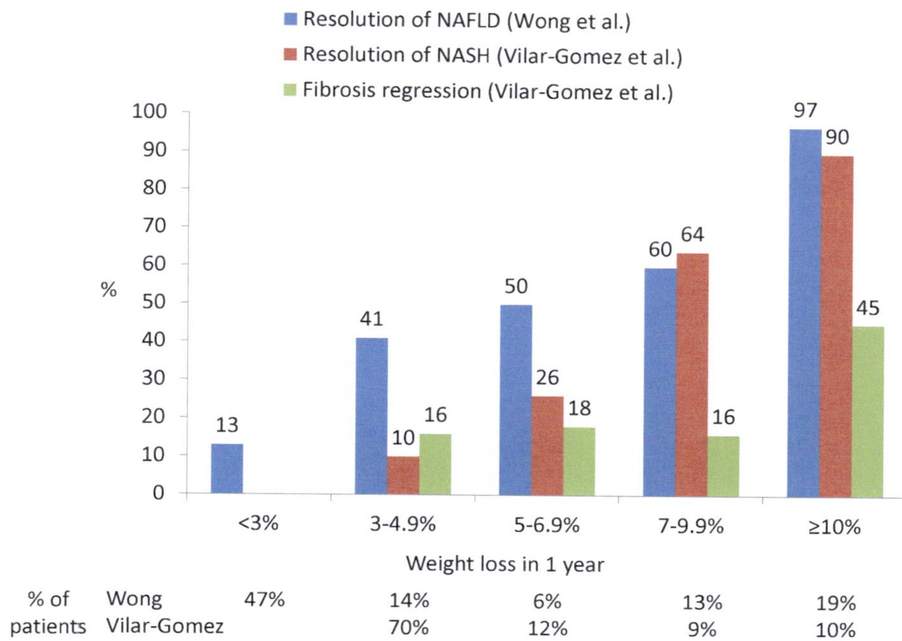

Fig. 12.1 **Relationship between weight reduction in 1 year and improvement in NAFLD.** In the study by Wong et al. [9], 154 community NAFLD patients were randomized to a lifestyle intervention program (n = 77) or usual care (n = 77). Resolution of NAFLD was defined as an intrahepatic triglyceride content of <5% by proton-magnetic resonance spectroscopy at 1 year. In the study by Vilar-Gomez et al. [10], 293 NAFLD patients received lifestyle advice and underwent liver biopsy at baseline and 1 year. Patients in the first category in Vilar-Gomez's study had weight reduction <5%

Research Network, modest drinking was also less likely to have NASH and liver fibrosis [17]. In another community cohort, modest drinkers had lower blood levels of endotoxin, which was in turn linked to NAFLD and liver injury [18]. It should be noted that the protective effect of modest alcohol consumption has not been consistently shown across studies. The assessment of alcohol consumption is subject to recall bias, and the association may be confounded by other lifestyle factors.

Regular exercise is another integral component of healthy lifestyle. Both aerobic exercise and resistance training have been shown to reduce liver fat [19]. The time spent in exercise correlates with metabolic improvements [20]. In a recent meta-analysis, at least 60 min of moderate intensity physical activity per day is needed to eliminate the increased risk of death associated with high sitting time [21].

12.3 Pharmacological Treatment

The main challenge to lifestyle modification is long-term maintenance of weight loss, which is possible but only achieved by few [22]. Therefore, pharmacological treatment is still needed in some patients with confirmed NASH. For practical purpose, we classify potential agents based on their phase of development.

12.3.1 Existing Agents

12.3.1.1 Vitamin E

Vitamin E is an anti-oxidant that has been recommended as an acceptable treatment for NASH by the American and European guidelines (EASL) [23, 24]. In the Pioglitazone versus Vitamin E versus Placebo for the Treatment of Nondiabetic Patients with Nonalcoholic Steatohepatitis

(PIVENS) trial, 43% of the patients treated with vitamin E at a daily dose of 800 IU for 96 weeks had histological improvement (improvement by ≥1 point in the hepatocellular ballooning score; no increase in fibrosis score; either a decrease in the NAFLD activity score to <3 points or a decrease of ≥2 points, with ≥1 point decrease in either the lobular inflammation or steatosis score), compared with 19% of those receiving placebo (P = 0.001) [25]. Significant more patients had improvements in steatosis, lobular inflammation, hepatocellular ballooning and the total NAFLD activity score. Resolution of definite NASH was seen in 36% in the vitamin E group and 21% in the placebo group (P = 0.05). However, vitamin E did not lead to a greater improvement in liver fibrosis. Patients on vitamin E had greater reductions in aminotransferases. As expected, vitamin E had no impact on body weight, insulin sensitivity and the lipid profile.

The Treatment of NAFLD in Children (TONIC) study was conducted in children and adolescents aged 8–17 years [26]. Unlike the PIVENS study, recruitment of patients in the TONIC study was based on elevated alanine aminotransferase but not a diagnosis of NASH on histology. The primary outcome, sustained reduction in alanine aminotransferase to 50% or less of the baseline level or 40 U/L or less from 48–96 weeks of treatment, was achieved in 26% in the vitamin E group and 17% in the placebo group (P = 0.26). However, patients on vitamin E had greater reduction in the hepatocellular ballooning score and the NAFLD activity score. Resolution of NASH occurred in 58% in the vitamin E group and 28% in the placebo group (P = 0.006). Again, there was no significant difference in the change in fibrosis score. Similar results were observed in a meta-analysis of 5 randomized controlled trials including the PIVENS and TONIC studies [27].

Some studies, however, suggest that high dose vitamin E may increase all-cause mortality, although the results have been inconsistent [28]. Because liver fibrosis is one of the most important risk factors of HCC and adverse clinical outcomes in NAFLD patients, the risk-to-benefit ratio of a drug that has no impact on fibrosis is uncertain [29, 30].

12.3.1.2 Pioglitazone

Pioglitazone is a thiazolidinedione that activates peroxisome proliferator-activated receptor (PPAR)-gamma, which in turn increases the storage of fatty acids in adipocytes and thereby reduces circulating fatty acids. This is another treatment for NASH accepted by the American and European guidelines [23, 24]. Again, pioglitazone has been tested against placebo in the PIVENS study [25]. The primary histological outcome (described under the section on vitamin E) was achieved in 34% of NASH patients receiving pioglitazone at a dose of 30 mg daily and 19% of those receiving placebo (P = 0.04) [25]. Nevertheless, because the PIVENS study is a 3-arm study including pioglitazone, vitamin E and placebo, a P value of 0.04 for the primary outcome was considered insignificant after adjusting for dual comparisons. Compared with placebo, pioglitazone led to greater improvements in steatosis, lobular inflammation, hepatocellular ballooning and the total NAFLD activity score, but not fibrosis. Besides, when judged by the pathologist's global assessment, resolution of definite NASH was actually achieved in 47% in the pioglitazone group, 36% in the vitamin E group, and 21% in the placebo group. Pioglitazone also improved the transaminases level. As expected, insulin sensitivity improved with pioglitazone.

Four meta-analyses evaluated the effectiveness of thiazolidinediones in NASH [31–34]. Consistently, all included studies showed that thiazolidinediones can improve hepatic steatosis, lobular inflammation and hepatocellular ballooning. One of the meta-analyses included a subanalysis and showed that pioglitazone might improve fibrosis, but that analysis included only 137 patients treated with pioglitazone [32].

Thiazolidinediones commonly cause weight gain and may result in fluid retention and congestive heart failure [35]. Rosiglitazone, but not pioglitazone, also increases the risk of myocardial infarction and cardiovascular death [36, 37].

Pioglitazone may also increase the risk of bladder cancer [38].

12.3.1.3 Liraglutide

Liraglutide is a glucagon-like peptide-1 (GLP-1) agonist registered for the treatment of type 2 diabetes (at a dose of 1.2–1.8 mg daily) and obesity (at 3 mg daily). GLP-1 is an incretin secreted by the intestinal L cells in response to nutrients and exerts endocrine, gastrointestinal and central effects. It increases insulin and reduces glucagon secretion. It also delays gastric emptying and reduces the appetite, which together leads to reduced food intake and weight reduction.

In the Liraglutide Efficacy and Action in NASH (LEAN) study, 52 overweight NASH patients were randomized to receive liraglutide (1.8 mg daily) or placebo for 48 weeks [39]. The primary outcome of resolution of NASH with no worsening in fibrosis from baseline to week 48 was achieved in 9 of 23 (39%) patients in the liraglutide group and 2 of 22 (9%) patients in the placebo group. When the histological features were analyzed individually, more patients in the liraglutide group had improvement in steatosis and hepatocellular ballooning. Although liraglutide was not associated with improvement in fibrosis, fewer patients in the liraglutide group had worsening of fibrosis. Liraglutide improves insulin sensitivity in the liver and adipose tissue [40].

Liraglutide requires subcutaneous injection. Due to its mechanism of action, gastrointestinal side effects are common. It is therefore necessary to start liraglutide at 0.6 mg daily and slowly titrate to the target dose.

12.3.2 Agents in Phase 3 Development

12.3.2.1 Obeticholic Acid

Obeticholic acid is a potent farnesoid X receptor (FXR) agonist. Chenodeoxycholic acid is the natural ligand of FXR with the highest affinity, and obeticholic acid is 100 times more potent than chenodeoxycholic acid [41]. FXR is a nuclear receptor highly expressed in the liver, small intestines and kidneys. While its primary function is bile acid metabolism, it inhibits the expression of sterol regulatory element-binding protein 1c (SREBP-1c) and reduces hepatic lipogenesis [42]. It also modulates various lipoproteins and increases triglyceride clearance from the liver [43].

In the Farnesoid X nuclear receptor ligand obesticholic acid for non-cirrhotic, non-alcoholic steatohepatitis (FLINT) study, the primary outcome of a decrease in NAFLD activity score by ≥2 points with no worsening of fibrosis from baseline to week 72 was achieved in 45% of the patients receiving obeticholic acid and 21% of those receiving placebo [44]. Improvement in fibrosis was observed in 35% in the obeticholic acid group and 19% in the placebo group. However, obeticholic acid was associated with pruritus, increase in total and low density lipoprotein (LDL)-cholesterol, and decrease in high density lipoprotein (HDL)-cholesterol. Since dyslipidemia and ischemic heart disease are common in NASH patients [5], the long-term cardiovascular safety must be evaluated carefully. Currently, obeticholic acid is registered for the treatment of primary biliary cholangitis [45], and is currently evaluated in the phase 3 REGENERATE study.

Because FXR is expressed in different tissues, there has been interest in organ-specific FXR agonists. Recently, the effect of the non-steroidal, intestine-selective FXR agonist GS-9674 has been tested in cynomolgus monkeys fed with a high-fat, high-cholesterol diet [46]. GS-9674 upregulates the FXR targets *Shp* and *Fgf19*. Unlike obeticholic acid, GS-9674 reduces total cholesterol, LDL-cholesterol and serum apolipoprotein B, and increases hepatic expression of the LDL receptor. Its effect on NASH remains to be seen.

12.3.2.2 Elafibranor

Elafibranor is a dual agonist of peroxisome proliferator-activated receptors alpha and delta. In preclinical studies, activation of these nuclear receptors leads to favorable metabolic and anti-inflammatory effects [47, 48]. In the GOLDEN-505 study, NASH resolution without worsening of fibrosis occurred in 19% of patients taking elafibranor 120 mg daily for 1 year and 12% of those taking placebo [49]. Elafibranor also results in improved lipid profile and insulin sensitivity. A phase 3 trial is underway (NCT02704403).

12.3.2.3 Cenicriviroc

Cenicriviroc is a dual antagonist of chemokine receptor types 2 and 5 (CCR2/CCR5). The receptors are found on Kupffer cells and hepatic stellate cells, and preclinical studies suggest its anti-inflammatory and anti-fibrotic activity [50, 51]. In the phase 2b CENTAUR study, cenicriviroc treatment for 1 year failed to achieve the primary outcome of a decrease in NAFLD activity score by ≥2 points with no worsening of fibrosis [52]. Nonetheless, one of the key secondary outcomes, improvement in liver fibrosis without worsening of NASH, was achieved in 20% in the treatment group, compared with 10% in the placebo group. Besides, cenicriviroc reduced the serum levels interleukin-6, C-reactive protein and fibrinogen, suggesting its action on inflammation that may not be reflected by crude histological assessment. A phase 3 study is planned.

12.3.2.4 GS-4997

GS-4997 is an inhibitor of apoptosis signal-regulating kinase 1 (ASK1). ASK1 is a member of the mitogen-activated protein kinase kinase kinase family and is involved in endoplasmic reticulum stress and apoptosis [53–55]. In a phase 2 study, GS-4997 reversed liver fibrosis in NASH patients after only 24 weeks of treatment [56]. Importantly, the finding was consistently demonstrated using hepatic collagen content by morphometry as well as liver stiffness measurement by magnetic resonance elastography. A phase 3 study is planned.

12.4 Bariatric Surgery

Bariatric surgery is currently the most effective weight reduction treatment in patients with morbid obesity. Because of the close link between NASH and obesity, it comes as no surprise that NASH can improve after bariatric surgery. In a prospective study from France, the majority of patients had histological improvements 1 year after bariatric surgery; 85% had resolution of NASH and 46% had improvement in fibrosis [57]. In a murine model of NASH, roux-en-Y bypass surgery improved hepatic mitochondrial function [58]. Bariatric surgery is also cost-effective in NASH patients with different fibrosis stages [59].

12.5 NAFLD-Associated HCC

Despite numerous new developments in NASH treatment, it should be emphasized that the treatments have been evaluated using biochemical, radiological or histological assessments. At the end of the day, what we want to achieve is to prevent cirrhosis, HCC and liver-related deaths. Currently, none of the new agents have been shown to prevent these outcomes. Although the latest phase 3 studies are designed to study liver-related outcomes, the composite endpoint will likely be largely driven by progression to cirrhosis, whereas the prevention of HCC and liver-related deaths will unlikely be shown based on the sample size and duration of assessment. Nonetheless, weight reduction and physical activity are associated with a lower HCC risk both in animal models and observational studies [60, 61]. Metformin and statin, both being important metabolic treatments in patients with NAFLD, also appear to prevent HCC, though a causal relationship cannot be firmly established based on observational data [62–65]. While it is unlikely that metformin and statin will be tested as chemopreventive agents in randomized controlled trials, their safety in patients with compensated liver disease is well established; the drugs should be used liberally in patients with metabolic indications.

References

1. Younossi ZM, Koenig AB, Abdelatif D, Fazel Y, Henry L, Wymer M. Global epidemiology of nonalcoholic fatty liver disease-Meta-analytic assessment of prevalence, incidence, and outcomes. Hepatology. 2016;64:73–84.
2. Wong VW, Wong GL, Yeung DK, Lau TK, Chan CK, Chim AM, et al. Incidence of non-alcoholic fatty liver disease in Hong Kong: a population study with paired proton-magnetic resonance spectroscopy. J Hepatol. 2015;62:182–9.
3. Wong RJ, Aguilar M, Cheung R, Perumpail RB, Harrison SA, Younossi ZM, et al. Nonalcoholic steatohepatitis is the second leading etiology of liver disease among adults awaiting liver transplantation in the United States. Gastroenterology. 2015;148:547–55.
4. Younossi ZM, Otgonsuren M, Henry L, Venkatesan C, Mishra A, Erario M, et al. Association of nonalcoholic fatty liver disease (NAFLD) with hepatocellular carcinoma (HCC) in the United States from 2004 to 2009. Hepatology. 2015;62:1723–30.
5. Wong VW, Wong GL, Yeung JC, Fung CY, Chan JK, Chang ZH, et al. Long-term clinical outcomes after fatty liver screening in patients undergoing coronary angiogram: a prospective cohort study. Hepatology. 2016;63:754–63.
6. Wong VW, Chitturi S, Wong GL, Yu J, Chan HL, Farrell G. Pathogenesis and novel treatment options for non-alcoholic steatohepatitis. Lancet Gastroenterol Hepatol. 2016;1:56–67.
7. Brunt EM, Wong VW, Nobili V, Day CP, Sookoian S, Maher JJ, et al. Nonalcoholic fatty liver disease. Nat Rev Dis Primers. 2015;1:15080.
8. Wong VW, Chu WC, Wong GL, Chan RS, Chim AM, Ong A, et al. Prevalence of non-alcoholic fatty liver disease and advanced fibrosis in Hong Kong Chinese: a population study using proton-magnetic resonance spectroscopy and transient elastography. Gut. 2012;61:409–15.
9. Wong VW, Chan RS, Wong GL, Cheung BH, Chu WC, Yeung DK, et al. Community-based lifestyle modification programme for non-alcoholic fatty liver disease: a randomized controlled trial. J Hepatol. 2013;59:536–42.
10. Vilar-Gomez E, Martinez-Perez Y, Calzadilla-Bertot L, Torres-Gonzalez A, Gra-Oramas B, Gonzalez-Fabian L, et al. Weight loss through lifestyle modification significantly reduces features of nonalcoholic steatohepatitis. Gastroenterology. 2015;149:367–378 e365; quiz e314–365.
11. Kirk E, Reeds DN, Finck BN, Mayurranjan SM, Patterson BW, Klein S. Dietary fat and carbohydrates differentially alter insulin sensitivity during caloric restriction. Gastroenterology. 2009;136:1552–60.
12. Shai I, Schwarzfuchs D, Henkin Y, Shahar DR, Witkow S, Greenberg I, et al. Weight loss with a low-carbohydrate, Mediterranean, or low-fat diet. N Engl J Med. 2008;359:229–41.
13. Ouyang X, Cirillo P, Sautin Y, McCall S, Bruchette JL, Diehl AM, et al. Fructose consumption as a risk factor for non-alcoholic fatty liver disease. J Hepatol. 2008;48:993–9.
14. Abdelmalek MF, Suzuki A, Guy C, Unalp-Arida A, Colvin R, Johnson RJ, et al. Increased fructose consumption is associated with fibrosis severity in patients with nonalcoholic fatty liver disease. Hepatology. 2010;51:1961–71.
15. Basciano H, Federico L, Adeli K. Fructose, insulin resistance, and metabolic dyslipidemia. Nutr Metab (Lond). 2005;2:5.
16. Dunn W, Xu R, Schwimmer JB. Modest wine drinking and decreased prevalence of suspected nonalcoholic fatty liver disease. Hepatology. 2008;47:1947–54.
17. Dunn W, Sanyal AJ, Brunt EM, Unalp-Arida A, Donohue M, McCullough AJ, et al. Modest alcohol consumption is associated with decreased prevalence of steatohepatitis in patients with non-alcoholic fatty liver disease (NAFLD). J Hepatol. 2012;57:384–91.
18. Wong VW, Wong GL, Chan HY, Yeung DK, Chan RS, Chim AM, et al. Bacterial endotoxin and non-alcoholic fatty liver disease in the general population: a prospective cohort study. Aliment Pharmacol Ther. 2015;42:731–40.
19. Keating SE, Hackett DA, George J, Johnson NA. Exercise and non-alcoholic fatty liver disease: a systematic review and meta-analysis. J Hepatol. 2012;57:157–66.
20. Oh S, Shida T, Yamagishi K, Tanaka K, So R, Tsujimoto T, et al. Moderate to vigorous physical activity volume is an important factor for managing nonalcoholic fatty liver disease: a retrospective study. Hepatology. 2015;61:1205–15.
21. Ekelund U, Steene-Johannessen J, Brown WJ, Fagerland MW, Owen N, Powell KE, et al. Does physical activity attenuate, or even eliminate, the detrimental association of sitting time with mortality? A harmonised meta-analysis of data from more than 1 million men and women. Lancet. 2016;388:1302–10.
22. Wing RR, Phelan S. Long-term weight loss maintenance. Am J Clin Nutr. 2005;82:222S–5S.
23. Chalasani N, Younossi Z, Lavine JE, Diehl AM, Brunt EM, Cusi K, et al. The diagnosis and management of non-alcoholic fatty liver disease: practice guideline by the American Association for the Study of Liver Diseases, American College of Gastroenterology,

and the American Gastroenterological Association. Hepatology. 2012;55:2005–23.
24. European Association for the Study of the Liver, European Association for the Study of Diabetes, European Association for the Study of Obesity. EASL-EASD-EASO Clinical Practice Guidelines for the management of non-alcoholic fatty liver disease. J Hepatol. 2016;64:1388–402.
25. Sanyal AJ, Chalasani N, Kowdley KV, McCullough A, Diehl AM, Bass NM, et al. Pioglitazone, vitamin E, or placebo for nonalcoholic steatohepatitis. N Engl J Med. 2010;362:1675–85.
26. Lavine JE, Schwimmer JB, Van Natta ML, Molleston JP, Murray KF, Rosenthal P, et al. Effect of vitamin E or metformin for treatment of nonalcoholic fatty liver disease in children and adolescents: the TONIC randomized controlled trial. JAMA. 2011;305:1659–68.
27. Sato K, Gosho M, Yamamoto T, Kobayashi Y, Ishii N, Ohashi T, et al. Vitamin E has a beneficial effect on nonalcoholic fatty liver disease: a meta-analysis of randomized controlled trials. Nutrition. 2015;31:923–30.
28. Miller ER 3rd, Pastor-Barriuso R, Dalal D, Riemersma RA, Appel LJ, Guallar E. Meta-analysis: high-dosage vitamin E supplementation may increase all-cause mortality. Ann Intern Med. 2005;142:37–46.
29. Younossi ZM, Stepanova M, Rafiq N, Makhlouf H, Younoszai Z, Agrawal R, et al. Pathologic criteria for nonalcoholic steatohepatitis: interprotocol agreement and ability to predict liver-related mortality. Hepatology. 2011;53:1874–82.
30. Ekstedt M, Hagstrom H, Nasr P, Fredrikson M, Stal P, Kechagias S, et al. Fibrosis stage is the strongest predictor for disease-specific mortality in NAFLD after up to 33 years of follow-up. Hepatology. 2015;61:1547–54.
31. Angelico F, Burattin M, Alessandri C, Del Ben M, Lirussi F. Drugs improving insulin resistance for non-alcoholic fatty liver disease and/or non-alcoholic steatohepatitis. Cochrane Database Syst Rev. 2007:CD005166.
32. Boettcher E, Csako G, Pucino F, Wesley R, Loomba R. Meta-analysis: pioglitazone improves liver histology and fibrosis in patients with non-alcoholic steatohepatitis. Aliment Pharmacol Ther. 2012;35:66–75.
33. Musso G, Cassader M, Rosina F, Gambino R. Impact of current treatments on liver disease, glucose metabolism and cardiovascular risk in non-alcoholic fatty liver disease (NAFLD): a systematic review and meta-analysis of randomised trials. Diabetologia. 2012;55:885–904.
34. Singh S, Khera R, Allen AM, Murad MH, Loomba R. Comparative effectiveness of pharmacological interventions for nonalcoholic steatohepatitis: a systematic review and network meta-analysis. Hepatology. 2015;62:1417–32.
35. Lago RM, Singh PP, Nesto RW. Congestive heart failure and cardiovascular death in patients with prediabetes and type 2 diabetes given thiazolidinediones: a meta-analysis of randomised clinical trials. Lancet. 2007;370:1129–36.
36. Nissen SE, Wolski K. Effect of rosiglitazone on the risk of myocardial infarction and death from cardiovascular causes. N Engl J Med. 2007;356:2457–71.
37. Lincoff AM, Wolski K, Nicholls SJ, Nissen SE. Pioglitazone and risk of cardiovascular events in patients with type 2 diabetes mellitus: a meta-analysis of randomized trials. JAMA. 2007;298:1180–8.
38. Lewis JD, Habel LA, Quesenberry CP, Strom BL, Peng T, Hedderson MM, et al. Pioglitazone use and risk of bladder cancer and other common cancers in persons with diabetes. JAMA. 2015;314:265–77.
39. Armstrong MJ, Gaunt P, Aithal GP, Barton D, Hull D, Parker R, et al. Liraglutide safety and efficacy in patients with non-alcoholic steatohepatitis (LEAN): a multicentre, double-blind, randomised, placebo-controlled phase 2 study. Lancet. 2016;387:679–90.
40. Armstrong MJ, Hull D, Guo K, Barton D, Hazlehurst JM, Gathercole LL, et al. Glucagon-like peptide 1 decreases lipotoxicity in non-alcoholic steatohepatitis. J Hepatol. 2016;64:399–408.
41. Pellicciari R, Costantino G, Camaioni E, Sadeghpour BM, Entrena A, Willson TM, et al. Bile acid derivatives as ligands of the farnesoid X receptor. Synthesis, evaluation, and structure-activity relationship of a series of body and side chain modified analogues of chenodeoxycholic acid. J Med Chem. 2004;47:4559–69.
42. Xiong X, Wang X, Lu Y, Wang E, Zhang Z, Yang J, et al. Hepatic steatosis exacerbated by endoplasmic reticulum stress-mediated downregulation of FXR in aging mice. J Hepatol. 2014;60:847–54.
43. Fuchs M. Non-alcoholic fatty liver disease: the bile acid-activated farnesoid x receptor as an emerging treatment target. J Lipids. 2012;2012:934396.
44. Neuschwander-Tetri BA, Loomba R, Sanyal AJ, Lavine JE, Van Natta ML, Abdelmalek MF, et al. Farnesoid X nuclear receptor ligand obeticholic acid for non-cirrhotic, non-alcoholic steatohepatitis (FLINT): a multicentre, randomised, placebo-controlled trial. Lancet. 2015;385:956–65.
45. Nevens F, Andreone P, Mazzella G, Strasser SI, Bowlus C, Invernizzi P, et al. A placebo-controlled trial of obeticholic acid in primary biliary cholangitis. N Engl J Med. 2016;375:631–43.
46. French D, Liles JT, Liu H, Huntzicker EG, Djedjos CS, Kremoser C, et al. Pharmacodynamic effects of the non-steroidal farnesoid X receptor (FXR) agonist GS-9674 in high fat, high cholesterol diet fed cynomolgus monkeys. Hepatology. 2016;64(Suppl):71A.
47. Pawlak M, Lefebvre P, Staels B. Molecular mechanism of PPARalpha action and its impact on lipid metabolism, inflammation and fibrosis in non-alcoholic fatty liver disease. J Hepatol. 2015;62:720–33.
48. Odegaard JI, Ricardo-Gonzalez RR, Red Eagle A, Vats D, Morel CR, Goforth MH, et al. Alternative M2 activation of Kupffer cells by PPARdelta ameliorates obesity-induced insulin resistance. Cell Metab. 2008;7:496–507.

49. Ratziu V, Harrison SA, Francque S, Bedossa P, Lehert P, Serfaty L, et al. Elafibranor, an agonist of the peroxisome proliferator-activated receptor-alpha and -delta, induces resolution of nonalcoholic steatohepatitis without fibrosis worsening. Gastroenterology. 2016;150:1147–1159 e1145.
50. Lefebvre E, Moyle G, Reshef R, Richman LP, Thompson M, Hong F, et al. Antifibrotic effects of the dual CCR2/CCR5 antagonist cenicriviroc in animal models of liver and kidney fibrosis. PLoS One. 2016;11:e0158156.
51. Puengel T, Krenkel O, Mossanen J, Longerich T, Lefebvre E, Trautwein C, et al. The dual Ccr2/Ccr5 antagonist cenicriviroc ameliorates steatohepatitis and fibrosis in vivo by inhibiting the infiltration of inflammatory monocytes into injured liver. J Hepatol. 2016;64(Suppl):S160.
52. Sanyal A, Ratziu V, Harrison S, Abdelmalek M, Aithal GP, Caballeria J, et al. Cenicriviroc vs placebo for the treatment of non-alcoholic steatohepatitis with liver fibrosis: results from the year 1 primary analysis of the phase 2b CENTAUR study. Hepatology. 2016;64(Suppl):1118A.
53. Ichijo H, Nishida E, Irie K, ten Dijke P, Saitoh M, Moriguchi T, et al. Induction of apoptosis by ASK1, a mammalian MAPKKK that activates SAPK/JNK and p38 signaling pathways. Science. 1997;275:90–4.
54. Tobiume K, Matsuzawa A, Takahashi T, Nishitoh H, Morita K, Takeda K, et al. ASK1 is required for sustained activations of JNK/p38 MAP kinases and apoptosis. EMBO Rep. 2001;2:222–8.
55. Nishitoh H, Matsuzawa A, Tobiume K, Saegusa K, Takeda K, Inoue K, et al. ASK1 is essential for endoplasmic reticulum stress-induced neuronal cell death triggered by expanded polyglutamine repeats. Genes Dev. 2002;16:1345–55.
56. Loomba R, Lawitz E, Mantry PS, Jayakumar S, Caldwell SH, Arnold H, et al. GS-4997, an inhibitor of apoptosis signal-regulating kinase (ASK1), alone or in combination with simtuzumab for the treatment of nonalcoholic steatohepatitis (NASH): a randomized, phase 2 trial. Hepatology. 2016;64(Suppl):1119A.
57. Lassailly G, Caiazzo R, Buob D, Pigeyre M, Verkindt H, Labreuche J, et al. Bariatric surgery reduces features of nonalcoholic steatohepatitis in morbidly obese patients. Gastroenterology. 2015;149:379–88. quiz e315–376
58. Verbeek J, Lannoo M, Pirinen E, Ryu D, Spincemaille P, Vander Elst I, et al. Roux-en-y gastric bypass attenuates hepatic mitochondrial dysfunction in mice with non-alcoholic steatohepatitis. Gut. 2015;64:673–83.
59. Klebanoff MJ, Corey KE, Chhatwal J, Kaplan LM, Chung RT, Hur C. Bariatric surgery for nonalcoholic steatohepatitis: a clinical and cost-effectiveness analysis. Hepatology. 2016.
60. Kushi LH, Doyle C, McCullough M, Rock CL, Demark-Wahnefried W, Bandera EV, et al. American Cancer Society Guidelines on nutrition and physical activity for cancer prevention: reducing the risk of cancer with healthy food choices and physical activity. CA Cancer J Clin. 2012;62:30–67.
61. Piguet AC, Saran U, Simillion C, Keller I, Terracciano L, Reeves HL, et al. Regular exercise decreases liver tumors development in hepatocyte-specific PTEN-deficient mice independently of steatosis. J Hepatol. 2015;62:1296–303.
62. Donadon V, Balbi M, Mas MD, Casarin P, Zanette G. Metformin and reduced risk of hepatocellular carcinoma in diabetic patients with chronic liver disease. Liver Int. 2010;30:750–8.
63. Chen HP, Shieh JJ, Chang CC, Chen TT, Lin JT, Wu MS, et al. Metformin decreases hepatocellular carcinoma risk in a dose-dependent manner: population-based and in vitro studies. Gut. 2013;62:606–15.
64. El-Serag HB, Johnson ML, Hachem C, Morgana RO. Statins are associated with a reduced risk of hepatocellular carcinoma in a large cohort of patients with diabetes. Gastroenterology. 2009;136:1601–8.
65. Hsiang JC, Wong GL, Tse YK, Wong VW, Yip TC, Chan HL. Statin and the risk of hepatocellular carcinoma and death in a hospital-based hepatitis B-infected population: a propensity score landmark analysis. J Hepatol. 2015;63:1190–7.

MIX
Papier aus verantwortungsvollen Quellen
Paper from responsible sources
FSC® C105338

If you have any concerns about our products,
you can contact us on
ProductSafety@springernature.com

In case Publisher is established outside the EU,
the EU authorized representative is:
Springer Nature Customer Service Center GmbH
Europaplatz 3, 69115 Heidelberg, Germany

Printed by Libri Plureos GmbH
in Hamburg, Germany